WOMEN, HEALTH AND THE MIND

Edited by

Dr Lorraine Sherr
Royal Free
and
University College Medical School, London, UK

Dr Janet S. St Lawrence
Centers for Disease Control and Prevention, Atlanta, USA

JOHN WILEY & SONS, LTD
Chichester • New York • Weinheim • Singapore • Toronto

Other Wiley Editorial Offices

John Wiley & Sons, Inc., 605 Third Avenue,
New York, NY 10158–0012, USA

WILEY-VCH Verlag GmbH, Pappelallee 3,
D-69469 Weinheim, Germany

Jacaranda Wiley Ltd, 33 Park Road, Milton,
Queensland 4064, Australia

John Wiley & Sons (Asia) Pte Ltd, 2 Clementi Loop #02–01,
Jin Xing Distripark, Singapore 129809

John Wiley & Sons (Canada) Ltd, 22 Worcester Road,
Rexdale, Ontario M9W 1L1, Canada

Library of Congress Cataloging-in-Publication Data
Women health and the mind/edited by Lorraine Sherr, Janet S. St Lawrence.
  p. cm.
  Includes bibliographical references and index.
  ISBN 0–471–99879–6 (alk. paper)
    1. Women—Health and hygiene—Psychological aspects. 2. Women—Mental
  health. 3. Clinical health psychology. I. Sherr, Lorraine. II. St Lawrence, Janet S.
    [DNLM: 1. Women's Health. 2. Women—psychology. WA 309 W8709 2000]
  RA564.85.W6645 2000
  613′.04244 21—dc21

99–040817

British Library Cataloguing in Publication Data
A catalogue record for this book is available from the British Library

ISBN   0–471–99879–6

Typeset in 10/12pt Palatino by Florence Production, Stoodleigh, Devon
Printed and bound in Great Britain by Biddles Ltd, Guildford and King's Lynn
This book is printed on acid-free paper responsibly manufactured from sustainable
forestry, in which at least two trees are planted for each one used for paper
production.

To

Cookie Garvey, Margie Smith, Cynthia Salten, Sharon Davidson, Wendy Scolnik, Valerie Brasse, Rhona Lunsky, Sandra Wagner and Marion Adler.

Lorraine Sherr

To

My mother, Edith Bardella Strommer, who spent her lifetime promoting women's rights to gender equity in education and employment; and to her granddaughters, Julia and Sara who were among the beneficiaries of her life-long dedication.

Janet St Lawrence

CONTENTS

Women and Reproductive Health

Women and Physical Health

Women, Health Promotion and Health Life-styles

ABOUT THE AUTHORS

Margarita Alegría, Ph.D., is Professor of Health Services Research and Director of the Center for Sociomedical Research and Evaluation at the School of Public Health, University of Puerto Rico. She has conducted several major studies of mental health care, consequences of drug use and HIV risk behaviours with low-income populations. She also collaborates with the International Consortium of Psychiatric Epidemiology, comparing cross-national patterns of mental health service delivery. She has published in the areas of mental health services research, conceptual and methodological issues with minority populations, and HIV risk behaviours.

Marrie H.J. Bekker works at the Departments of Clinical Health Psychology and Women's Studies of Tilburg University in The Netherlands. She obtained a master's degree in Clinical Psychology at the University of Amsterdam, where she completed her Ph.D. in 1991. She has researched and published on a breadth of topics addressing health and gender, such as women's syndromes like agoraphobia and eating disorders (dissertation); sexual inequality in the training of clinical psychologists; psychological consequences of DES; body-image and body-experience; menopause; virginity, sexuality and mental health in Islamic girls in The Netherlands; and health effects of gender roles in women and men. She is the chair of the Dutch Foundation of Women & Health Research and co-ordinates the further development of the European Association of Women & Health Research (EAWHR). Her current research projects concern gender-related stress, in particular health effects of sex-specific stressors associated with multiple roles, and the relationship between gender, body-awareness and body-image.

Lisa Belcher Ph.D. is a community psychologist in the Division of HIV/AIDS Prevention at the US Centers for Disease Control and Prevention. She received her Ph.D. from Georgia State University, Atlanta, in 1997. Dr Belcher has worked in the field of sexual risk reduction and behavioural intervention research for several years, and has authored and co-authored several papers in this area. Her major research interests include the effectiveness of brief intervention in reducing HIV risk behaviour, the interaction of sexually transmitted disease and HIV infection, women's sexual risk related to the use of crack cocaine, and behavioural interventions with persons living with HIV/AIDS.

Julia C. Berryman B.Sc. Ph.D. C Psychol AFBPsS is a Senior Lecturer in Psychology at the Department of Adult Education at the University of Leicester. She has researched and published widely in the areas of developmental psychology, sex and gender, parenthood and parenting. She set up the Parenthood Research Group at Leicester University and has investigated a variety of aspects of parenthood and parenting. She directed the Leicester Motherhood Project and the Leicester Mother and Child Project, two projects which formed part of a longitudinal study of women of all ages, designed to examine the effect of age and parity on women's experiences of motherhood and on child outcomes. She is co-author of the book *Older Mothers – Conception, Pregnancy and Birth after 35* (Berryman, J.C., Thorpe, K.C. & Windridge, K.C. (1995). London: Pandora).

Ernest Brahn M.D. is a Professor of Medicine in the Division of Rheumatology at the UCLA School of Medicine in Los Angeles, California. He received his medical degree from the University of Chicago and completed an Internal Medicine Residency at the University of California School of Medicine, San Francisco, USA. He did a Rheumatology/Immunology research fellowship at Harvard Medical School, Brigham and Women's Hospital, Boston where he then joined the faculty.

Glorisa Canino, Ph.D., is a Professor of Pediatrics and Director of the Behavioral Sciences Research Institute at the University of Puerto Rico, Medical Sciences Campus. She is principal or co-principal investigator of several grants funded by the National Institute of Mental Health and National Institute of Drug Addiction. She has published extensively in the areas of psychiatric epidemiology, cross-cultural instrument development and psychometrics and methodological challenges faced by the cross-cultural researcher.

Ruth C. Cronkite carries out work and research at the Department of Health Services Research and Development associated with Stanford University School of Medicine.

Denise T.D. de Ridder is associate professor at the Department of Health Psychology, Utrecht University, The Netherlands. She specializes in research on stress, coping, and self-regulation in chronic health problems, including topics such as adherence from a self-regulation perspective, self-regulation in chronically ill people, and the role of positive beliefs in adaptation to chronic illness. She is a member of the Editorial Board of *Psychology, Health, and Medicine* and a number of Dutch psychology journals. She teaches in the advanced Psychology and Health courses for Ph.D. students of Utrecht University.

Bathsheba Doran read English at Cambridge and went on to be in the first year of the new graduate course in Women's Studies at Oxford University, UK. After graduating she spent a year working for the independent television company *Planet 24*. She now writes for the stage and BBC radio and television and teaches Media at the University of Surrey.

Louise Dye Ph.D. is a lecturer in Biological Psychology in the School of Psychology, University of Leeds. Her research interests cover the menstrual cycle in relation to both cognitive performance and subjective experience. She is particularly interested in eating behaviour in relation to hormonal state and has written widely on appetite control and food cravings. She held a Royal Society European Science Exchange Programme Fellowship at the Ruhr University Bochum, Germany.

Gloria D. Eldridge received her Ph.D. in Clinical Psychology in 1991 from the University of Manitoba in Winnipeg, Manitoba, Canada. Following her Ph.D., she was Behavioral Science Consultant to a joint University of Manitoba/University of Nairobi project on "Strengthening STD/HIV Control in Kenya". For the past 6 years, she has been Project Director in the Community Health Program in the Department of Psychology at Jackson State University, Jackson, Mississippi, USA. Her research interests include prevention of sexually transmitted infections (STI) and HIV in vulnerable populations in the United States and in the developing world. Her current research focuses on applying behavior skills training, motivational enhancement, and relapse prevention to embed HIV/STI-prevention into drug treatment programs and programs for incarcerated women and men.

James M. Fitterling is Chief of the Chemical Dependence Treatment Program at the G.V. (Sonny) Montgomery Veterans Affairs Medical Center and Assistant Professor in the Department of Psychiatry and Human Behavior at the University of Mississippi Medical Center, Jackson, Mississippi, USA. He received his Ph.D. in Clinical Psychology with a specialization in behavior therapy from Georgia State University in Atlanta, Georgia, USA. His research and clinical interests include motivational enhancement, conditioned drug cue reactivity, HIV prevention, homelessness, and community-based approaches to substance abuse treatment.

Dolores Gallagher-Thompson Ph.D. ABPP is a licensed psychologist with over 15 years' experience who practices primarily as a geropsychologist doing research, teaching, and clinical care in several different academic and service environments. At present she is responsible for development of training programs in geriatrics/gerontology at the Veterans Affairs Palo Alto Health Care System in Palo Alto, California, USA, and is associate director of the Geriatric Research, Education and Clinical Center there. She is also an Associate Professor of Research at the Stanford University School of Medicine in the Department of Psychiatry and Behavioral Sciences. She has been a funded researcher from the NIA and NIMH since 1983, focusing on bereavement, treatment of late-life depression, and the development of interventions to reduce distress in family caregivers.

Rosemary Gillespie is a senior lecturer in sociology and women's studies at the University of Portsmouth. Her main research interests are gender and the body and femininity and identity. She is currently researching voluntary childlessness in women. She has published in each of these areas, and has co-edited with Graham Moon *Society and Health: An Introduction to Social Science for Health Professionals*.

Judith Greenberg Ph.D., received her doctorate from the University of California, San Diego. For 10 years, she has been a research sociologist at the Centers for Disease Control and Prevention, Division of Sexually Transmitted Diseases Prevention, focusing on the design and evaluation of interventions for groups at high risk. She has numerous publications from this work. Dr Greenberg previously directed a community agency serving victims of childhood sexual abuse and their families and was instrumental in establishing a state intervention program for male adolescent perpetrators. A major research interest is preventing or reducing sexual-risk behaviour in teen girls who have experienced childhood sexual abuse.

Jennifer Grossman M.D. is a Clinical Instructor in the Department of Medicine, Division of Rheumatology at UCLA School of Medicine, Center for Health Sciences in Los Angeles, California, USA. She obtained her undergraduate degree from Williams College, Williamstown, Massachusetts, and her medical degree from the University of Rochester, Rochester, New York. She completed a residency in Internal Medicine and a fellowship in Rheumatology at UCLA. Her research interests include the genetic influences on systemic lupus erythematosus, as well as quality of care for patients with rheumatic diseases.

Karla A. Henderson is Professor and Chair in the Department of Recreation and Leisure Studies at the University of North Carolina at Chapel Hill. She has actively been researching issues pertaining to women and leisure over the past 15 years. She is co-author of a book *Both Gains* *and Gaps – a Feminist Perspective on Women and Leisure*. In addition, she has written extensively about research methods and women in the outdoors. When not involved in scholarly pursuits she enjoys music, marathon running and reading just for fun.

Eileen Hoffman is Assistant Professor of Medicine at the Mount Sinai School of Medicine and Associate Director for Education at the Mount Sinai Women's Health Program in New York City, USA. A group delivering comprehensive primary care to women, the Women's Health Program also educates and trains physicians, and performs research in women's health. She is founding board member of the American College of Women's Health Physicians; an organization dedicated to the development of an interdisciplinary primary care speciality in women's health. Dr Hoffman speaks and writes extensively on reforming medical education and restructuring the delivery of clinical services to provide better health care to women. She also addresses the challenges and opportunities of managed care for women's health. She has chaired a session of the American Psychological Association's Women's Health Conference on these issues and is an adviser to the Jacob's Institute for Women's Health Symposia. She is author of the commissioned paper on "The Women-Centered Health Care Team" which puts forth a new model of delivery based on women as a defined population. She has also published on the implications for the training of primary care physicians imposed by managed care.

Darrelle Koonce-Volwiler Ph.D. is a second year Post-Doctoral Fellow at Stanford University, USA, and the VA Palo Alto Health Care System. She currently works at the VA Clinic of Monterey where she coordinates the local branch of a research project for female care givers of family members with dementia. Her clinical and research interests include behavioral medicine (prevention and treatment of psychological symptoms associated with chronic illness), and geropsychology (working with older adults on psychological issues).

Charlea Massion graduated with a degree in Human Biology from Stanford University, attended medical school at Case Western Reserve University School of Medicine, and completed a family practice residency at Duke University Medical Center. Currently a family physician at the Santa Cruz Medical Clinic in Santa Cruz, CA, USA and an Assistant Clinical Professor, Division of Family and Community Medicine at Stanford University School of Medicine, Charlea is on the Founding Board and currently on the Board of Directors of the American College of Women's Health Physician.

Christine L. McKibbin Ph.D. is a Postdoctoral Fellow in the Department of Endocrinology, Gerontology, and Metabolism within the Stanford University School of Medicine and is affiliated with the Older

Adult and Family Research and Resource Center within the Veterans Affairs Palo Alto Health Care System. Dr. McKibbin's research interests include psychosocial correlates of care giver mental and physical health, women's health, as well as health care utilization.

Paula Nicolson Ph.D. is a senior lecturer in health psychology at the School for Health and Related Research at Sheffield University, UK. Her research interests are on the social organisation of health care organisations, particularly gender and inter-professional relations and women's health. She is author of *Gender, Power and Organisation: A Psychological Perspective* published in 1996 by Routledge, and with Christopher Welsh is working on a study of inequality in medical education. Routledge published her most recent book *Post Natal Depression* in 1998.

John Richardson Ph.D. is Professor of Psychology in the Department of Human Sciences, Brunel University. His research has concerned a wide variety of topics in cognitive psychology, but he is particularly interested in the applications of cognitive psychology to neuropsychology, health psychology, and educational psychology. He is the editor of *Cognition and the Menstrual Cycle* (New York: Springer-Verlag, 1992).

Patrizia Romito is a psychologist at the Department of Psychology, University of Trieste, Italy. She holds a Ph.D. in Psychology and another in Women and Children Health. She has researched and teaches in the area of women's health, of motherhood and more particularly on post-natal depression, and of social policies concerning parenthood and employment. In the last few years, her main field of research and activism has become male violence against women and children and the response of social institutions. She is currently coordinating two European projects on this topic and organizing teaching and training for social and health workers and university students.

Janet S. St Lawrence Ph.D. is Chief of the Behavioral Interventions and Research Branch in the Division of STD Prevention at the Centers for Disease Control and Prevention in Atlanta, GA, USA. She completed her doctoral training in clinical psychology and has been actively involved in HIV/AIDS research since the mid 1980s. After 20 years as a Professor and Director of the Community Health Program in Mississippi, she moved to CDC in 1996.

Susan Shaw is a professor in the Department of Recreation and Leisure Studies at the University of Waterloo in Ontario, Canada. She has a Ph.D. is Sociology from Carleton University Ottawa, and taught for eight years at Dalhousie University in Nova Scotia before moving to Waterloo in 1991. Dr Shaw's research has focused on gender and leisure, including the gendered nature of leisure and the family. Most recently she has been investigating ways in which leisure practices act to re-inforce or challenge societal ideologies of femininity and masculinity.

Lorraine Sherr Ph.D. is a Clinical Psychologist and Reader in Health Psychology at the Royal Free and University College Medical School, London, UK. She has carried out research in women and health as well as a number of studies on HIV and AIDS. She is the editor of *Psychology Health and Medicine* and the *International Journal AIDS Care*. She has worked on a variety of research projects at national, European and international levels. She was appointed a Churchill Fellow for Life for work on AIDS and HIV infection in mothers and babies. She has written a number of texts, including *The Psychology of Pregnancy and Childbirth* (Blackwell Publications), *AIDS as a Gender Issue* (Taylor and Francis), *AIDS and Adolescents* (Harwood Academic), *Grief and AIDS* (John Wiley & Sons), *AIDS and the Heterosexual Population* (Harwood Academic). She has chaired the British Psychological Society committee on teaching of psychology to other professions as well as the special interest group in AIDS. She has co-ordinated and contributed to a number of European projects covering diverse topics such as ethics, discrimination and HIV disease, ante-natal HIV screening and policy, and the megapoles study on Health Promotion across Europe.

Carina Bildt Thorbjörnsson is a registered psychologist, with a degree from the Department of Applied Psychology at Uppsala University, and has been working at the National Institute for Working Life in Sweden since 1993. She has mainly been interested in psychosocial factors in relation to low back pain among women and men, but is also interested in the mechanisms in occurrence of health problems in general. Within her Ph.D. work she has been looking at the develop-ment of methods to collect information about psychosocial working conditions, as well as conditions in family life. For over a year she has been involved in developing the research program "Gender, work and health" at the institute.

Jane M. Ussher Ph.D. is an academic Psychologist with a background in Clinical Psychology and an expertise in women. She is currently at the Centre for Critical Psychology in Sydney, Australia. Her research work covers a wide range of feminist and women's issues. She has published widely in peer-reviewed journals and has written numerous texts including *The Psychology of the Female Body* (Routledge, 1989), *Women's Madness – Misogyny or Mental Illness?* (Harvester Wheatsheaf, 1991), *Fantasies of Femininity – Reframing the Boundaries of Sex* (Penguin, 1997), *Body Talk – the Material and Discursive Regulation of Sexuality, Madness and Reproduction* (Routledge).

Section 1

WOMEN TODAY

Chapter 1

Women's Health as a Medical Specialty and a Clinical Science

Eileen Hoffman M.D.

Mount Sinai School of Medicine, New York, USA

and

Charlea Massion M.D.

Stanford University School of Medicine

Women's health has inherited a model of health care that reflects both the Cartesian duality of mind and body, and a philosophy of medical science based on biological reductionism that views the body as a machine and the whole as merely a sum of the parts. As two practising physicians with over 40 years of clinical experience between us, we will explore the context of current women's health care and describe our vision for women's health in the millennium. We will focus on our own country, the United States, but believe that the concepts are universal.

Why do we need a new, interdisciplinary vision of women's health? All our health care systems are built on an outdated concept of women's lives. Today's professional medicine took form in the mid-nineteenth century, when women were considered "bodies built around a uterus". In the nineteenth and early twentieth centuries, if women survived being

Women, Health and the Mind
Edited by L. Sherr and J.S. St Lawrence. © 2000 John Wiley & Sons, Ltd

born and childhood infections, their primary cause of death was child-birth. Most of women's morbidities were also reproductively related, e.g. incontinence of urine and stool from childbirth injuries, prolapse of the uterus from multiple birthing (making some women housebound), and chronic pelvic pain from untreated venereal infections that led some women to become morphine addicts. For these problems, the field of obstetrics and gynaecology was an appropriate response by professional medicine. Outside obstetrics and gynaecology, however, men were the norm around which the rest of modern medicine evolved. Women were invisible elsewhere in health care and in medical research.

Women's invisibility has hindered and continues to impair equal quality of health care. This gender bias amplifies gender invisibility. For example, all major clinical trials of coronary artery disease have studied men, although heart disease is the leading cause of death in both men and women. We have learned that coronary artery disease progresses one way in a woman's oestrogen-rich environment and another way in a man's testosterone-rich environment. Oestrogen is anti-atherogenic. Studies show that oestrogen given to women with known coronary artery disease can reduce the risk of a second heart attack by 47% (O'Keefe et al., 1996)!

The example of coronary artery disease has parallels in all other organ systems. The belief that chest pain is benign in women has influenced generations of physicians. Even today, physicians frequently are untrained in how coronary artery disease can manifest in women. Consequently, women are less aggressively diagnosed and treated. In an editorial about gender bias in the management of heart disease, Bernadine Healey, a cardiologist who was also Director of the National Institutes of Health, coined the phrase the "Yentl syndrome" (Healy, 1991). In the "Yentl syndrome", women must appear just like men to get equal treatment. However, to get an equal quality of care, women actually need to be treated as women.

Unequal care for women has existed for hundreds of years. In Ehrenreich's & English's 1972 landmark book, *For Her Own Good*, they describe this tension as "one hundred and fifty years of quiet warfare between women and 'expert professionals' . . ." In the United States, in the 1970s this tension exploded into a women's health movement much stronger than its predecessors. Angry over medical professionals' influence over women's bodies and minds, women's health activists advocated that women empower themselves through self-help and consciousness-raising groups and by opening feminist women's health centres. Many women cut their teeth on this movement as activists, consumers, counsellors and organisers. Some even went on to become medical "experts" themselves.

In the 1970s, women's health activists diverted women from traditional physicians and hospitals towards health care organisations created by feminists, including abortion clinics, prenatal centres, contraception clinics, and feminist women's health centres. These services applied a competitive pressure to traditional health care institutions and triggered more responsiveness to health care consumers. As the number of women in medicine and other positions of influence increased, researchers became more interested in issues that were important to women. Also, with more women clinicians, gender-congruent care has become more accessible.

In the 1990s, male-modelled medicine began to transform into a women-centred science through research, new models of clinical practice, and collaboration with new organisations such as the American College of Women's Health Physicians (ACWHP), the American Medical Women's Association (AMWA), and the National Academy of Women's Health Medical Educators (NAWHME).

FROM REPRODUCTIVE RIGHTS TO EQUITY IN HEALTH CARE

The women's health movement reflected the advancement of women in other areas of society such as medicine, business, politics, and government. The presence of women in Congress, at the National Institutes of Health (NIH), and in advocacy groups such as the Society for the Advancement of Women's Health Research catalysed institutional changes. In the United States, pressure from these groups resulted in a 1990 General Accounting Office (GAO) audit that documented, in highly publicised hearings, the failure of the NIH to implement its own 1986 policy requiring inclusion of women in clinical trials. On the heels of this highly visible exposé, the American Medical Association Council on Ethical and Judicial Affairs admitted that gender bias in clinical decision-making was restricting women's access to and use of medical care (Council on Ethical and Judicial Affairs, 1991). Seemingly overnight, women's health activism catapulted from reproductive rights to a comprehensive range of women's health issues.

The "40-something" activists now took on heart disease as they had attacked reproductive issues 20 years earlier. Women baby boomers were incensed by the exclusively male-based research agenda. Whether this outrage was about exclusion or about data derived from men that could not be extrapolated to women, the stage was set to see "women as different" in a positive manner. The women's health movement had previously taken a gender-neutral stance while seeking equal opportunity in the marketplace and under the law. Could equality not be based on sameness? As the focus on women's health care shifted from abortion rights to heart disease and other issues, women realised that equal quality of health care requires an appreciation of and respect for sex and gender differences. Official responses to the GAO report included introduction and passage of the Women's Health Equity Act; creation of the Office of Women's Health at the NIH, appointment of Bernadine Healey to direct the NIH, and, eventually, funds for the Women's Health Initiative, the largest clinical trial ever undertaken.

However, in order to improve women's health, advances in medical research must be translated into improvements in health care delivery. Consequently, Congress mandated an evaluation of clinical training in women's health, both in undergraduate medical schools and the medical specialty training programmes in all disciplines. Recommendations stressed the need for "innovative approaches that cross institutional boundaries" (Council on Graduate Medical Education, 1995) and the establishment of "a place in academic medicine dedicated to advancing the art and science of women's health" (Office of Women's Health and Minority Affairs, 1996). To establish an interdisciplinary field of women's health, a professional organisation was needed to bridge the traditional boundaries among existing medical specialties and in academic medicine. To meet this need, eight women physicians from a spectrum of medical specialties founded the ACWHP in March 1996.

LEARNING FROM WOMEN'S STUDIES

In the medical sciences, women's health is analogous to women's studies in the social sciences, providing an academic base for faculty development and professional advancement based on interdisciplinary scholarship. This structure facilitates all individual contributions to "woman-centred" scholarship, while sustaining collaborations with other academic departments (Rosser, 1994). The presence of women's health physicians does not eliminate the need for internists, gynaecologists, family practitioners and other specialists anymore than women's studies eliminated sociologists, psychologists, art historians, or political scientists. A specialty in women's health assures the growth of this interdisciplinary field and encourages the integration of new knowledge and skills into all areas of medicine.

Residency programmes in women's health will provide medical students with a direct route into specialty training. The medical specialty of women's health also provides a model for efficient use of faculty resources by academic health centres. The current multidisciplinary programmes in women's health waste valuable resources. In the multidisciplinary model, clinicians with a mutual interest in women's health are brought together in the same physical location, but maintain their professional boundaries and traditional clinical roles. This model aggregates contiguous and complementary skills, but leaves major interdisciplinary gaps (see Figure 1.1 as an example of a multidisciplinary model). Faculties still retain their primary allegiances to their department-of-origin. This department also decides on promotions and mandates research and teaching assignments. Contributing departments also often duplicate educational programmes. In contrast, a true interdisciplinary model will create physicians who integrate disciplines,

MULTIDISCIPLINARY

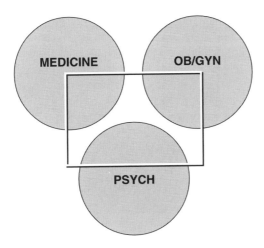

Figure 1.1   Contiguous areas with interdisciplinary gaps – breadth

INTERDISCIPLINARY

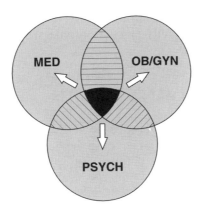

Figure 1.2   Narrow areas of overlap collectively defining the field – depth

such as medical with reproductive health, and mind with body (see Figure 1.2). All information is viewed through a gender lens focused on the whole woman. The synergy of interdisciplinary efforts, whether in treating battered women with chronic pain, women with diabetes and bulimia, or women with premenstrual heart arrhythmias, will define the field of women's health (see Figure 1.3). Women's health faculties will perform interdisciplinary research, teaching, and practice. They will develop and provide educational experiences for under-graduate medical students, for residents, and for specialists in other

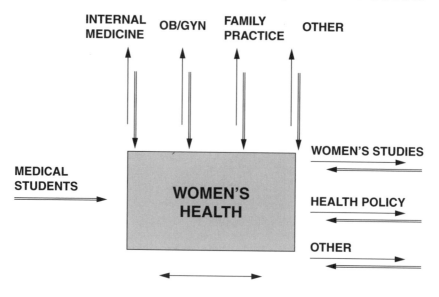

Figure 1.3 Women's economic and political power and market demands

fields, e.g. an integrated basic science course in gender-based biology, a core clerkship in women's primary care, and an ambulatory women's health experience for family practice, internal medicine, and obstetrics–gynaecology residents.

DEFINING WOMEN'S HEALTH

Listing the competencies needed to deliver comprehensive care to women is a strategic goal for existing medical specialties, but the field of women's health must be defined more precisely. The current definition of the NIH Office of Women's Health focuses on how women deviate from a male norm, i.e. "diseases, disorders and conditions that are unique to, more prevalent among, far more serious in women, or for which there are different risk factors or interventions for women than men" (Rosser, 1993). During its early development, women's studies had a similar "male-as-norm" platform. However, with evolution of the field, women's studies became defined on its own terms. This also will be necessary in women's health.

Male-modelled medicine often masquerades behind gender neutrality. For example, the current Agency for Health Care Policy and Research guidelines for the detection and treatment of depression in primary care (Agency for Health Care Policy and Research, 1996) fail to mention incest, battery, or sexual violence as sex-specific risk factors for women's depression. There is also no discussion of sex differences in the psychopharmacology of antidepressants. Although we are just beginning to understand the social and political differences that make depression twice as frequent in women as in men, if the gender-specific aspects of depression are omitted, how can women achieve equal quality of care?

Merely including women in research, without adjusting the study design and without attending to gender during analysis of the data, is an inadequate solution in medical research. A glaring example of this inadequacy is a 1996 publication entitled "Hostility predicts restenosis after PTCA" (Goodman et al., 1996). Hostility predicted restenosis after angioplasty only in men. Women, who had significantly fewer "high hostility" scores (14 versus 52%), had higher rates of restenosis (43 versus 33%). This study identified an emotional disturbance that increases cardiovascular disease risk in men, while failing to capture any emotional disturbance that results in similar risks for women. However, in the title the authors implied that hostility predicts restenosis for both men *and* women.

Gender differences in coronary artery disease have been demonstrated in other species. Those studies show that social status is an important modulator of disease severity. For example, in *Cynomolgus* monkeys, the most severe coronary lesions are seen in the most dominant males and in the most submissive females (who also have the lowest oestrogen levels) (Shively et al., 1997).

The American College of Women's Health Physicians defines women's health as "a sex- and gender-informed practice centred on the whole woman in the diverse context of her life grounded in an interdisciplinary sex- and gender-informed biopsychosocial science". This definition goes beyond reproduction, and beyond deviation, to a woman-centred paradigm that appreciates the variation in biology and sociology that is intrinsic in studying men and women.

WOMEN'S HEALTH AS A CLINICAL SCIENCE

Historically, medicine viewed women's differences as solely related to reproduction. In Darwinian analysis, women were considered devolved or "frozen in evolutionary time" because of their biological role. The predominant scientific paradigm purported that the uterus and ovaries ruled every woman's life! This focus on reproductive health influenced the development of obstetrics and gynaecology in the early twentieth century. However, from a twenty-first century perspective, what differentiates women is *not* their reproductive role *per se* or the assumption that all else is similar in men and women, but that the ability to reproduce has biological, psychological, and sociological impacts on women's health and illness.

The transition from obstetrics–gynaecology to comprehensive women's health parallels the transition of physics from Newton's mechanistic perspective to contemporary chaos theory and complexity.

Complex systems have basic components that follow basic laws. The complexity, however, is in the organisation and myriad ways that the components can interact and create systems that have different functions. The clinical science of women's health will help us to understand the amazingly complex and adaptive properties of the human organism from the "viewpoint of women". Just as the new physics includes, but does not replace, the reductionistic perspective of Newtonian mechanics, women's health includes, but does not replace, obstetrics–gynaecology.

Women's health is a science with five primary elements that assume a mind–body fusion and an appreciation of ecological impact:

1. *Pregnancy*: beyond pregnancy's relationship to increased or decreased risks for certain diseases are the biological adaptations or maladaptions to pregnancy that put women at specific risk for illness or make them especially healthy. For example, acute heart attack is seen during the peri-partum period. Coronary angiography demonstrates atherosclerosis in fewer than half of these cases (Roth and Elkayam, 1996). Most peri-partum heart attacks are related to changes that cause rupture of the artery walls or blood clots and arterial spasm. The risk for thrombosis (blood clot) is greater in the peri-partum because of the acute decline in t-Pa inhibitor, a natural anticoagulant, after placental separation. Naturally occurring vascular phenomena in women provide a model to investigate the pathogenesis and treatment of circulatory disease in women.

2. *Systemic effects of ovarian hormones*: reproductive hormones affect all organ systems. For example, oestrogen is anti-atherogenic. Oestrogen alters lipids, has antioxidant and antiplatelet functions, improves muscle tone in the heart and circulatory systems, and improves function in the tissue that lines all arteries. Another example is that progesterone raises the seizure threshold. For epileptic women who have anovulatory cycles, adding progesterone can eliminate seizures that occur on "therapeutic" doses of anticonvulsants (Herzog, 1986). Therapeutic advances for both women and men follow sex-specific applications of all research findings!

3. *Menstrual cycle chronobiology*: many illnesses are affected by the menstrual cycle, e.g. asthma, migraine, diabetes, pneumothorax, appendicitis, rheumatoid arthritis, and vasodepressor syncope. In premenopausal women, menstrual cycle timing of mastectomy may affect survival (Hrushesky, 1996). Using bras that detect temperature, investigators found higher temperatures in cancerous breasts across the entire menstrual cycle. Normal breasts only had higher temperatures in the luteal phase (Simpson et al., 1995). Menstrual cycle chronobiology illustrates that knowledge of complex interrelationships is required to provide good clinical care to women. Outcome data cannot be interpreted with any accuracy if the women in clinical trials are not identified as premenopausal, perimeno-

pausal, postmenopausal, anovulatory, on hormone therapy, or on oral contraceptives.

4. *Sex differences at the molecular level*: recent work in genetic imprinting reveals the sex-specific nature of DNA itself. Genetic imprinting is defined as the parental-dependent transmission of genetic traits. This phenomenon can best be appreciated in experiments of nature. For example, the hydatidiform mole contains DNA only from the father and is expressed as placental proliferation and invasiveness. The dermoid cyst, on the other hand, has DNA derived only from the mother and expresses every embryonal cell line, but without placental development, vascular invasion, or orderly tissue development. Furthermore, parental genetic material interacts with the sex of the fetus. For example, the gene for spinal cord malformation, carried by the maternal line, will usually produce anencephaly in a female fetus but spina bifida in a male fetus.

5. *Gender differences at the sociocultural level*: in addition to using women's biology as the foundation of women's health, women's life experiences are essential components of a sex- and gender-informed science. Violence, for example, is a tragically common aspect of many women's lives and has a dramatic impact on women's health. In a prospective study of primary care patients, victimisation was significantly associated with lower self-perceptions of health and with higher physician visits and outpatient expenses (Koss et al., 1991). In fact, violence was a stronger predictor of physician visits and outpatient costs than were age and other common health hazards. A history of abuse has also been linked to subsequent aberrations in physiological arousal and neuroendocrine responses.

TOWARD WOMAN-CENTRED SCIENCE

Woman-centred medicine implies a "woman-as-norm" foundation. For example, in a fanciful yet scientifically well-grounded paper, Profet recasts menstruation as a biological defence against reproductive tract diseases caused by bacteria clinging to sperm (Profet, 1993). Instead of a failed opportunity for conception or "the womb weeping for a baby" as menstruation has been described, Profet sees menstruation as an adaptive design for female health and fertility. Current data show that white blood cells found in menstrual blood are important in vaginal immunity (Hill and Anderson, 1992). The rarity of CD4 cells in the normal vagina may explain why women are at increased risk of HIV infection when traumatic bleeding occurs during intercourse or when coexisting infections damage the integrity of vaginal cells.

Women's normal biology is instructive for understanding commonly occurring complex phenomena. For example, spontaneous angiogenesis, i.e. growth of new arteries and veins, is uncommon in the adult except during wound healing and tumour growth. However, in the female reproductive tract, this angiogenic activity regularly occurs during many phases of the menstrual cycle and during implantation of the placenta during pregnancy. These easily accessible tissues can elucidate the mechanisms involved in menorrhagia, endometriosis, and perimenopausal, intermenstrual, and oral contraceptive-induced bleeding, as well as tumour growth and vascular proliferation in both sexes (Rogers et al., 1992).

THE PRO/CON DEBATE

It is a false dichotomy and a disservice to women to think that a specialty in women's health excludes improvements in family practice, internal medicine, obstetrics–gynaecology and all other current medical specialties. Both a specialty in women's health *and* improved care by all existing specialties are needed. Internists, gynaecologists and family physicians all need improved training in women's health (Johnson, 1992, in Johnson et al., 1992). No one specialty yet focuses its mission on advancing the art and science of comprehensive women's health.

The evolution of a medical specialty often begins by identifying a population that needs improved services. The science then follows. For example, departments of surgery resisted emergency medicine, the most recently evolved medical specialty in the United States, and medicine claimed it did not represent new or unique knowledge. Yet, over the last 20 years, we have all benefited from the advances made by physicians trained in emergency medicine and dedicated to patients in need of emergency care. As with emergency medicine, some physicians are now aware how poorly the current health care system serves women and of the variable quality of services offered by different providers. Both emergency medicine and women's health began their efforts with those already working in the field, upgrading their skills and improving quality by transferring state-of-the-art knowledge into clinical practice, setting standards, and training new practitioners.

Proponents of a new field must articulate its necessity and project a vision for its evolution. Sceptics and those who expect to lose professional "turf" and dollars will cling to the status quo. Resistance will also come from the historical, political and sociological discomfort that has existed in differentiating women from men. Women, however, are more prepared than ever to speak to that difference. This shared vision between consumers and health providers will surely overcome professional self-interest by physicians and others who feel bound to the current inadequate model of women's health.

The driving force behind this transformation in health care services for women is the dramatic change in women's lives during this century. Seventy-five percent of women in the United States are in the paid labour force, and by the year 2000, 50% of the paid labour force will be female. Women are no longer economically dependent solely upon men. Most, however, remain in the paid labour force while mothering. Also, most women will live many years after menopause.

The development of obstetrics–gynaecology was an appropriate response by professional medicine to the needs of early twentieth century women, whose major morbidities and mortality were from reproductive causes and who rarely lived beyond their fertile years. Women's health as a medical specialty responds to the lives of women entering the twenty-first century, many of whom spend their reproductive years preventing or limiting pregnancy and who live 30–50% of their life span beyond the menopause. The American College of Women's Health Physicians follows seven guiding principles (ACWHP, 1997):

1. *Women-centred care*: Women's health is a distinct field of biomedical, psychological, and sociological knowledge and skills based on the study of women's experiences.
2. *Respectful use of power*: The respectful use of power is the capacity to produce positive and empowering change. Throughout the health care system, power affects women's assessment and treatment and her interactions with others. Effective education, trustworthy research and constructive organisational functioning thrive in environments in which power is used respectfully.
3. *Diversity*: The recognition and appreciation of diversity is the key to the development of progressive models of research, medical education, patient care and organisational development. Parsimonious theories that attempt to describe all people are unrealistic and ultimately inaccurate. ACWHP is committed to recognising the diversity among women and the differences and similarities between women and men from a positive perspective.

   Theories and methods of research, medical education, patient care, and organisational development must reflect an awareness and appreciation of the realities and perspectives of students, patients, colleagues and research participants who differ in culture, ethnicity, socio-economic status, sexual orientation, physical and emotional abilities, and other socially-constructed or biologically-determined categories.
4. *Activism*: Many of the health problems of girls and women are influenced by the broader political and economic contexts of their lives. It is important to recognise that political and economic systems have the power to diminish or eliminate health problems or to create, exacerbate or ignore them. Therefore, beyond providing health care for individuals, there is a need to accept responsibility to exercise influence in the service of girls and women in these broader arenas.
5. *Eclectic healing practices*: Healing takes many forms. The biomedical model has been and will continue to contribute strongly to healing

techniques. However, it has limits. On behalf of our patients, we take a pragmatic, rather than a dogmatic, approach to healing. Support for research to evaluate the safety and effectiveness of alternative and complementary healing practices is needed. This knowledge needs to be integrated into teaching, research, and clinical recommendations.

6. *Complexity*: Health is a function of the interactions among biological, psychological, familial, ethnic, social, cultural, environmental, occupational, and spiritual factors and, sometimes, chance. Health problems cannot be accurately and effectively detected, diagnosed, or resolved separately from the complex context in which they occur. Interdisciplinary knowledge and skills with sensitivity to all these factors are essential to the art and science of women's health.

7. *Individual and organisational well being*: Individual and collective success occurs best in the context of respectful connection and caring. Interactions characterised by interdependence, mutuality and reciprocity support individual well being, as well as organisational success. Informed care should be dedicated to practices that 1) empowers or enables others' achievements, 2) encourages one's own personal growth and professional accomplishments, and 3) enhances team spirit and collaboration.

All health professions need a better paradigm for learning about women's health and illness and for guiding their work with women. Simply increasing the list of competencies of traditionally trained physicians is an inadequate solution. New structures are needed within medicine, nursing, mental health and all allied health sciences that not only contain a "woman-as-norm" curricular content but that reflect the complex interrelationships between molecules, cells, organ systems, body, mind, culture, and the health professions. As the power of women increases and is expressed throughout all our social, political, and economic institutions, we can expect new structures, including a medical specialty in women's health, to be created. Imagine what Charlotte Perkins Gilman, an early twentieth century woman who describes her mistreatment by misogynist physicians in her book, *The Yellow Wallpaper*, would say if she could see women's health care on the brink of the twenty-first century!

REFERENCES

Agency for Health Care Policy and Research (1996). *Depression in Primary Care: Detection, Diagnosis, and Treatment*. DHHS. PHS. HRSA.

American College of Women's Health Physicians (1997). *American College of Women's Health Physicians Guiding Principles*. ACWHP, 1111 N. Plaza Drive, Suite 550, Schaumburg, Illinois 60173, USA or ACWHP website, <www.Acwh.org.>

Council on Ethical and Judicial Affairs, American Medical Association (1991). Gender disparities in clinical decision making. *New England Journal of Medicine, 266*, 559–561.

Council on Graduate Medical Education (1995) *Fifth Report: Women & Medicine*. DHHS. USPHS. HRSA. July.

Ehrenreich & English (1972). *For Her Own Good*. New York: Doubleday.

Goodman, M., Quigley, J., Morgan, G., Meilman, H., & Sherman, M. (1996). Hostility predicts restenosis after percutaneous transluminal coronary angioplasty. *Mayo Clinic Proceedings, 71*, 721–734.

Healy, B. (1991). The Yentl syndrome. Editorial. *New England Journal of Medicine, 325*, 274–276.

Herzog, A.G. (1986). Intermittent progesterone therapy and frequency of complex partial seizures in women with menstrual disorders. *Neurology, 36*, 1607–1610.

Hill, J.A., & Anderson, D.J. (1992). Human vaginal leukocytes and the effects of vaginal fluid on lymphocyte and macrophage defense functions. *American Journal of Obstetrics and Gynecology, 166*, 720–726.

Hrushesky, W.J. (1996). Breast cancer timing of surgery, and the menstrual cycle: call for prospective trial. *Journal of Women's Health, 5*, 555–566.

Johnson, K., Harrison, M., & Wallis, L. (1992). Johnson, K., PRO. Women's health: developing a new interdisciplinary specialty. CON. Harrison, M., Women's health as a specialty: a deceptive solution. Commentary. Wallis, L., Women's health: a specialty? Pros and cons. *Journal of Women's Health, 1*, 95–108.

Koss, M.P., Koss, P.G., & Woodruff, J. (1991) Deleterious effects of criminal victimization on women's health and medical utilization. *Archives of Internal Medicine, 151*, 342–347.

Office of Women's Health and Minority Affairs (1996). *Conference on Women's Health and Cultural Competency in Medical Education*. DHHS. USPHS. HRSA.

O'Keefe, J.H. Jr, Conn, R.D., Lavie, C.J., & Bateman, J. (1996). New Paradigms for Coronary Artery Disease. *Mayo Clinic Proceedings, 1*, 957–965.

Profet, M. (1993). Menstruation as a defense against pathogens transported by sperm. *The Quarterly Review of Biology, 68*, 335–381.

Rogers, P.A.W., Abberton, K.M., & Susil, B. (1992). Endothelial cell migratory signal produced by human endometrium during the menstrual cycle. *Human Reproduction, 7*, 1061–1066.

Rosser, S.V. (1993). A model for a specialty in women's health. *Journal of Women's Health, 2*, 99–104.

Rosser, S.V. (1994) *Women's Health – Missing From U.S. Medicine*. Indiana: Indiana University Press.

Roth, A., & Elkayam, U. (1996). Acute myocardial infarction associated with pregnancy. Review. *Annals of Internal Medicine, 125*, 751–762.

Shively, C.A., Leber-Laird, K., & Anton, R.F. (1997). Behavior and phys-
    iology of social stress and depression in female *Cynomolgus* monkeys.
    Biological Psychiatry, 41, 871–882.
Simpson, H.W., McArdle, C., Pauson, A.W., Hume, P., Turkes, A., &
    Griffiths, K.A. (1995). A noninvasive test for the precancerous breast.
    European Journal of Cancer, 31, 1768–1772.

Chapter 2

The Gendered Body: Body and Gender and the Inter-relationships with Health

Marrie H.J. Bekker

Tilburg University, The Netherlands

The body is the center of health and illness experiences. Gender identity is also primarily based on the body. It goes without saying that many sex differences in the domain of health are due to the fact that men and women have different bodies: some diseases or health-related phenomena such as reproduction simply occur in one sex only. Breast cancer and prostate cancer for example are inextricably bound up with one gender.

This relatively simple relationship between biological sex and health covers only a small part of the many associations between these two. First, many diseases or health-related phenomena do not occur in one sex only but in both sexes – more precisely, more in one and less in the other. Here, the relationships between sex and health immediately become more complex and gender presents itself. For example, should we explain the earlier mortality in men due to cardiovascular diseases by sex-specific physical characteristics, by sex-specific daily life influences, by gender differences in symptom perception or illness behavior,

Women, Health and the Mind
Edited by L. Sherr and J.S. St Lawrence. © 2000 John Wiley & Sons, Ltd

or by differential diagnostic processes? Second, due to sociocultural (gender) differences in the meaning of (sex-specific) parts of the body, e.g. female breasts or male prostates, sex-bound diseases or health-related phenomena have different implications for both sexes. The experience and implications of breast cancer, for example, can only be adequately understood if the sociocultural meanings of female breasts are taken into consideration. Third, sociocultural sex differences in socialization processes and daily life imply sex differences in relating to and experiencing the body; this gendered body experience influences health.

The focus of this chapter is mainly on this third relationship between biological sex, gender, body and health. Its aim is to examine the most salient differences between men and women in our culture in experiencing their bodies, and to explore what these differences might imply for male and female health and, hence, for gender-sensitive health care. First, the above-mentioned relationships between biological sex, gender, body and health will be inventoried and described more precisely by means of a model. Second, the psychological literature will be scrutinized to examine one part of the model in greater detail: sex differences in experiencing the body. The implications of gender-specific body experiences for the domain of health will also be discussed. Here, the focus will be on body image, -esteem and -satisfaction on the one hand and body awareness on the other. Then, the discussion will be raised to a more general level addressing the relationship between gender, the body and autonomy, again in relation to health. Finally, conclusions will be drawn regarding health care and future research.

BIOLOGICAL SEX, BODY, GENDER, AND HEALTH; A MODEL

Being male or being female is a core aspect of our bodies as well as our identities, that thoroughly influences all domains of life including health. As the author's Multi-Facet Gender and Health Model shows (see Figure 2.1), several relationships can be distinguished between biological (bodily) sex differences, gender and sex differences in health. First of all, having a male or female body means, of course, that some diseases can and others cannot affect a person, simply because of their exclusive occurrence in sex-specific parts of the body. Reproduction-associated health risks are a clear example. Another relationship between biological sex and health exists because of the mediation of several sex-bound physical health influences, such as hormones, that also produce sex differences in health.

People's health is strongly influenced by their direct environment and daily life situation which, again, are different for men and women and contain numerous sex-specific stressors. Processes of sex-typing and gender-identity development result in the continuous

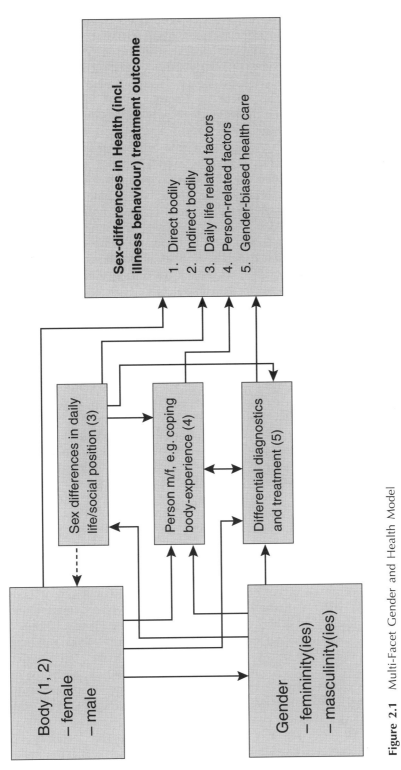

Figure 2.1 Multi-Facet Gender and Health Model

reproduction of a world in which both sexes occupy different social positions: they differ in professions, number of hours working in paid jobs, time spent on child care and care for other people, and amount of leisure time and types of leisure activities. All these differences seem relevant for sex differences in health protection and risk. For instance, Frankenhaeuser & Lundberg (in Lundberg, 1996) concluded that, in women, stress caused by domestic responsibilities contributed to a lack of unwinding at home after work. According to Lundberg (1996), women's elevated psychophysiological arousal from work stems from role conflicts and overload and might induce psychosomatic symptoms such as cardiovascular and musculoskeletal disorders. Other authors emphasize the health-protecting effects of combining work and care, which is so often practiced by women, for instance a longer life expectancy (Hibbard & Pope, 1991; Kotler & Wingard, 1989; Waldron & Jacobs, 1989). In summary, the many sex differences in daily life resulting from gender differences in social positions imply differences between men and women in health, including illness behavior, incidence of diseases and treatment outcome. Simultaneously, gendered daily life results in sex-specific bodily functioning which, in turn, also leads to sex differences in health.

The development of gender differences in men and women not only results in the "choice" of different daily lives, all with their own health-relevant characteristics; gender also implies that men and women have different personalities coping and body experiences and attitudes. We have to remember here that gender is what culture makes out of the "raw material" of biological sex (Oakley, 1972; Unger & Crawford, 1996) and that the body is so prone to cultural meanings of masculinity and femininity. When we take this paradox into consideration, it is amazing that the most important measures of gender identity in psychology only focus upon one's psychological characteristics and totally obscure the gendered ways in which people experience their bodies, perceive their inner bodily states, and "make" an outward appearance "out of their raw material". Because culture shapes gender and gender shapes body experiences, male and female body experiences vary across cultures. For example, Richters (1997) referring to the anthropological work of Becker (1995) contrasts Western culture, where the female body has become an object of individual control and will power (see also Bordo, 1993), with the Fiji islands, where a well-fed male or female body means that others take care of you. On the Fiji islands, the body seems to be an instrument for cultivating social relations, not for cultivating one's own outward appearance as an esthetic object. In the case of illness, the body, being owned by the community, has to be healed by the community too. Healing is done by conflict solving and rearranging the social order, a totally different way from that which is common in Western medicine.

In the processes of evaluating, maintaining and regaining health, others, especially health care workers, can be crucial. They talk with patients about their health problems, decide about diagnoses and propose treatment procedures. At the interpersonal level, biological sex is an important cue for how to behave (Unger & Crawford, 1996). Results of various studies indicate that the biological sex of the patient plays an important role in all stages of health care, mediated by cognitive processes within health care workers such as sex role stereotyping. For instance, sex-specific interaction patterns in doctor–patient conversations appear to influence the labeling of the patient's "problem" (Davis, 1988; Meeuwesen, 1988; Weijts, 1993). This interpersonal, differential effect of biological sex on diagnostics is also active on the level of treatment. A well-known example is the gender-bias that is supposed to play a role in the management of cardiovascular diseases (e.g. Healy, 1991). A study by Van der Waals (1995), another example, showed that male doctors prescribed benzodiazepines more often to female patients than to male patients.

Gender determines sex differences in health not only via different body experiences in women and men and via sex-specific social positions. Gender also constructs differences in self-presentation and presentation of complaints and thus contributes to gender bias in diagnostics and treatment. Meeuwesen (1988), for example, found that when they visit their general practitioner women talk more about their life in general than do men.

In summary, the outcome variable in the Multi-Facet Gender and Health Model, sex differences in health (including sex differences in prevalence of illnesses, illness behavior, implications of illnesses, treatment outcome, etc.), can be determined by multiple factors: direct (1) and indirect (2) bodily factors play a role; numerous biopsychosocial factors resulting from sex-specific daily life (3) form a substantial background; gendered person-related factors, e.g. coping and body experiences (4) leave their marks; and, finally, gender-bias in health care (5) is contributing.

Having inventoried facets of the relationships between biological sex, gender, and health, I will further scrutinize one part of the model in greater detail. In the next section, I will examine gendered body experiences and attitudes that are described in Western psychological literature, together with their implications for sex differences in health-related phenomena.

BODY EXPERIENCES BY MEN AND WOMEN IN WESTERN CULTURE

The Role of Outward Appearance

Notwithstanding the centrality of body experience in health-related phenomena, its relationship with health has received relatively little attention. An exception, however, is the area of eating disorders, the prevalences of which are extremely different for both sexes [American Psychiatric Association (APA), 1994]. Therefore, sex differences in body experience are a primary focus of studies on eating disorders. How is body experience conceptualized in these studies?

In general, body experience, in these studies mainly labeled *body image*, is constricted to the perceptual, attitudinal and emotional aspects of (possibly) being fatter than one should be according to the current cultural ideal of slenderness. Because the cultural pressure of slenderness almost exclusively concerns the female sex, the (perceived) discrepancy between actual and ideal body weight and shape implies *body dissatisfaction* (Fallon & Rozin, 1985; Keeton et al., 1990; Thompson & Psaltis, 1988), and mainly affects women (e.g. Boskind-White & White, 1983; Garner et al., 1985; Hawkins & Clement, 1980; Huon & Brown, 1989; Orbach, 1978; Stice, 1994). Female body dissatisfaction has been considered a serious threatening factor for self-esteem (Silberstein et al., 1987) and has been identified as a predictor of eating disorders (e.g. Noordenbos, Acda & Borreson-Gresko, 1999; Stice, 1994). In addition, fear of physical unattractiveness appeared as one of the dimensions of feminine gender role stress (Gillespie & Eisler, 1992), stress resulting from a rigid adherence to the traditional feminine gender role. Martz et al. (1995) concluded from their studies that feminine gender role stress might be the missing link between cultural values of femininity, particularly having to be slim, and vulnerability for eating disorders.

Although many authors agree that body image, and thus body dissatisfaction, are multidimensional constructs (Ben-Tovim & Walker, 1991, 1992; Cash & Brown, 1989), the dimensions under study usually refer to weight or dieting only. Only in a small number of studies have aspects such as fitness also been considered (e.g. Cash & Brown, 1989).

In the few studies concerning body experience that were done outside the context of eating disorders, broader concepts of body experience have been used. Nevertheless, the majority of these studies also focused on the impact of differing sociocultural pressures brought to bear on men and women, in particular the importance of female outward appearance, or slenderness. Franzoi & Shields (1984) found that male and female body esteem can be discussed in terms of three primary dimensions that are different for either sex. For women, these were the dimensions of sexual attractiveness, i.e. body aspects dealing with facial attractiveness and sexuality; weight concern, i.e. body parts and functions associated with controlling food intake; and physical condition, i.e. dealing with attitudes toward physical qualities such as stamina and strength. For men, the dimensions were physical attractiveness, i.e. satisfaction with facial and body features determining how "good-looking" a male is; upper body strength, i.e. attitudes toward upper body parts and functions that can be altered through anaerobic exercise; and physical condition, i.e. evaluating satisfaction with how well the body works and its general strength. Notice that, for both sexes, only one dimension referred to an aspect of body experience other than appearance-related aspects. Franzoi et al. (1989) investigated body awareness in both sexes (considered here, again, as awareness of outward bodily characteristics!) and found that females – when attentive to their bodies – experienced more negative feelings than males. Moreover, the awareness of the women appeared to be more directed toward specific body parts or functions than to the body as a whole, which was the case for the men. The results of this study indicate that neither the degree of body awareness nor its importance differed for both sexes. However, males' degree of body awareness was positively related to body esteem, while females' body experience was positively related to beliefs about the importance of physical criteria in judging their body dimensions. Ben-Tovim & Walker (1991) also aimed to explore normal women's *attitudes toward their own bodies*, especially to generate a profile of those body-related attitudes that a majority of women feel to be important. The authors claim that the six subscales of their *Body Attitudes Questionnaire* (BAQ), including Feeling Fat, Disparagement, Strength, Salience, Attractiveness and Lower Body Fat, identify a broader range of specific body attitudes than had previously been assessed. Their comparison of BAQ scores of normal females from a community sample with those of patients with anorexia nervosa revealed that the latter had negative feelings toward every aspect of body functioning and appearance (disparagement) and not only, as is commonly described, toward their own weight and shape.

It is remarkable how dominant outward appearance is in these conceptions of body image and attitudes. Even concepts such as body dissatisfaction and body esteem are dominated by dissatisfaction about and esteem of the body-as-an-external-esthetic-object, in particular of its weight and shape. This is surprising given the possibility to evaluate the body by using other aesthetic criteria such as expressivity or other dimensions such as alienation (see Bekker et al., 1996), fitness, strength, health and adequacy with respect to its numerous functions (see Franzoi, 1995) such as sleeping, eating, seeing, hearing, smelling, sexuality, reproduction and sports. It is difficult to determine whether the preoccupation with outward appearance, particularly with weight and shape, reflects the minds of the researchers, the subjects under study, the fact that most of the studies were done in the context of eating disorders (which are generally assumed to be strongly determined by an obsession with the current female beauty ideal of slenderness) and/or a general obsession or one-sidedness within our culture.

With respect to health, several implications of this unidimensional body experience can be mentioned. First, as has already been elaborated before, obsessional attempts to achieve a slim body can deteriorate into eating disturbances. Second, other health-relevant types of behavior associated with eating and hence with calorie intake can also be affected by the weight and shape obsession. One of them is the level of physical activity. Silberstein et al. (1988) found that women, more than men, exercised to control their weight. These findings were confirmed by McDonald & Thompson (1990) and by Van Steen & Bekker (submitted). Women exercised more than men for weight control reasons and this motive was positively associated with dissatisfaction with the body. One might wonder how a potentially positive female health behavior, exercising, is predominantly motivated by the wish to change the body into a culturally accepted shape. Due to biological factors, the ideal presented in the media is hard to achieve; the percentage of fat in women's bodies is 25%, whereas in men's bodies it is 15%, so women naturally "deviate" from the ideal of thinness. If weight loss and toning up body shape remain the primary motivation for women to exercise, women are more likely to stop physical exercise when the desired effect is not achieved (Van Steen & Bekker, submitted).

Another health-relevant behavior that is clearly associated with eating and calorie intake, is smoking. Smoking seems to keep body weight down, which may contribute to beginning smoking among adolescents, especially females (Camp et al., 1993). Moreover, women appear to be less interested in giving up smoking than men. One of the reasons is that they are more concerned about weight gain after quitting (Sorensen & Pechacek, 1987).

As numerous authors have pointed out, many women experience body dissatisfaction due to the (perceived) discrepancy between the cultural ideal and the actual body weight and shape. What, beside eating-related behaviors, are the implications of body dissatisfaction for health behavior? Dissatisfaction implies negative affect, and negative affect is related to a wide range of disturbances such as alcoholism, depression and poor health. Taylor (1995) concludes that individuals who are chronically high in negative affect may be more likely to become sick and also to show distress, physical symptoms and illness behavior even when they are not sick. One might wonder what specific health effects can be added that are related to the dissatisfaction concerning the body. It might, for instance, be harder for women than for men to show their bodies to the doctor, which might influence their illness behavior.

One final remark in this section concerns the research on body image and esteem. Apparently, women and men have reacted so differently to body image and esteem measures in various studies that results have been presented for one sex only, or different dimensions or subscales for men and women have been used separately. Of course, this might adequately reflect the situation as it is: women and men in our current culture have quite different experiences in the domain of outward appearance. However, these current measures do not allow any comparison of the sexes. Therefore, with colleagues, I initiated a study to compare the two sexes on body experience dimensions with highly similar meanings for both men and women (Bekker et al., 1999). We identified three subscales with similar meanings for men and women, namely Body Acceptance, Appearance Appraisal by Others, and

Physical Strength. Men scored significantly higher than women on body acceptance and on appearance appraisal by others, but no sex difference was found on physical strength. For men and women separately, we found different correlations between their scores on the body experience subscales and various health measures. We therefore think that the use of such a body experience measure allowing comparisons between both sexes might be fruitful for future health research.

What about Body Awareness?

Psychological literature shows a large discrepancy in the amount of attention paid to experiencing the outward body (appearance) compared with inner body experiences. At this point, we turn to the other psychological tradition aimed at body-related subjectivity, the area of internal *body awareness* and *symptom perception* (see Pennebaker, 1982). Here, the inner body is the core issue, as far as it is perceived, interpreted and made a motive by the subject for showing illness behavior.

In the tradition of symptom perception research, sex differences and gender-related issues have also been subjected to investigation. For instance, Gijsbers van Wijk (1995) studied sex differences in morbidity and symptom perception, taking the female excess report of physical symptoms as a starting point. She found a higher female somitization score in primary care patients which could be explained by, among other factors, a heightened selective attention to bodily states. Within the same theoretical framework, Gijsbers van Wijk & van Vliet (1989) argued that women compared to men are more aware of their bodies and therefore perceive more physical symptoms. As a consequence, women also show more preventive behavior such as visiting their general practitioner (see also Hibbard & Pope, 1986).

An important implication of this point of view is that the higher report of physical symptoms by women that is generally found in research, together with their higher medical consumption (see Verbrugge, 1989), might be substantially explained by a higher awareness of bodily signals and the perception of more physical symptoms. Women, from this perspective, are not "the sicker sex"; they just notice more bodily signals and/or interpret their bodily signals more in terms of physical symptoms. As a result, they will show more preventive illness behavior than men do, which is a sex difference that has nothing to do with actual illness.

Gijsbers van Wijk (1995) mentioned several aspects of the female body, of sex-specific daily life, and of girls' socialization processes that might play a role in the presumed higher body awareness of women. For example, female reproductive processes such as the menstrual cycle produce a host of internal information that is absent in men. Having a job might imply that one is exposed to an environmental condition that yields more external information than being at home, a daily life situation which is more frequently experienced by women than by men. Following Pennebaker's (1982) competition of cues model, the sex differences in employment rate, considered here as sex differences in exposure to external information (women less, men more), might also contribute to differences in symptom perception: women more, men less. Regarding sex role socialization, Gijsbers van Wijk referred, among other things, to the "boys don't cry doctrine" that might result in a higher threshold for detecting somatic sensations.

Of course, body awareness as a concept is difficult to measure. In particular, distinguishing internal awareness from the report of somatic signals is an important problem. Additionally, not much is known at present about sex differences in body awareness nor about their determinants. For example, we do not know whether the assumption that housekeeping implies exposure to less and employment implies exposure to more external information, holds water. Furthermore, women can definitely have specific bodily experiences that might predispose them to a higher body awareness, e.g. menstruation, but men seem to have other, presumably also body-awareness-increasing, experiences, such as their higher involvement in sports and physical activity. Also, sexually, men generally still seem to show more proactive, initiating behavior, and to explore more different behavioral alternatives. The higher involvement of men in domains such as physical exercise, sports and sexuality might mean that they, rather than women, develop a higher general body awareness. Another, maybe more plausible, option is that body awareness varies with the (sex-specific) social domain with which several bodily functions are associated; perhaps women are more aware of their bellies and breasts (naturally), due to conception, menstruation, pregnancy, lactation, etc., whereas men have greater awareness of their muscular strength, physical coordination and condition, because of their higher involvement in sports.

Much more research is needed to gain insight into the relationships between gender, body awareness and sex-specific daily life situations. Subcultural differences and life span effects also seem relevant. Furthermore, the relationships between body awareness and symptom perception deserve further exploration.

Following the state of the art in the psychological literature, in which body-related concepts are so strictly separated into concepts referring to the inner body and concepts referring to outward appearance, several additional questions come to mind. How are body awareness experiences related to appearance-related ones? Particularly, what are the relationships between women's presumed heightened body awareness and the above-mentioned empirical findings concerning orientation to outward appearance and body image, esteem and satisfaction? Does a stronger orientation to outward appearance of women compared to men imply that women are less aware of their inner bodies? Clinical observations (Bekker, 1986; Vandereijcken, 1996) indicate that, in bulimic women, dieting and an obsession with slenderness and calorie intake are associated with a diminished ability to recognize internal signals such as hunger, saturation and specific food preferences. Or is the relationship between orientation on outward appearance and internal body awareness the reverse: the stronger this orientation, the more body awareness?

To my knowledge, only one study examined both types of body experiences in relation to each other. Franzoi (1995) labeled the concepts referring to outward body experiences as "body-as-object": an object of discrete parts that others evaluate esthetically. "Body-as-process" is the label that Franzoi used to mention inner body experiences or "to conceptualize it [the body] as a dynamic *process* where function is of greater consequence than beauty" (p.417). Franzoi elaborated how, starting at a young age, females are taught that their body-as-object is significant in how others judge their overall value. Men, on the other hand, "are typically trained for a world of action . . . where the ability of the body to adeptly move through physical space is stressed more than how it looks as a stationary object" (p.419). Although recognizing that there will be considerable overlap in body orientation between women and men, he described the resulting gender differences in body orientation in terms of Freedman (1990) as the "ornamental feminine ideal" and the "instrumental masculine ideal". Results of the study showed that, regardless of gender, young adults had less positive attitudes toward their body parts (body-as-object) than toward their body functions (body-as-process). Furthermore, women who had adopted more masculine attributes seemed to be less susceptible to the feminine body-as-object "beauty trap". Franzoi (1995) concluded that female body esteem might be restructured if women and others pay more attention to their body-as-process.

In summary, it is clear that experiences related to the body as an esthetic object are a part of body-related subjectivity on which many psychological studies have focused, whereas cognitive-emotional processes related to the inner body have not been studied extensively. This comes as no surprise; the predominantly female domain of outward appearance, weight and shape has a high clinical and health–psychology relevance.

The association with health problems might obscure the fact that women also gain pleasure (see Coward, 1984) and autonomy (Davis, 1995) from actively manipulating their outward appearance or deciding to let others, e.g. cosmetic surgeons, do it for them. Nevertheless, the dark side seems to fit rather well into the old feminist complaint that female bodily experiences are highly influenced by power inequality between the sexes and by patriarchal dispossession. Let me quote here the well-known statement by Berger (1972): "Men look at women. Women are being looked at, and that is how they look at themselves: as subjects that are being looked at." From the dispossession point of view, greater attention to the female body as a process and greater awareness of its functioning might imply greater bodily autonomy for women and might indeed bring about the process of restructuring female body esteem mentioned by Franzoi (1995). In the next section, women's relationship to their bodies will be further elaborated from the perspective of power, autonomy and control.

GENDER, THE BODY, AND AUTONOMY

More than 25 years have passed since publication of *Our Bodies, Ourselves* by the Boston Women's Health Collective. This important and influential collective emphasized, among other things, that our female bodily experiences were highly influenced by patriarchal dispossession and that many women had become alienated from their own bodies. The Boston Collective encouraged women to get acquainted with their own bodies once again, to regain the feeling of owning their own bodies and to realize self-determination in health decisions, in sexuality and in reproduction issues. In the previous section of this chapter, women's relationships toward their own bodies still appeared to be a matter of concern; yet data about changes in this domain over time are lacking. Do women nowadays experience more autonomy in the areas of health decisions, sexuality and reproduction?

First, it is necessary to recognize worldwide differences between women's opportunities to make their own decisions in body-related domains. In Eastern Europe and Africa, for example, it is hardly possible to speak of autonomy regarding women and health matters. Second, if one tries to determine whether Western women nowadays have more autonomy in the area of health, sexuality and reproduction, an ironic picture emerges. Women definitely do have more contraceptive choices, it is easier for them to have an abortion and they generally seem to experience more sexual pleasure. More options are also available in the domain of outward appearance, due to the new developments in cosmetic surgery. Western bodily self-determination can also be considered to have increased because of the option of in vitro fertilization and other fertility-increasing procedures and new screening techniques. One may wonder, however, whether new reproductive technology and cosmetic surgery are positive contributions to women's bodily self-determination (see also Bekker, van Vliet & Kolk, 1999).

Self-determination by women is only one side of the increasing possibilities of medical technology for women. For example, it has become complicated to make choices about conception and about prenatal screening with the aid of new medical technologies. Also with respect to cosmetic surgery, it is one-sided to analyse the new possibilities in terms of increased autonomy, given the cultural pressure upon women to adapt to the female beauty standards (see also Van Lenning, 1997). In summary, when highlighting and using self-determination as a criterion, it seems to be very difficult to analyze whether women's autonomy concerning bodily issues has genuinely improved in the last few decades.

CONCLUSIONS

In this chapter, the relationships between biological sex, gender, body and health were presented in a model developed by the author and one part of the Multi-Facet Gender & Health Model was described in greater detail using the psychological literature concerning body experience, gender and health. Although there are huge differences among women and among men in how they experience their bodies, the culture-bound differences between both sexes appeared to be impressive and relevant for health and health care. One of the most salient sex differences in body experience in our culture is directly associated with Western values of femininity and concerns about the importance of outward appearance for women. Although women may gain autonomy or pleasure in manipulating their outward body and appearance, negative health consequences have also been identified. Objectifying one's own body can imply losing contact with the inner body. Comparing one's own outward body with the cultural ideal of female beauty can lead to body dissatisfaction and thus negative affect and negative self-esteem. Consequences in terms of eating disturbances, smoking, and illness behavior have been described.

Experiencing the body as a process and being attentive to its functions seem to be more promising ways of relating to the body; it guarantees more contact with one's own inner body and thus more autonomy in bodily matters. Female and male body awareness and their relationships with health are relatively under-investigated so far and deserve more attention. The same is true for female and male health-related body experiences in other cultures and subcultures. More knowledge of these areas can help in realization of a gender-sensitive health care in a multicultural society.

REFERENCES

American Psychiatric Association (APA) (1994). *Diagnostic and Statistic Manual of Mental Disorders*, 4th Edition. Washington DC: APA.

Becker, A.E. (1995). *Body, Self, and Society. The View from Fiji.* Philadelphia: University of Pennsylvania Press.

Bekker, M.H.J. (1986). Eten en opgegeten worden. Aspecten van eetverslaving in relatie tot kijken, bekeken worden en verschijnen. *Tijdschrift voor Vrouwenstudies, 7(3)*, 356–365.

Bekker, M.H.J., Heck, G.L. Van, & Vingerhoets, A.J.J.M. (1996). Gender-identity, body-experience, sexuality and the wish for getting children in DES-daughters. *Women and Health, 24*, 65–82.

Bekker, M.H.J., & Van Lenning, A., Vanwesenbeeck, I., & Vossen, R. (submitted). The relationship of body-experience with gender, health, sexuality and childhood – and puberty experiences in Dutch students.

Bekker, M.H.J., van Vliet, K.P., & Kolk, A.M. (1999). Realising gender-sensitive health care: the role of research. In: Kolk, A.M., Bekker, M.H.J., & van Vliet, K.P., (Eds.) *Advanced Studies in Women and Health Research; Toward Gender-Sensitive Strategies*, pp. 15–25. Tilburg: Tilburg University Press.

Ben-Tovim, D.I., & Walker, K. (1991). The development of the Ben-Tovim Walker Body Attitudes Questionnaire (BAQ), a new measure of women's attitudes towards their own bodies. *Psychological Medicine, 21*, 775–784.

Ben-Tovim, D.I., & Walker, K. (1992). A quantitative study of body-related attitudes in patients with anorexia and bulimia nervosa. *Psychological Medicine, 22*, 961–969.

Berger, J. (1972). *Ways of Seeing*. London: Penguin.

Bordo, S. (1993). *Unbearable Weight. Feminism, Western Culture, and the Body*. Berkeley: University of California Press.

Boskind-White, M., & White, W.C. (1983). *Bulimarexia: The Binge/Purge Cycle*. New York: Norton.

Boston Women's Health Collective (1971) *Our Bodies, Ourselves*. London: Penguin.

Camp, D.E., Klesges, R.C., & Relyea, G. (1993). The relationships between body weight concerns and adolescent smoking. *Health Psychology, 12*, 24–32.

Cash, T.F., & Brown, T.A. (1989). Gender and body images: stereotypes and realities. *Sex Roles, 21*, 361–373.

Coward, R. (1984). *Female Desire. Women's Sexuality Today*. London: Paladin Books.

Davis, K. (1988). *Power Under the Microscope*. Dordrecht: Foris Publications.

Davis, K. (1995). *Reshaping the Female Body. The Dilemma of Cosmetic Surgery*. New York: Routledge.

Fallon, A.E., & Rozin, P. (1985). Sex differences in perceptions of desirable body shape. *Journal of Abnormal Psychology, 94*, 102–105.

Franzoi, S.L. (1995). The body-as-object versus the body-as-process: Gender differences and gender considerations. *Sex Roles, 33*, 417–437.

Franzoi, S.L., & Shields, S. (1984). The Body Esteem Scale: multidimensional structure and sex differences in a college population. *Journal of Personality Assessment, 48*, 173–178.

Franzoi, S.L., Kessenich, J.J., & Sugrue, P.A. (1989). Gender differences in the experience of body awareness: An experiential sampling study. *Sex Roles, 21*, 499–515.

Freedman, R. (1990). Cognitive behavioral perspectives on body-image change. In Cash, T.F. & Prozinsky, T. (Eds.) *Body Images: Development, Deviance and Change*, pp. 272–295. New York: Guildford Press.

Garner, D.M., Rockert, W., Olmsted, M.P., Johnson, C., & Coscina, D.V. (1985). Psychoeducational principles in the treatment of bulimia and anorexia nervosa. In Garner, D.M., & Garfinkel, P.E. (Eds.), *Handbook of Psychotherapy for Anorexia Nervosa and Bulimia* (pp. 513–572). New York: Guilford.

Gijsbers van Wijk, C.M.T. (1995). *Sex Differences in Symptom Perception; A Cognitive-Psychological Approach to Health Differences Between Men and Women*. Thesis, Universiteit van Amsterdam.

Gijsbers van Wijk, C.M.T., & van Vliet, K.P. (1989). "Het zieke geslacht". Over sekseverschillen in symptoomperceptie, medische consumptie en morbiditeit. *Gedrag en Gezondheid, 17*, 59–68.

Gillespie, B.I., & Eisler, R.M. (1992). Development of the Feminine Gender Role Stress scale: A cognitive/behavioral measure of stress, appraisal, and coping for women. *Behavioral Modification, 16*, 426–438.

Hawkins, R.C., & Clement, P.F. (1980). Development and construct validation of a self-report measure of binge eating tendencies. *Addictive Behaviors, 5*, 219–226.

Healy, B. (1991). The Yentl syndrome. *New England Journal of Medicine, 325*, 274–276.

Hibbard, J., & Pope, C.R. (1986). Another look at sex differences in the use of medical care: illness orientation and the types of morbidities for which services are used. *Women & Health, 11*, 21–36.

Hibbard, J., & Pope, C.R. (1986). Another look at sex differences in the use of medical care: illness orientation and the types of morbidities for which services are used. *Women & Health, 11*, 21–36.

Huon, G.F., & Brown, L.B. (1989). Assessing bulimics' dissatisfaction with their body. *British Journal of Clinical Psychology, 28*, 283–284.

Keeton, W.P., Cash, T.F., & Brown, T.A. (1990). Body image or body images? Comparative, multidimensional assessment among college students. *Journal of Personality Assessment, 54*, 213–230.

Kotler, P., & Wingard, D. (1989). The effect of occupational, marital and parental roles on mortality: the Alameda study. *American Journal of Public Health, 79*, 607.

Lundberg, U. (1996). Influence of paid and unpaid work on psychophysiological stress responses of men and women. *Journal of Occupational Health Psychology, 1*, 117–130.

Martz, D.M., Handley, K.B., & Eisler, R.M. (1995). The relationship between feminine gender role stress, body image, and eating disorders. *Psychology of Women Quarterly, 19*, 493–508.

McDonald, K., & Thompson, J.K. (1990). Eating disturbance, body image dissatisfaction, and reasons for exercising: gender differences and correlational findings. *International Journal of Eating Disorders, 11*, 289–292.

Meeuwesen, L. (1988). *Spreekuur of Zwijguur; Somatische Fixatie en Sekse-Asymmetrie Tijdens het Medisch Consult*. Nijmegen: KUN.

Noordenbos, G., Acda, S., & Borreson-Gresko, R. (1999). Strategies for the prevention of anorexia and bulimia nervosa. In Kolk, A., Bekker, M., & van Vliet, K. (Eds.) *Advances in Women and Health Research; Towards Gender-sensitive Strategies*, pp. 123–137. Tilburg: Tilburg University Press.

Oakley, A. (1972) *Sex, Gender and Society*. London: Temple Smith.

Orbach, S. (1978). *Fat is a Feminist Issue; The Anti-diet Guide to Permanent Weight Loss*. London: Paddington Press.

Pennebaker, J.W. (1982). *The Psychology of Physical Symptoms*. New York: Springer Verlag.

Richters, A.J.M. (1997). Lichaamsbeleving als sociaal-culturele constructie. In Lagro-Janssen, T., & Noordenbos, G. (Eds.), *Sekseverschillen in Ziekte en Gezondheid*. Nijmegen: Sun.

Silberstein, L.R., Striegel-Moore, R.H., & Rodin, J. (1987). Feeling fat: A woman's shame. In Lewis, H.B. (Ed.), *The Role of Shame in Symptom Formation*. New York: Lawrence Erlbaum Associates.

Silberstein, L.R., Striegel-Moore, R.H., Timko, C., & Rodin, J. (1988). Behavioral and psychological implications of body dissatisfaction: do men and women differ? *Sex Roles, 19*, 219–232.

Sorensen, G., & Pechacek, T.F. (1987). Attitudes toward smoking cessation among men and women. *Journal of Behavioral Medicine, 10*, 129–138.

Stice, E. (1994). Review of the evidence for a sociocultural model of bulimia nervosa and an exploration of the mechanisms of action. *Clinical Psychology Review, 14*, 633–661.

Taylor, S.E. (1995). *Health Psychology*. New York: McGraw-Hill.

Thompson, J.K., & Psaltis, K. (1988). Multiple aspects and correlates of body figure ratings: a replication and extension of Fallon and Rozin (1985). *International Journal of Eating Disorders, 7*, 813–818.

Unger, R.K., & Crawford, M. (1996). *Women and Gender; A Feminist Psychology*. New York: McGraw-Hill.

Vandereijcken, W. (1996). *Eeetstoornissen: Over anorexia nervosa en bulimia nervosa*. Wormer: Inmerc.

Van der Waals, F.W. (1995). *Sex Differences in Benzodiazepine Use*. Doctoral Dissertation, University of Amsterdam.

Van Lenning, A. (1997). Utopian bodies and their shadows. In van Lenning, A., Bekker, M.H.J., & Vanwesenbeeck, I. (Eds.), *Feminist Utopias in a Postmodern Era*. Tilburg: Tilburg University Press.

Van Steen, S., & Bekker, M.H.J. (submitted). Satisfaction, body attitudes and reasons for exercise: gender differences and correlates.

Verbrugge, L.M. (1989). The twain meet: empirical explanations of sex differences in health and mortality. *Journal of Health and Social Behavior, 30*, 282–304.

Waldron, I. & Jacobs, J.A. (1989). Effects of multiple roles on women's health – Evidence from a national longitudinal study. *Women and Health, 15*, 3–19.

Weijts, W. (1993). *Patient participation in gynaecological consultations. Studying interactional patterns*. Maastricht: RUL.

Chapter 3

Gender, Power and the Health Care Professions

Paula Nicolson

Sheffield University, UK

Women are entering the health professions in increasing numbers. This chapter examines the psychological impact of the male-dominated work setting on women in the health organisations. It is particularly concerned with the emotional health of those women who achieved, or aspire to achieve, professional and organisational power.

The achievement and maintenance of power in organisations is increasingly a gender battle and it is almost always the case that women are in some way subordinate in these contexts (Bleier, 1984; Leonard, 1984). This chapter, however, is not about the identification, political and social challenges of inequality. This topic has been taken up effectively elsewhere (Davidson & Cooper, 1992; Hansard Society Commission, 1990). It is about the *psychological consequences* of gender and power imbalances for senior and ambitious middle-ranking women in health care management and professional life (Marshall, 1984; Nicolson, 1996; White et al., 1992).

THE FIGHT FOR EQUALITY

Work organisations have become a major site of gender politics for professional women and men over the last 20 years. While equal

Women, Health and the Mind
Edited by L. Sherr and J.S. St Lawrence. © 2000 John Wiley & Sons, Ltd

opportunities policies and affirmative action in the selection and training of women in the professions has had a qualified impact (Aitkenhead & Liff, 1990), increased career opportunities appear to have made the psychological context of the organisation more stressful for women (Davidson & Cooper, 1992; Marshall, 1984; McKenzie-Davey, 1993).

While women and men have always coexisted in various capacities in extended families, their relationships in the work place are relatively new. Women in Western society have entered the work place in increasing numbers only since the late 1950s and their entry has been rapid. However their work has not been and is unlikely to be on equal or gender-free terms. Typical of female work is that it is often part-time and in stereotyped occupations, such as clerical, secretarial, nursing, health care, teaching, child care, social work, sales and manu-facturing [Organisation for Economic Co-operation and Development (OECD), 1979]. These occupations provided some opportunity for professional career progression, but men entering these professions consistently rise to the top relatively quickly while women remain in the junior posts (Reskin & Padavic, 1994). There is also a close rela-tionship between relatively low pay and "typically female" occupations, such as teaching and nursing, that has persisted (Pillinger, 1993).

Although men have traditionally succeeded over women in terms of pay, seniority and status, women are now entering the preservations of male power in health professions such as medicine, health service management, clinical psychology and related areas of academia. For instance, while women make up three-quarters of the British National Health Service and at least half of their potential users, the service remains under the control of men. This is exemplified in hospital medi-cine where the overwhelming number of consultants are men (i.e. 83%) [Women in Medicine Collective (WIM), 1998]. Thus the picture is far from one of equality and women are no longer content; which has consequences for gender relations.

Women have trained as doctors in increasing numbers since the 1970s. However there has been relatively little change in the relative propor-tions of women and men at the top of the profession in either the United Kingdom or United States (Department of Health, 1991/2; Silver, 1990). Within the branches of the medical profession in which status and remuneration are high (e.g. surgery) there is only limited improve-ment in the proportion of female consultants) [3% in 1990 (Department of Health, 1991/2) to 4% in 1998 (WIM, 1998)]. Even in psychiatry, in which the patient group has low status and there are few opportuni-ties for lucrative private practice in the United Kingdom, only around 25% of consultants were female at the start of the decade (Department of Health, 1991/2) with the proportions slightly improved to 31% by 1998 (WIM, 1998).

Women, like men, enter medicine full of motivation and expectations about their career potential. A small number succeed and reach senior levels. The majority does not. What happens to women who distinguish themselves and those who continue to try against the odds? Successful and aspiring women may differ from others in several ways. They differ from their peers who enter the professions but who are sidetracked or drop out. They are separated from women who choose not to enter professional life in the first place but opt for the more traditional family/non-career employment route. They also differ from those women who choose semi-professional work such as administration or being a secretarial/personal assistant. Most significant is that they are unlike their work peers who are men. Being so different has major psychological consequences. There are few role models at hand, not only at work but also to provide inspiration about all other aspects of life. Patriarchal structures, firmly established in the organisational context of the health care professions, resist women's progress. But male success has psychological implications for women's emotional health, and achieving against such odds has an impact on women's daily life. The general theme of this argument is not new (see Marshall, 1984; McKenzie-Davey, 1993) but nevertheless is neglected. The more opportunities there are for women to achieve, the more scrutiny of women's career accomplishments is required so that success may be sustained.

In 1971, DeLamater and Fidell wrote about the problems of professional women as having a "cumulative impact as she moves from childhood to occupational employment" (DeLamater & Fidell, 1971, p.7). They described how girls are socialised into being people-oriented and dependent, while work and particularly success at work was perceived to be masculine and, as such, undesirable for women. They suggest that "socialisation to traditional feminine values results in lower occupational aspirations for women" (DeLamater & Fidell, 1971, p.7). What has changed since that time is that many women's aspirations have been raised.

Barriers to success have a psychological impact, and women pay the price – either in loss of career potential or in more personal ways. This is different from the experience of men. While it is not true that all ambitious men succeed, the majority of people who *do* succeed are men. The personal and professional costs of career failure are recognised as attacking masculine identity, but there is little theorisation of the influence of career success or failure on feminine identity. Masculinity is equivalent to success, achievement and power, while femininity is largely still perceived by men and women in the outdated traditional way, as dependent passivity. This has implications for self-esteem, gender relations at home and at work, and is critical for women who challenge traditional gender expectations. Thus, although the potential cost of thwarted ambition is painful for men and may skew their own self-evaluation, the lack of a similar career-expectation model for women denies them a framework through which to explain their experiences and emotions to themselves and others.

A woman who fails to achieve promotion or appointment to a senior management or consultant post is seen, and probably sees herself, as *lucky to get that far*. This is particularly significant because of the way women have had to struggle for success and develop intricate coping and image management strategies that appear to be essential to organisational achievement (see Cassell & Walsh, 1991; Marshall, 1984).

FEMININITY AND PROFESSIONAL LIFE

There is conflict and contradiction between the experience of being a woman and the social construction of femininity that explicitly prioritises the non-assertive and non-rational part of human action and emotion (see Bem, 1974; Broverman et al., 1970; Nicolson, 1992). The dilemma for many professional women is how to negotiate and give meaning to their sense of femininity and gender identity in the world of power and intellect, when that world has defined them as outside the main professional arena.

In order to survive in senior roles, women need to (re)claim their *right* to the world of intellect, authority and power that is denied to them under social practices that define the normal woman as "emotional", "nurturing" and "passive". The difficult, unfeminine harridan is perceived as disturbing the rightful territory of men. It is stressful to be marginal to patriarchy and the successful woman is often marginalised because she is unfeminine as a consequence of having to "toughen herself up" to succeed in existing male strongholds.

From birth women and men are compelled to seek confirmation of gender identity (Archer, 1989). From the time we recognise we are female or male and even before we are sure we know how those in each category are meant to behave, all human individuals actively pursue the project of "becoming gendered" (Coward, 1993). Women's bodies, with the capacity for child bearing and breastfeeding, are clearly different anatomically and biologically from men's. These anatomical and biological differences are the source of different behaviours associated with reproductive function. This is not in dispute.

FEMININITY AND THE BODY

What is problematic however, is the various ways in which the female body has been positioned as being subordinate to that of the male rather than being different (Ussher, 1989). This is often achieved in relation to women's reproductive *capacities* by a patriarchal science that operationalises female differences as if they were deficiencies. For example, the menstrual cycle has often been socially represented as a disability, a myth that has permeated popular knowledge. It is particularly important in professional life, because the belief that women are intellectually weak at certain "times of the month" has been used implicitly and explicitly against women aspiring to senior roles. Who would want therapy from a psychologist suffering from premenstrual tension? The idea of the surgeon bursting into tears during the difficult part of the operation is horrific. However, consistent evidence that only around 5–10% (Warner & Walker, 1992) of the female population has menstrual disorders continues to be ignored in favour of these misogynist images. However, not having menstrual periods is no safeguard for the image of the competent woman. Older postmenopausal women who brought up their children or who have simply taken longer to decide upon a career path are also discriminated against for their lack of youth and femininity – the counterpart of their lack of fertility (Gannon, 1994; Ussher, 1989).

Masculinity, on the other hand, is positioned as positive and competent in youth, middle and old age. This is not to say that all men are destined to be successful in their professional lives, far from it. Masculinity is about competition, often to the "death" of the rival. It is not uncommon for newly appointed senior managers to openly express hostility to rivals, particularly towards those in slightly junior positions who might be "in waiting". Whereas the older woman is seen mainly in terms of her faded femininity, the older man, if he is no longer in the running for power, is seen as wise and experienced.

THE BODY AT WORK

As women demanded increased access to power, the power structure used the "beauty myth" to undermine women's advancement (Wolf, 1991, p.20).

Women, valued by men and women alike according to cultural standards of "beauty", are traditionally seen as valuable in relation to their reproductive capacity (Buss, 1994). According to Wolf, there is still no other way of judging women's worth, which presents a major dilemma for women who wish to be successful at work and to be valued at all stages of their career and life cycles. The "beauty myth" discussed by Wolf represents an important cultural focus in relation to the female body. Men value women for their beauty (associated with youth and reproductive capacity). Men have the economic power, which means that women need to compete with other women on beauty terms in order to achieve scarce male attention and ultimately to survive. As they get older, their value is less. This results in multi-million dollar industries aimed at sustaining and enhancing female beauty, which themselves have a culturally vested interest in maintaining this beauty requirement. All of these influence women's everyday experiences in the work place. Women have to be attractive, but if they are too sexually attractive they are dangerous and/or dismissed as mere objects of male desire (Nicolson, 1996; Ussher, 1989). If they rebel and refuse to compete in the beauty game they are seen as ugly harridans.

The 1980s in Europe and the United States introduced the decade of "power dressing". Power dressing, or wearing business suits, might have been the "answer" for aspiring professional women who wished to be attractive rather than sexy. Faludi (1992) discussing the repercussions associated with John Molloy's (1977) *The Woman's Dress for Success Book* said:

> ... for the next three years, women's magazines recycled scores of fashion stories that endorsed not only the suits but also the ambitions they represented – with headlines like YOUR GET-AHEAD WARDROBE, POWER! and WHAT TO WEAR WHEN YOU'RE DOING THE TALKING. (Faludi, 1992, p.210)

As both Faludi and Wolf point out, there was a fashion industry and media backlash against power dressing, although many women who wore suits (a uniform similar to that of professional men) felt comfortable and that it suited their behaviour and aspirations. Women were accused of looking masculine, although the suits women wore were "masculine only in so far as it established for women something recognisable as professional dress" (Wolf, 1991, p.45). Wearing more traditionally feminine clothes, particularly those that accentuate female characteristics (tight jumpers, short skirts) leaves the woman in danger of provoking sexual harassment (Nicolson, 1996; Wolf, 1991) and not being taken seriously as a professional.

All women and men create and recreate their images throughout their careers. Undergraduates with pink spiky hair wearing jeans do not become senior health professionals without changing their image to a more conservative one. The emphasis as women and men enter the professional world is upon specifying their *difference*, although this in turn reproduces inequalities. It is clear what the professional man is expected to be, but the professional woman is left floundering with the strong possibility of falling into the perception that she does not look the part.

What is the significance of the difference between the ways in which the female and male bodies need to be represented? Despite understanding the politics and economics of gender and the implicit sexualised relations, there are important unconscious aspects of gender similarities and differences that provide symbolic meaning to the bodies of women and men.

PROFESSIONAL SOCIALISATION AND ORGANISATIONAL CULTURE

Even though interactions between society and self occur early in a person's life (Leonard, 1984; Mead, 1934), socialisation, and transmission of cultural values from one generation to the next, is a continuing process throughout the life cycle. Society and its social institutions are microcosmic representations of wider cultural contexts that are hierarchical and patriarchal. Entering professional life is akin to the general socialisation process.

Entry into a health care profession is the beginning of a specific socialisation process and professional organisations operate to ensure that new members are aware of the rules and values that ensure perpetuation of the dominant culture within that organisation. That is not to say that cultures are intractable or inescapable, nor that individuals and groups never resist socialisation. However, the cultural mores of the organisation pre-date the individual employee and operate to restrict entry and career progress and influence behaviour in all the operations of the organisational culture.

Entry into a male-dominated profession, such as medicine, is likely to be a severe culture shock for women early in their careers, so much so that they may fail to perceive the extent of male domination that occurs at different levels of visibility. The psychological consequences of patriarchy for professional women are detrimental to both mental and physical health. This is for both indirect reasons, such as ignoring women's special needs in relation to domestic commitments and traditional styles of social interaction, and for direct reasons such as overt sexism and sexual harassment. This "toxic context" constrains women's experience and although some women may achieve success, they pay a dearer price for their attainment than their male equivalents.

For women there are three main stages of socialisation into a patriarchal organisational culture:

1. *Shock* on entry into the system that frequently occurs in delayed stages, because of a previous lack of awareness of sexism that resulted from school success, high motivation, and an idealised view of their potential. This shock frequently leads to:
2. *Anger, and/or protest* and a decision to leave or the development of a coping strategy/compromise referred to as gender management strategies (Cassell & Walsh, 1991; Marshall, 1984, 1994). The decision to leave might be masked (consciously or unconsciously) by a decision to have children, focus on the family or work part-time, thereby "dropping out" of the fast track.
3. *Internalisation of values.* This process – which leads to the ultimate acceptance of the patriarchal culture – operates differently for women who opt out than for those who opt in. The former group re-evaluate themselves negatively against the prevailing criteria. Thus they might say that "family comes first", or "women aren't made for the pressures of senior management" or "I have failed" or even "who wants to work with such people/in that way?" The second group, who take up the challenge of patriarchy are the future "Queen Bees" who see themselves as exceptions to the rules that subordinate and disparage women (see Marshall, 1984; McKenzie-Davey, 1993; White

et al., 1992). Yet, all women, however successful, operate within a toxic context, negative attention, and derision that reinforces the objectification of women and hinders their progress as professionals.

The *toxic context* of a patriarchal organisation may permit equal opportunity policies but resists changes that enable women and other minority groups to have the same opportunities as those that are available to men. Professional organisations, top heavy with men, may pay lip-service to increasing recruitment and promotion opportunities for women. However, the existence of such "policies" makes it more difficult for women to negotiate their careers or to challenge the "system". It is currently fashionable to deride feminism as humourless "political correctness". Young women with good qualifications and expectations of career success firmly believe they have reached the "post-feminist" utopia that will enable their efforts to be judged on merit rather than on gender, and feminist critiques or actions are seen as lacking "style" and relevance (see Faludi, 1992).

Working with women as equals disrupts masculine subjectivity. That is not to say that all men are misogynist. One of the findings from my study of doctors, lecturers and medical students (Nicolson & Welsh, 1992) was the way that senior men's perspectives on gender discrimination were polarised. They were either supportive of equal opportunities or angry about sexual harassment of women by men or they saw sexual harassment and the pursuit of equal opportunities as trivial or a joke. Other men in the study were careless about equal opportunities issues, revealing underlying prejudice in the expression of their views.

It is difficult for men to *experience* women who are 'other' than them as equal, and the pressure to recognise women as equals and/or superiors that is caused by both policy and the characteristics of ambitious and capable women precipitates anxiety, guilt and envy in the men. There are undeniably visible differences between women and men's expectations, attitudes and behaviour in relation to work organisations, and these distinctions solidify as individuals rise up the hierarchy. Men either push for career success and achieve seniority or they come to terms with having underachieved or deviated from social expectations. Women's experience is more complex. Socialisation into femininity is not as clear cut as masculinity and women do not have expectations of certain achievement. Thus women who find the going too tough may resign from the organisation or those who drop out of the fast track do so with fewer regrets than men (see Marshall, 1994). Women who succeed in the professions are more likely to experience an *increase* in problems and stress than if they opt out (Davidson & Cooper, 1992), and the more senior a woman becomes the more she is likely to be stressed at work than is a man of equivalent seniority (Cushway, 1991). There are good social reasons why women find the high-flying life difficult, particularly if they are mothers (see Cooper & Lewis, 1993). However, there are additional difficulties for senior women, particularly in relation to the management of *psychological boundaries* between self, social context and, in particular, their sense of gender subjectivity. To be doing "male" things in patriarchal organisations does not preclude the desire to be feminine and to enjoy being a woman and being seen as a woman with a sexual, intellectual and emotional presence that is feminine.

DOING WHAT WOMEN DO BEST

Both women and men negotiate boundaries between self, other, organisation and culture. Women in a patriarchal context need to be able to distinguish between their sense of subjectivity/self, cultural and interpersonal expectations, and the meaning given to their organisational contribution by *others because they are women*. It is difficult to have control over the latter, but it is vital to recognise through the process of reflexivity that those meanings exist and those boundaries are dynamic and shift from occasion to occasion.

There is no persuasive evidence of essential, immutable female characteristics that make deference a prerequisite for women's biographical development. However as Bell & Newby (1976, p.152) noted over 20 years ago, sexual stratification is about "the relationships between the sexes rather than the attributes of one sex or the other". While Bell & Newby focused their attention on husbands and wives, a similar perspective is crucial for understanding relationships between the sexes in organisations, where people frequently spend years coexisting, competing, supporting and forming relationships with others who just happen to work together rather than choosing to share their lives. Bell & Newby identify the "relational and normative means by which men (particularly husbands) maintain their traditional authority over women (wives), and . . . the strategies they employ in attempting to ensure the *stability* of their power" (Bell & Newby, 1976:, p.152). They argue that many wives believe their husbands have and ought to have more power than they do and traditional values lend support to the hierarchical nature of the relationship between husband and wife as being natural and immutable.

The existence of a tradition whereby men hold professional power serves to legitimate it and, for many women, this becomes manifest in their deference to a senior manager/professional who is also a man. Individual women who achieve power in their own right have challenged this, but their challenge does not deprive men of apparent legitimate authority in the eyes of both the men and other women. Many women, even senior and aspiring women, still exhibit non-assured, deferential qualities.

It is alarming to observe how professional women's accounts of their subjectivity in organisational life concur with this image (Tanton, 1994). Women display deference because of ongoing patterns of subordination of women/girls to men/boys, which is part of a relationship pattern based on power dynamics in the family, on socialisation and on cultural belief systems that are inescapable without taking on the mantle of an outcast. It is not difficult to see or reflect upon the way that being seen and treated as subordinate and gaining recognition through deference may set up a template for social relations, both in the family and in professional organisations. If women feel insecure about their talents and abilities because of socialisation and gender/power relations inherent in the dominant culture, they develop a range of coping/survival strategies to deal with this insecurity (see Cassell & Walsh, 1991; Marshall, 1984). This involves their attempting to negotiate their subjectivity and interpersonal relationships as though they were *other* than women. A

> ... requirement of woman's social role is that she must always be *connected* to others and shape her life according to a man. A woman's status will derive from that of her mate. Indeed her very sense of self and well being may rely on their connection. (Eichenbaum and Orbach, 1982, p.29)

A woman not connected with a man who presents herself as independent is treated with suspicion whether that independence is at home or at work. The sexualised nature of the work relationship carries over from heterosexual connectedness where women identify with their immediate bosses or senior men. However, this connectedness is often the means of acting out a deferential relationship because the man is the superordinate one.

Eichenbaum & Orbach (1982) suggest that deference and connectedness to others naturally leads on to "another psychological concomitant of women's social role: that of having emotional antennae. A woman must learn to anticipate others' needs" (Eichenbaum & Orbach, 1982, p.29). Subjectivity for women appears to contain far greater complexity than subjectivity for men, and for women in senior management roles in the health care professions, this complexity is exaggerated by the apparent stepping outside the boundaries of feminine behaviour.

ISOLATION

> *Intimacy* is a key in a world of connection where individuals negotiate complex networks of friendship, minimise differences, try to reach consensus, and avoid the appearance of superiority, which would highlight differences. In a world of status, *independence* is key, because a primary means of establishing status is to tell others what to do, and taking orders is a marker of low status. Though all humans need both intimacy and independence, women tend to focus on the first and men on the second. (Tannen, 1993, p.26)

Even though it is unlikely that *all* women and *all* men's behaviour and needs are demarcated in such a way, there is increasing support for the view that psychological and social factors conspire to achieve these gender differences. The specific difficulty that this imposes upon the lives of senior professional women is that while they are likely to develop skills that resemble those of male executives (see Marshall, 1984; McKenzie-Davey, 1993; White et al., 1992), there is something missing. There is no one with whom they are able to share intimacy. There are few opportunities for pragmatic relationships in corporate life of the same quality as men who relate to other men. While they are likely to achieve independence, there is nothing to moderate it and instead of being independent, they are lonely and isolated.

Sheppard (1992) found that female managers perceived themselves to be isolated in a variety of contexts, and much of this related to the way that organisational culture reflects male styles and interactional patterns. "Women can't take for granted with whom they can associate, as they perceive political consequences that may devolve from even the most casual or informal contacts" (Sheppard, 1992, p.156). They have to be careful of relationships with men that may be misconstrued as sexual or that might be misconstrued as supportive instead of career-oriented friendships. More important in their sense of isolation, was that women managers needed to detach themselves from being identified with women in clerical and secretarial posts and those in junior roles in the organisation. Thus the life of a female senior health care professional is exceptionally hard because she is both deprived and has to deprive herself of most opportunities for intimacy and connectedness (Tanton, 1994).

To cope with isolation and loneliness, barriers have to be erected. Men have opportunities to receive support from women to overcome the potential for desolation and emotional bleakness that strong barriers and the maintenance of power precipitate. Women do not have the same opportunities because they cannot afford to obtain support from junior women. This is partly because they need to be seen as being different from the junior women and partly because junior women's expectations of them are likely to weigh them down as much as support them.

CONCLUSIONS

To cope with being a woman in a man's world, women have to manage boundaries between themselves and other women, themselves and men, and themselves and the patriarchal organisation culture. Are they selling out? Are they losing their femininity? Are they exploiting their sexuality? Are they doing their job well? These issues have to be managed constantly if the woman professional is to survive emotionally. She has constantly to redefine her own boundaries. Promotion and success mean personal growth and that is the benefit of rewarded talent

and ambition. However, for women, out of place in patriarchal organisations, it is imperative that they reassess their relationship with
themselves and reflect on their experience and to find a means of maintaining and enhancing ego–strength.

REFERENCES

Aitkenhead, M., & Liff, S. (1990). The effectiveness of equal opportunities policies. In Firth-Cozens, J., & West, M.A. (Eds.), *Women at
Work*. Milton Keynes: Open University Press.

Archer, J. (1989). Childhood gender roles: structure and development.
The Psychologist, 9, 367–370.

Bell, C., & Newby, H. (1976). Husbands and wives: the dynamics of
the deferential dialectic. In Barker, D., & Allen, H. (Eds.), *Dependence
and Exploitation of Women in Work and Marriage*. London: Longman.

Bem, S.L. (1974). The measurement of psychological androgyny. *Journal
of Consulting and Clinical Psychology, 42*, 155–162.

Bleier, R. (1984). *Science and Gender: A Critique of Biology and Its Theories
on Women*. Oxford: Pergamon.

Broverman, I.K., Broverman, D.M., Clarkson, F.E., Rosenkrantz, P.S., &
Vogel, S.R. (1970). Sex role stereotypes and clinical judgments of
mental health. *Journal of Consulting and Clinical Psychology, 34*, 1–7.

Buss, D.M. (1994). The strategies of human mating. *American Scientist,
82*, 238–249.

Cassell, C., & Walsh, S. (1991). Towards a woman-friendly psychology
of work: gender, power and organisational culture. Paper presented to the British Psychological Society's Annual Occupational
Psychology Conference, Liverpool University.

Cooper, C., & Lewis, S. (1993). *The Workplace Revolution: Managing
Today's Dual Career Families*. London: Kogan Page.

Coward, R. (1993). *Our Treacherous Hearts*. London: Faber and Faber.

Cushway, D. (1991). Stress in clinical psychologists. Paper presented at
the British Psychological Society's Annual Conference, Bournemouth.

Davidson, M.J., & Cooper, C.L. (1992). *Shattering the Glass Ceiling: The
Woman Manager*. London: Paul Chapman Publishing Ltd.

DeLameter, J., & Fidell, L.S. (1971). On the status of women. In Fidell,
L.S., & DeLameter, J. (Eds.), *Women in the Professions: What's All the
Fuss About?* London: Sage.

Department of Health (1991/2). Medical and dental staffing prospects
in the NHS in England and Wales 1990. *Health Trends, 23(4)*, 132–141.

Eichenbaum, L., & Orbach, S. (1982). *Outside in. Inside Out*. Harmsonds-
worth: Penguin.

Faludi, S. (1992). *Backlash*. London: Vintage.

Fidell, L.S., & DeLameter, J. (1991). Editorial. In Fidell, L.S., &
DeLameter, J. (Eds.), *Women in the Professions: What's All the Fuss
About?* London: Sage.

Gannon, L. (1994). Sexuality and the menopause. In Choi, P.Y.L., & Nicolson, P. (Eds.), *Female Sexuality: Psychology, Biology and Social Context*. Hemel Hempstead: Harvester Wheatsheaf.

Hansard Society Commission (1990). *Women at the Top*. London: Hansard Society.

Leonard, P. (1984). *Personality and Ideology*. Basingstoke: Macmillan.

Marshall, J. (1984). *Women Managers: Travellers in a Male World*. New York: Wiley.

Marshall, J. (1994). Why women leave senior management jobs. In Tanton, M. (Ed.), *Women in Management*. London: Routledge.

McKenzie-Davey, K. (1993). Women balancing power and care in early career: am I feminine or just one of the lads? Presented at the BPS Psychology of Women Section Annual Conference, University of Sussex.

Mead, G.H. (1934). *Mind, Self and Society*. Chicago: University of Chicago Press.

Molloy, J.T. (1977). *The Woman's Dress for Success Book*. New York: Warner Books.

Nicolson, P. (1992). Towards a psychology of women's health and health care. In Nicolson, P. & Ussher, J. (Eds.), *The Psychology of Women's Health and Health Care*. Basingstoke: Macmillan.

Nicolson, P. (1996). *Gender, Power and Organisation: A Psychological Perspective*. London: Routledge.

Nicolson, P., & Welsh, C.L. (1992). *Gender Inequality in Medical Education. Preliminary Report to Trent Regional Health Authority*. Sheffield: Trent RHA.

Organisation for Economic Co-operation and Development (OECD) (1979). *Equal Opportunities for Women*. Paris: OECD.

Pillinger, J. (1993). *Feminising the Market*. Basingstoke: Macmillan.

Reskin, B.F., & Padavic, I. (1994). *Women and Men at Work*. London: Pine Forge Press.

Sheppard, D. (1992). Women managers' perceptions of gender and organisational life. In Mills, A.J., & Tancred, P. (Eds.), *Gendering Organisational Analysis*. London: Sage.

Silver, G. (1990). Monopoly of middle-aged men. Editorial. *The Lancet*, *335*, 1149–1150.

Tannen, D. (1993). *You Just Don't Understand: Women and Men in Conversation*. London: Virago.

Tanton, M. (1994). *Women in Management*. London: Routledge.

Ussher, J.M. (1989). *The Psychology of the Female Body*. London: Routledge.

Warner, P., & Walker, A. (1992). Menstrual Cycle Research – Time to take stock. Editorial. *Journal of Reproductive and Infant Psychology*, *10*, 63–66.

White, B., Cox, C., & Cooper, C. (1992). *Women's Career Development: A Study of High Flyers*. Oxford: Blackwell Business.

Women in Medicine Collective (WIM) (1998). *Careers for Women in Medicine: Planning and Pitfalls*. London: WIM.

Wolf, N. (1991). *The Beauty Myth*. London: Vintage.

Chapter 4

Women and Clinical Trials

Lorraine Sherr

Royal Free and University College Medical School, London, UK

In medical trials women fare differently from men. This chapter will assess the roots of this variation, its academic basis, scientific justification, effects, and consequences. Many questions will be addressed that currently cannot be answered. For example, will the variations persist while researchers stand on the sidelines observing the phenomenon or will vigorous reaction redress the imbalance? From where will the adjustment come, and will the mechanisms for change transfer to new conditions or will the obligatory learning curve of omission, reaction and commission be present in new conditions? Both the facts and the awakening of researchers to this imbalance can be observed within the health literature generally and in medical trials specifically. This chapter will attempt to explore, by way of a number of examples, the movement in and out of the spotlight for women according to various clinical trials, treatment conditions and political backgrounds. Two examples of medical conditions will be used as examples. Coronary heart disease provides a good focus to explore a major life-threatening issue and AIDS, as a relatively new disease which emerged after the "awakening" of gender imbalances in clinical trials, will provide insight into how new diseases fare according to gender perspectives.

Theoretically observation of the phenomenon of women in clinical trials is interesting (Stewart, 1997a; Whiteside et al., 1997). Gender imbalances are clearly articulated in recent literature. Stewart (1997b) noted that women accounted for 5% of research subjects in Canada and 15%

Women, Health and the Mind
Edited by L. Sherr and J.S. St Lawrence. © 2000 John Wiley & Sons, Ltd

in the United States. She pointed out that approaches that exclude women in an attempt to "protect them" from research risk actually enhance their risk because findings from male-based studies are simply transferred to women with scant appreciation for gender-specific effects. Gender studies are needed to explore conditions that are unique to women (such as ovarian cancer), conditions that are more prevalent in women, those that may be more serious in women and those that are simply different in women. Whenever trends are studied, these comparisons reveal systematic data and systematic differences that ought to trigger research into specific projects and funding to ensure that gender issues are addressed. For example the male:female ratio of prevalence is greater in ischaemic heart disease while the female:male ratio is greater in cardiovascular disease, hypertension and mental illness diagnoses. Lung cancer has shown a dramatic increase within the female population since 1969, probably accounted for by the increases in female smoking, specifically female teenage smoking, on the one hand and decreases in male smoking on the other. Indeed, the prevalence of lung cancer among women now exceeds that of breast cancer, yet Stewart (1997a) reports that men are 1.6 times more likely to have their sputum analysed. In terms of other health inequalities she also points out that women on dialysis in the United States, Canada, Scandinavia and Italy are at least 30% less likely to receive a transplant than are men.

The early feminist approach to these problems was to highlight the gaps and to deplore the situation. Many examples of the neglect of women could be gathered and the situation could arise where medical treatment of women for some conditions continued for decades, based on male evidence-based studies. Yet is there a theoretical framework that could conceptualise the process. Bereavement theories may provide one such framework. Early bereavement theories provided a stage like process to understand and integrate reactions (Kubler Ross, 1969). An initial shock is followed by denial, then by anger and depression, and finally by reconstitution. Similarly, early revelations of the status of women within clinical trials went through shock and denial phases, followed by angry outbursts, where the inequalities were listed (e.g. see Stewart, 1997a,b). In some areas, apathy has followed, yet others see a vibrant reconstitution that may allow for redress and witness a surge of women's studies or a new approach to the inclusion of women within clinical trials towards the latter half of this century. Critics of the stage model for bereavement point to the inadequacies of such a formulation and tend to favour a more task-oriented approach. Such approaches overcome the rigidity of stage models and address action via outstanding tasks. Perhaps this is a more constructive way to approach the problem of women in clinical trials. What are the tasks and how have they been addressed? Clearly the first task of articulating and gesticulating about the differences has passed. Anger and outrage within the women's movement served to trigger change. What is the nature of the change?

In the case of cardiovascular disease, change is slow but noticeable. An analysis of the studies over time shows gradual inclusion of women (Morisky et al., 1983), first in their role as wives (Knutsen and Knutsen, 1991) and finally in their own right (Glasgow et al., 1995). How was this brought about? Often the movement was paralleled by the emergence of female principal investigators (Stamler et al., 1989). So women were triggering study of women by women (and for women). The movement also reflects a political change, in which to overlook women became frowned upon and in which budget lines allowed for token and at times specific inclusion of women. Was this a policy of positive discrimination and did it work? The test would not be the simple increase of women-based studies but a balanced integration driven by evidence rather than political correctness or pique. Indeed, in the United Kingdom, funding has just now been received to commence a women's study within the British Heart Study after some 20 years of investigating men (Ebrahim & Wincup, pers. comm.). Women-specific initiatives are also emerging in the United States (Manson et al., 1995) and other centres.

Acquired immunodeficiency syndrome (AIDS) and human immunodeficiency virus (HIV) infection provides another mirror to explore women in clinical trials. Here the epidemic commenced with a male focus in research despite the fact that women were always part of the epidemic (Diaz et al., 1995). The geographical and socio-economic position of these women probably compounded the gender bias of research (Amoro, 1993). Women affected by HIV were mainly concentrated among poor, disenfranchised and marginalised social groups. Males were disproportionately concentrated among the wealthy nations in higher educational and political positions. The first era of HIV research overlooked women (Hankins et al., 1994 ; Sherr, 1993). Yet this was quite quickly addressed as the role of women in clinical trials was taken to another extreme. Women-specific trials (notably ACTG 076 and the use of anti-retroviral treatment to prevent vertical transmission during pregnancy) provided a fascinating platform at the heart of women's issues, addressing their core role in reproduction and perhaps pitting this role and associated infant considerations against their own disease management. In developing countries access to treatment is almost exclusively reserved for pregnant women, either within clinical trials or within compassionate release programmes. How has this fared and what does the future hold?

CARDIOVASCULAR DISEASE

Coronary heart disease accounts for high levels of mortality and morbidity. Many countries responded with a sophisticated set of interventions aimed at primary prevention by modifying risk factors. Interventions appraised in the literature include counselling, education, pharmacological treatments and risk factor reduction. The data has been reviewed and analysed in a series of meta-analyses. For the purposes of this chapter, the most recent and most comprehensive review, (Ebrahim & Davey Smith, 1997) will be examined from a gender perspective. Essentially, we will explore the selected studies by gender of investigator as well as gender of subjects (see the Acknowledgement, p. 55). This review examined all the literature and selected 14 trials of multiple risk factor intervention of which nine provided disease events and risk factor changes as outcome measures and five only risk factor change. Table 4.1, adapted from Ebrahim & Davey Smith, provides data only on the gender of participants.

The table summarises the key methodologically sound studies in the area. Of note is the fact that the majority of subjects were male. Five of the studies were based on men only and eight included both males and females. No studies were based on women only. Of the eight studies that included females, they were only present in equal proportion when randomised population based strategies were used (Imperial Cancer Research Fund OXCHECK Study Group, 1994). Otherwise men predominated (Lindholm et al., 1995, in which 87% were male) or women were only included if they were partners to men (Knutsen & Knutsen, 1991, who included wives and the Family Heart study which included female partners).

The early studies comprised male subjects exclusively. The introduction of females arose when it became unavoidable (i.e. in studies that utilised randomised selection at a population level where the presence of women was not in question). Initially, this was by relationship (when studies included wives); then, as later trends emerged, the inclusion of women was noted. Not a single study in this systematic review revealed a women-only study.

A similar evaluation was carried out by Rochon et al. (1998). These authors evaluated all randomised controlled trials and meta-analyses of any myocardial infarction drug treatment study published in five leading medical journals between 1992 and 1996. Their review located 102 papers that met inclusion criteria and 43 were studied in depth. They noted that even though women were included in clinical trials, gender results were only provided in 32% of the studies and only five studies mentioned gender differences in the discussion section. These findings showed poor representation and utilisation of women's data irrespective of specific gender policies in the institutions from which the studies emanated. McDermott et al. (1995) explored gender issues in three major medical publications for the years 1971, 1981 and 1991, resulting in a detailed review of 444 articles to evaluate changes over time. Clinical trials doubled over time and randomised controlled trials increased from 31 to 76% at the expense of non-randomised controlled trials. Studies that explicitly excluded women decreased from 11 to 3%. In 1991, 7% of studies were of male subjects only. Only 0.7% were specific to men's health while 12% were specific to women's health. Between 1971 and 1991, they noted no change in female first authors

Table 4.1 Trials in cardiovascular prevention by gender

Study	Place	Sample	Subject gender	PI[†] Female?	Variables explored
Multiple risk factor trials with risk factor change and disease event outcome available					
WHO Factor Study, 1982, 1989 (WHO, 1989)	5 European cities	63 732	Men only	×	Risk reduction relating to diet, smoking, weight, exercise, antihypertensive drugs, mass media
Wilhelmsen et al. (1986)	Gote-burg, Sweden	30 022	Men only	×	Risk reduction relating to diet, smoking, antihypertensive drugs, cholesterol lowering drugs
Hjermann et al. (1981)	Oslo	1232	Men only	×	Diet and smoking
Multiple Risk Factor Intervention Trial Research Group (1982)	USA	12 866	Men only	×	Risk reduction related to diet, smoking, weight, antihypertensive drugs
Strandberg et al. (1991), Miettinen et al. (1985)	Finland	1222	Men only	×	Risk reduction related to diet, smoking, exercise, antihypertensive drugs, cholesterol lowering drugs
Hypertension Detection and Follow-up Programme Cooperative Group (1979)	USA	10 940	Men and women	×	Antihypertensive drugs, general health advice
Morisky et al. (1983)	USA	400	Men and women	×	Risk reduction related to weight, antihypertensive drugs, general health advice
Lindholm et al. (1995)	Sweden	681	87% Men and 13% women	×	Risk reduction counselling, videos, group discussion, risk management, food purchasing, exercise
Imperial Cancer Research Fund OXCHECK Study Group (1994)	UK	6124	44% Men and 56% women	×	Diet, smoking, weight, alcohol, exercise, high and raised blood pressure protocols

(*continued overleaf*)

Table 4.1 (*continued*)

Study	Place	Sample	Subject gender	PI[†] Female?	Variables explored
Multiple risk factor trials in which changes in risk factors were included					
Stamler et al. (1989)	USA	201	Men and women	✓	Diet, weight, exercise, alcohol
Baron et al. (1990)	UK	368	Men and women	×	Nurse conducted diet, weight, smoking, exercise, alcohol – results by gender
Knutsen and Knutsen (1991)	Tromso	2182	1373 Men, 809 wives	✓	Doctor and dietician counselling, diet, smoking and exercise
Family Heart Study Group (1994)	UK	12 472	7460 Men, 5012 female partners	×	Nurse counselling, diet, weight, smoking, exercise, alcohol
Glasgow et al. (1995)	USA	1977	Men and women	?	Stage of change model, smoking and diet

[†] Principal investigator.

and concluded that the exclusion of women from directing clinical trials contributes to the paucity of data on women's health.

AIDS

Human immunodeficiency virus (HIV) has been established as an infectious agent for only 15 years. Discovery and isolation of HIV as the causative agent in the mid 1980s means that AIDS emerged after the initial gender awareness movement. With a new disease and a new opportunity, how did the international research community respond? Figure 4.1 illustrates the results of a Medline search. For this search the terms AIDS and HIV were entered over four time periods: 1976–84, 1985–89, 1990–94, and 1995–98. The key word "Women" was entered for the same periods. A "combine sets" instruction revealed how often women appeared in these HIV and AIDS studies and the results are set out in the figure. This reveals that in the first period, women appeared in 0.6% of relevant studies. The figure increased to 1.5% for the next period, 3.9% for the third period and 5.4% for the final period. Yet the course of the epidemic witnessed a nine-fold increase in studies on women over that duration.

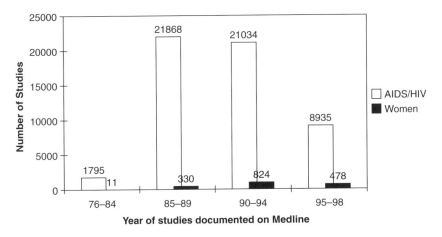

Figure 4.1 Studies on AIDS/HIV reported in Medline from 1976 to 1998, and women-specific studies of AIDS/HIV in the same period.

Recognition of the absence of comprehensive data on women led to an upsurge of interest, a number of critical reviews (Hankins, 1990), and a number of women-specific studies [Women and Infant Transmission Study (WITS) – see Rodriguez et al. (1996)]. The HIV Epidemiology Research Study (HERS) (Smith, 1998) is a multi-site, prospective cohort study of HIV-infected women and uninfected women reporting HIV risk behaviour (Cohen et al., 1998) in the United States, Canada, and Europe.

Examining reports from clinical trials adds an interesting new dimension. A similar Medline search for the same four time periods added the word "trial" as an additional key word. Of 125 trials noted in 1985–89, two mention women; of 332 trials in 1990–1994, eight mention women; and of 219 trials recorded from 1995–1998, 17 mention women. The time trend was from 1.6 to 2.4 to 7.8%. Often natural history investigations as well as intervention trials specifically excluded women, frequently because of potential biological confounds such as lactation or pregnancy. The problem with this approach is that it not only limits insight into interventions for women, but also fails to provide treatment data for lactating or pregnant women. The question of including pregnant women in clinical trials has been raised in the literature by Kornblum (1994), who noted that very specific women-based questions become exclusion criteria for studies but challenging issues for treatment.

The issue of women's participation in clinical trials has been addressed in several research studies. In the United States Diaz et al. (1995) interviewed 4604 people with AIDS. Trial participation was noted by 10% of the sample with significant differences in enrolment according to race/ethnicity, gender, exposure mode and income. Stone et al. (1997)

repeated a similar study of 260 people with HIV disease, also in the United States, and found that 22.3% had participated in a clinical trial and that women, patients of colour and drug users were significantly less likely to have participated. When trials for women are made specifically available, they also raise complex moral and ethical questions often related to the locations of such trials, the kind of treatment arms utilised, and the availability of compounds shown to be efficacious after the trial period ends (Lurie and Wolfe, 1997).

THE WAY FORWARD

The gender imbalance in clinical trials is prevalent and persistent. Concerted action to promote women-focused studies is needed (Matthews et al., 1998) and the inception of such approaches can provide a future pathway for understanding women's health. In the examples cited here, the study of new diseases did not take old lessons into account. Their courses seem to be fairly similar. As with HIV disease, specific action was needed before women were included in clinical trials. Gender may well coexist with other factors that contribute to an increased chance of exclusion or overlooking women in clinical trials. When colour, race, poverty and gender are combined, the exclusion effects are even more obvious (Mouton et al., 1997). Sadly, like many conditions, HIV disease affects women but is also bound up with poverty and deprivation (Pinn, 1996).

The study of new diseases does not seem to benefit from the lessons learned from old conditions. The passage of time may help, but it also brings problems such as the increased population of elderly women (Butler et al., 1995) which changes the population profiles. The increased presence of women researchers often creates a trigger point for women's issues to be placed on the research agenda. Direct political lobbying and subsequent earmarked funding also may play a role. Studies of politicised conditions such as HIV and AIDS utilised such processes to improve the inclusion and understanding of women (Williams, 1992), but the study of other diseases still lags behind. Evidence-based medicine in general highlights the evidence-based ignorance about women in many areas of health care.

Insight needs to be sophisticated and innovative to address the inclusion of women in clinical trials (Moore and Bernard, 1997) as bias continues to be present (Berg, 1997). Innovative ways to address the problems, remedy the imbalance and meet the health needs of women by gender-specific analyses of clinical trials need to be implemented as a standard for new research, new diseases and new challenges (Gerace et al., 1995; Rosendorf et al., 1993). The cycle of repetition needs to be broken.

ACKNOWLEDGEMENT

Many thanks for Professor Shah Ebrahim for supplying data on gender of researchers and providing an overview for this chapter.

REFERENCES

Amaro, H. (1993). Reproductive choice in the age of AIDS policy and counselling issues. In Squire, C. (Ed.), *Women and AIDS: Psychological Perspectives* (pp. 20–41). London: Sage Publications.

Baron, J.A., Gleason, R., Crowe, B., & Mann, J.I. (1990). Preliminary trial of the effect of general practice based nutritional advice. *British Journal of General Practice, 40(333)*, 137–141.

Berg, M.J. (1997). Status of research on gender differences. *Journal of the American Pharmacological Association (Washington), NS37(1)*, 43–56.

Butler, R.N., Collins, K.S., Meier, D.E., Muller, C.F., & Pinn, V.W. (1995). Older women's health: "taking the pulse" reveals gender gap in medical care. *Geriatrics, 50(5)*, 39–40, 43–46, 49.

Cohen, C.J., Iwane, M.K., Palensky, J.B., Levin, D.L., Meagher, K.J., Frost, K.R., & Mayer, K.H. (1998). A national HIV community cohort: design, baseline, and follow-up of the AmFAR Observational Database. American Foundation for AIDS Research Community-Based Clinical Trials Network. *Journal of Clinical Epidemiology, 51(9)*, 779–793.

Diaz, T., Chu, S.Y., Sorvillo, F., Mokotoff, E., Davidson, A.J., Samuel, M.C., Herr, M., Doyle, B., Frederick, M., & Fann, S.A. (1995). Differences in participation in experimental drug trials among persons with AIDS. *Journal of Acquired Immune Deficiency Syndromes & Human Retrovirology, 10(5)*, 562–568.

Ebrahim, S., & Davey Smith, G. (1997). Systematic review of randomised controlled trials of multiple risk factor interventions for preventing coronary heart disease. *British Medical Journal, 314*, 1666–1674.

Family Heart Study Group (1994). Randomised controlled trial evaluating cardiovascular screening and intervention in general practice principal results of British Family heart study. *British Medical Journal, 308*, 313–320

Gerace, T.A., George, V.A., & Arango, I.G. (1995). Response rates to six recruitment mailing formats and two messages about a nutrition program for women 50–79 years old. *Controlled Clinical Trials, 16(6)*, 422–431.

Glasgow, R.E., Terborg, J.R., Hollis, J.F., Severson, H.H., & Boles, S.M. (1995). Take heart: results from the initial phase of a work-site wellness program. *American Journal of Public Health, 85(2)*, 209–216.

Hankins, C. (1990). Women and HIV infection and AIDS in Canada – should we worry? *Canadian Medical Association Journal, 143*, 1171–1173.

Hankins, C., Lamont, J., & Handley, M. (1994). Cervicovaginal screening in women with HIV infection – a need for increased vigilance. *Canadian Medical Association Journal, 150*, 681–686.

Hjermann, I., Velve Byre, K., Holme, I., & Leren, P. (1981). Effect of diet and smoking intervention on the incidence of coronary heart disease. Report from the Oslo Study group of a randomised trial in healthy men. *Lancet, Dec. 12, 2 (8259)*, 1303–1310.

Hypertension Detection and Follow-up Program Cooperative Group (1979). Five-year findings of the hypertension detection and follow-up program. I. Reduction in mortality of persons with high blood pressure, including mild hypertension. *Journal of the American Medical Association, 242(23)*, 2562–2571.

Imperial Cancer Research Fund OXCHECK Study Group (1994). Effectiveness of health checks conducted by nurses in primary care: results of the OXCHECK study after one year. *British Medical Journal, 308(6924)*, 308–312.

Knutsen, S., & Knutsen, R. (1991). The Tromso survey the family intervention study the effect of intervention on some coronary risk factors and dietary habits. A 6 year follow up. *Preventive Medicine, 20*, 197–212.

Kornblum, A. (1994). Trial and error: should pregnant women be research subjects? *Environmental Health Perspectives, 102(9)*, 752–753.

Kubler Ross, E. (1969). *On death and dying.* New York: Macmillan.

Lindholm, L., Ekbom, T., Dash, C., Eriksson, M., Tibblin, G., & Schersten, B. (1995). The impact of health care advice given in primary care on cardiovascular risk. *British Medical Journal, 310*, 1105–1109.

Lindholm, L.H., Ekbom, T., Dash, C., Isacsson, A., & Schersten, B. (1996). Changes in cardiovascular risk factors by combined pharmacological and non-pharmacological strategies: the main results of the CELL Study. *Journal of Internal Medicine, 240(1)*, 13–22.

Lurie, P., & Wolfe, S.M. (1977). Unethical trials of interventions to reduce perinatal transmission of the human immunodeficiency virus in developing countries. *New England Journal of Medicine, 337(12)*, 853–856.

McDermott, M.M., Lefevre, F., Feinglass, J., Reifler, D., Dolan, N., Potts, S., & Senger, K. (1995). Changes in study design, gender issues, and other characteristics of clinical research published in three major medical journals from 1971 to 1991. *Journal of General Internal Medicine, 10(1)*, 13–18.

Manson, J.E., Gaziano, J.M., Spelsberg, A., Ridker, P.M., Cook, N.R., Buring, J.E., Willett, W.C., & Hennekens, C.H. (1995). A secondary prevention trial of antioxidant vitamins and cardiovascular disease in women. Rationale, design, and methods. The WACS Research Group. *Annals of Epidemiology, 5(4)*, 261–269.

Matthews, K.A., Shumaker, S.A., Bowen, D.J., Langer, R.D., Hunt, J.R., Kaplan, R.M., Klesges, R.C., & Ritenbaugh, C. (1998). Women's health initiative. Why now? What is it? What's new? *American Psychologist, 52(2)*, 101–116.

Miettinen, T. A., Hutunen, J.K, Naukkarinen, V., Strandberg, T., Mattila, S., Kumlin, T., & Sarna, S. (1985). Multifactorial primary prevention of cardiovascular diseases in middle aged men. Risk Factor change, incidence, and mortality. *Journal of the American Medical Association*, *254*, 2097–2102.

Moore, D.L., & Bernard, S. (1997). The impact of managed care on women's health research: innovation versus renovation. *Journal of the American Medical Women's Association, 52(2)*, 83–84.

Morisky, D., Levine, D., Green, L., Shapiro, S., Russell, R., & Smith, C. (1983). Five year blood pressure control and mortality following health education for hypertensive patients. *American Journal of Public Health*, *73*, 153–162.

Mouton, C.P., Harris, S., Rovi, S., Solorzano, P., & Johnson, M.S. (1997). Barriers to black women's participation in cancer clinical trials. *Journal of the National Medical Association, 89(11)*, 721–727.

Multiple Risk Factor Intervention Trial Research Group (1982). Risk factor changes and mortality results. Multiple Risk Factor Intervention Trial Research Group. *Journal of the American Medical Association, 248(12)*, 1465–1477.

Pinn, V.W. (1996). The status of women's health research: where are African American women? *Journal of National Black Nurses Association, 8(1)*, 8–19.

Rochon, P.A., Clark, J.P., Binns, M.A., Patel, V., & Gurwitz, J.H. (1998). Reporting of gender-related information in clinical trials of drug therapy for myocardial infarction. *Canadian Medical Association Journal, 159(4)*, 321–327.

Rodriguez, E.M., Mofenson, L.M., Chang, B.H., Rich, K.C., Fowler, M.G., Smeriglio, V., Landesman, S., Fox, H.E., Diaz, C., Green, K., & Hanson, I.C. (1996). Association of maternal drug use during pregnancy with maternal HIV culture positivity and perinatal HIV transmission. *AIDS, 10(3)*, 273–282.

Rosendorf, L.L., Dafni, U., Amato, D.A., Lunghofer, B., Bartlett, J.G., Leedom, J.M., Wara, D.W., Armstrong, J.A., Godfrey, E., Sukkestad, E. (1993). Performance evaluation in multicenter clinical trials: development of a model by the AIDS Clinical Trials Group. *Controlled Clinical Trials, 14(6)*, 523–537.

Sherr, L. (1993). HIV testing in pregnancy. In Squire, C. (Ed.) AIDS and Women. London: Sage.

Smith, D. (1998). The HIV Epidemiology Research Study, HIV Out-Patient Study, and the Spectrum of Disease Studies. *Journal of Acquired Immune Deficiency Syndromes & Human Retrovirology, 17 (suppl 1)*, s17–19.

Stamler, R., Stamler, J., Gosch, F.C., Civinelli, J., Fishman, J., McKeever, P., McDonald, A., & Dyer, A.R. (1989). Primary prevention of hypertension by nutritional-hygienic means. Final report of a randomized, controlled trial. *Journal of the American Medical Association, 262(13)*, 1801–1807. [Published erratum appears in *JAMA* (1989), *262(22)*, 31–32.]

Stewart, D. (1997a). The case for including women in health research. Paper presented at The International Congress of Women in the Health Care System, Vienna, March 1997.

Stewart, D.E. (1997b). Women's health comes of age. *Canadian Medical Association Journal, 157(12),* 1711–1712.

Stone, V.E., Mauch, M.Y., Steger, K., Janas, S.F., & Craven, D.E. (1997). Race, gender, drug use, and participation in AIDS clinical trials. Lessons from a municipal hospital cohort. *Journal of General Internal Medicine, 12(3),* 150–157.

Strandberg, T., Salomaa, V., Naukkarinen, V., Vanhanen, S., & Miettinen, T. (1991). Long term mortality after 5 year multifactorial primary prevention of cardiovascular disease in middle aged men. *Journal of the American Medical Association, 266,* 1225–1229.

Whiteside, C., Dessureault, S., Dickstein, J., Tibbles, L.A., Torrance, S., Boynton, E., Seeman, M., Siminovitch, K., & Stewart, D. (1997). Women in biomedical research—addressing the challenges. *Clinical & Investigative Medicine – Medecine Clinique et Experimentale, 20(4),* 268–272.

Wilhelmsen, L., Berglund, G., Elmfeldt, D., Tibblin, G., Wedel, H., & Pennert, K., (1986). The multifactor primary prevention trial in Goteborg, Sweden. *European Heart Journal, 7,* 279–288.

Williams, A.B. (1992). Women and the AIDS epidemic: no longer hidden. *Todays OR Nurse, 14(7),* 23–27.

WHO (1989). *World Health Organisation European Collaborative Group WHO European Collaborative Trial in the Multifactorial Prevention of Coronary Heart Disease.* Copenhagen: WHO.

Chapter 5

Private Violence, Public Complicity: The Response of Health and Social Services to Battered Women

Patrizia Romito

University of Trieste, Italy

Battered women present a challenge to health care. This chapter will analyse how social agencies and public health services, in particular, respond to battered women. The reason underlying interest in the responses of social agencies toward violence against women is clear. Violence only becomes visible when it is socially recognised as such. When a husband rapes his wife, for example, it is not considered to be sexual violence unless the law defines it so (as was the case in Great Britain until 1991 and as still is the case today in some parts of the United States). Analysis of how different agencies and social/health workers conceptualise violence against women and how they react to it is crucial to understanding how society faces male violence and how victims socially construct their experience.

The first feminist studies on wife battering suggested that social institutions were often blind and deaf to the demands for treatment, support

Women, Health and the Mind
Edited by L. Sherr and J.S. St Lawrence. © 2000 John Wiley & Sons, Ltd

and protection made by battered women. Women who were interviewed reported that doctors, psychologists, health and social workers, as well as judges and members of the police force, preferred to ignore violence against women and its consequences. At times these social agents attributed responsibility for the violence to the victims themselves. They would make them feel guilty for causing it and gave higher priority to the needs of other members of the family (children, the violent man) than to those of the female victims (MacLeod, 1987).

Initially this chapter will provide a summary of what is known about wife battering to assist in understanding the experiences and suffering that burden battered women as they seek help from social and health services. Next, a brief outline of the main theoretical approaches toward battering will be provided because theory assists in understanding which models are used as reference points by social and health workers, both implicitly or explicitly, when they interact with a woman who has been battered. Finally, an analysis of the responses of operators and social and health services will be provided. A number of categories of analysis will be proposed to understand better the response of social services. These categories are based on the results of a study undertaken between 1994 and 1998 in two regions of northern Italy in which 30 female victims of male violence were interviewed. The study also involved 35 male and female social/health workers (physicians, psychologists, social workers and nurses) and 16 members of the police force (flying squads). For further details regarding the methodology of the study, see Romito (1997) and Romito (1999).

DOMESTIC VIOLENCE

Domestic violence can include physical, sexual, psychological and financial assaults. Most battered women fall victim to several types of assault. Battering is endemic. Indeed, between 25 and 30% of women are victims of the physical and/or sexual abuse of a partner during the course of their lives. Between 3–15% had been abused during the 12 months preceding recruitment into the studies (Gillioz et al., 1997; Juristat, 1994; Mooney, 1993; Morris, 1997). Abuse often continues after separation from the abuser and may even escalate in frequency and degree. According to the United States Department of Justice (1983), a woman runs a higher risk of death if she leaves a violent man than if she stays with him (see also Wilson & Daly, 1993). Canadian police statistics show that 23% of women killed by their husbands were separated and 3% were divorced at the time of the murder (Juristat, 1994). Abuse is also frequently perpetrated during pregnancy (7–16% of women studied; see Campbell, 1998) and in the months following birth (see Carlson Gielen et al., 1994). Often, children are also involved. According to Canadian statistics, children were present during at least 40% of assaults on women by men and, in particular, during over half of the serious assaults in which women feared for their lives (Juristat, 1994). Many women who died at the hands of their partner were killed in front of their own children (Campbell, 1992). According to American data, representative of the nation as a whole, half of all violent husbands also assault their children, often very seriously (see Peled, 1997). Despite this, these same men often request custody of their children following separation. Studies show that when the children of such men stay with their fathers following a separation, they run a serious risk of physical and sexual abuse (Peled, 1997; Radford et al., 1997).

These data provide a summary of the frequency and characteristics of battering. In-depth research data on the nature of violence and the impact of battering on these women can be illustrated by the details from my own research. In my interviews, data on physical abuse reveal a wide range of injuries. Women reported being pushed with force by their partners or ex-partners, thrown down stairs, slapped, punched, kicked and bitten. They reported incidents of hitting with clubs, injury with knives, burning with cigarettes, running over by cars and strangulation attempts. Many were left with medium- and long-term physical consequences including nose, jaw, head, rib, arm and finger fractures. Two were partially disabled, one must wear a denture and one has a permanent ear drum injury.

> He yanked my hair, bit my finger, butted his cigarette out on my hand, a bit of everything. He squeezed my neck tight, gave me a black eye, a swollen nose, a broken finger, these were the lighter bashing. He would drag me about the house, kicked me even in the breasts and had a nasty habit of beating my head against the wall, I was full of bumps right here.
>
> My son always witnessed all my abuses. When he was 2 years old his father grabbed him by the head one day, bashed him, he could have broken his neck. The child wet his pants, then, whenever his father called him he would always wet his pants.

Psychological abuse perpetrated by partners can include insults, denigration, threats or assaults against autonomy. The male partner wants to control the woman, preventing her from going out, going to work or even using the telephone. The objective is to dominate her entirely, limiting or destroying her material and psychological autonomy to the point of "annihilating" her.

> Incredible psychological pressure, he told me I wasn't worth anything, that I looked terrible, fat, he made me feel incapable of doing anything, absolutely nothing, he told me "you'll end up walking the streets sooner or later".
>
> He threw away all my photos, of when I was a little girl, all the photos of my parents, he wanted to destroy my past. He made so much trouble that my parents didn't speak to me any more

and I was left isolated and that's what he wanted, that nobody talk to me. He could not stand my seeing my girl friends, he could not accept my having male colleagues at work, he wanted me to lose my job.

It is important to underline that many of the women interviewed in this and other studies claimed that psychological violence was even more destructive and devastating than physical abuse.

THE THEORIES: AN OUTLINE

The first theoretical approach to be considered is best described as "naturalistic". In its "psychopathological" version, of Freudian deriva- tion, domestic violence is attributed to the personality characteristics of a violent man and of a battered woman. That is, a male's behaviour is the product of deep anxiety and frustration. It is often women, as "castrators", who provoke him to become violent with their attitudes. Furthermore, women are described as feeling a "masochistic" satisfac- tion, which explains why they don't always break off such relationships. In its "biological" version, violence against women is considered a func- tion of natural selection explained by high male hormone levels (for a review, see Herzberger, 1996). The appeal of naturalistic theories seems inversely proportional to their scientific foundation. Indeed, despite criticism, both the psycho-pathological and biological versions continue to represent strong models. [Criticisms of these concepts and analyses of how psychoanalysis has contributed to covering up male violence against women, and in particular sexual abuse and incest, have been discussed by Amstrong (1996), Rush (1980, 1996) and Tavris (1992).]

The sociological approach has traditionally considered the patriarchal family as a system functional to human needs. Violence is seen as a sign of poor communication between its components. Here the object of research is "violence in the family" rather than "male violence against women or wives". The most notable authors, the Americans Gelles and Straus, tried to measure the spousal acts of violence during a series of studies. They found that women were equally or even more violent than their husbands and concluded that there is also a "syndrome of the bat- tered husband". These results are entirely contradictory to data from other studies however, that show that violence "in couples" is most often perpetrated by men towards women. The 1992 British Crime Survey, for example, found that at least 80% of all violent acts that occur among spouses are assaults by the husband or ex-husband on the wife (HMSO, 1993). The instrument used in the American studies – the Conflict Tactics Scales – presents gross methodological limitations. Such downfalls can explain the overestimate of female violence observed in those studies (see Nazroo, 1995). It should also be noted that the same authors later retracted, at least in part, their conclusions (Gelles, 1997).

In a clinical setting, we find that the systemic view represents the most frequent theoretical reference point for family therapy. According to the theory, violence is not "linear"; a better portrayal is that of a mutual–casual interaction process. As a consequence, what is said of victims of violence is that their own behaviour in the mutual–casual family system provoked the violence they experienced. Like psychoanalysis, the systemic approach has raised criticism, especially, but not exclusively, from feminist researchers (Bograd, 1984; Dell, 1989).

The feminist approach stems from a preliminary statement – an ethical statement – that male domination of women is unacceptable. This domination, at a material and symbolic level, brings with it numerous financial and psychological advantages for men. Violence is a tool to maintain this domination and the advantages deriving from it when other means of coercion and duress prove inadequate (Delphy, 1984; Delphy & Leonard, 1992). Feminist research has provided an understanding of the experience of being a victim of male violence. Feminist research challenged widespread stereotypes such as accepting violence as a consequence of social difficulties or viewing women victims as passive or even masochistic victims. It also illustrated the existence of a continuum between the different types of violence and between violence against women and children such as battering, femicide, marital rape, and sexual harassment and denounced the family as a privileged place where violence is practised (see Dobash & Dobash, 1979; Kelly, 1988; Kelly and Regan, 1993; Radford and Russell, 1992; Russell, 1990).

THE RESPONSE OF HEALTH AND SOCIAL SERVICES TO BATTERED WOMEN

Assaults by men – physical, sexual, and psychological – compromise the well-being and physical and mental health of women. Battered women are more often depressed and make more suicide attempts. They have more frequent visits to the Emergency Room, additional hospitalisations and increased use of outpatient health care facilities (see also Andrews & Brown, 1988; Bergman & Brismar, 1991; Fishbach & Herbert, 1997; Grisso et al., 1991; Heise et al., 1994). If battered when pregnant, women have an increased risk of having a stillborn baby (Dye et al., 1995).

How do services and social/health workers respond to this? Reviewing the literature and the results of my own research, a number of categories of responses can be formulated. The first important distinction is between appropriate and inappropriate responses. Inappropriate responses can be subdivided into three main categories: denial or non-acknowledgement of violence, refusal and abusive psychologisation.

Inappropriate Responses

Denial

Denial of violence can be passive or active. Passive denial, or non-acknowledgement, occurs when the people around a woman do not delve into the visible signs of violence or accept her unlikely justifications without difficulty. Non-acknowledgement of male violence is frequent. In the Emergency Room, nobody asks anything of women who display the consequences of abuse; when, for fear of retaliation by her partner or for shame, women tell unlikely stories, they are "believed" without a word.

> Whenever I went to the hospital with a broken arm I always used to say I had fallen, he broke it three times, once with a club ... I always said I had fallen on the stairs (Did they believe you?) Yes.

After analysing the patient files of Emergency Room admissions, Stark et al. (1983) found that for every case of violence acknowledged there were at least another eight highly probable cases. McLeer & Anwar (1989) arrived at similar conclusions. Indeed in the department studied, before the beginning of the interviews the victims of abuse represented 6% of women with trauma. After the introduction of a simple protocol in which each woman was directly asked whether and by whom she had been battered, the percentage acknowledging abuse increased to 30%. In Italy, 45% of Emergency Room doctors who were interviewed in Bologna claimed never to have had any professional contact with female victims of abuse, while the "Casa delle Donne" (a women's shelter) in Bologna had given refuge to 1246 "new cases" from 1992 to 1995 (Gonzo, 1997).

The staff of prenatal medicine departments appear equally oblivious. In one study, 16% of women who went to hospital for pregnancy check-ups had been abused by their partners, but only 20% of these cases were "acknowledged" by health workers (Dye et al., 1995). In another sample of pregnant women, 7% were abused and of these two-thirds asked for medical care following abuse. Only 3% of the victims of abuse discussed their experience during prenatal visits (Stewart & Cecutti, 1993).

Another example of denial is illustrated by the behaviour of certain family doctors or specialists whose advice is sought by women suffering psychological distress. Of the women I interviewed, one, who had been raped as a child by her brother, had spent at least 15 years of her life in a state of severe mental suffering: nervous breakdowns, panic attacks, depression, attempted suicide and alcoholism. She reached a stage of alcoholic coma before a physician asked her, for the first time, to discuss her problems.

Other data from the United States confirm the evidence given by the women who were interviewed in Italy. A number of studies at community mental health centres and inpatient facilities find that therapists and other service providers are aware of only a small proportion of their clients being victims of physical assault (Aldarondo & Straus, 1994). While studies of family therapy clients show rates of women's battering as high as 70% (O'Leary & Murphy, 1992), a survey of members of the American Association of Marriage and Family Therapy (AAMFT) found that 60% did not consider family violence to be a significant clinical problem in their practices. A survey of participants at an AAMFT convention found that 40% failed to recognise any evidence of wife assaults in vignettes that contained clear indicators of violence (quoted by Aldarondo & Straus, 1994). A study in a family therapy clinic suggested that more than half of all cases involving physical violence against women are not detected (O'Leary et al., 1992).

Refusal and Complicity of Violent Men

Battered women have often been considered responsible for the inadequate responses they receive from health services: after all, at times they prefer to hide their abuse or minimise it. However, when they do talk openly about it and make explicit requests to service providers (treatment, advice, support and information), they run the risk of receiving equally explicit refusals.

Refusal

The second category is that of refusal. Where violence is visible and the woman does not hide it and makes explicit requests for assistance, she often finds herself receiving negative answers because of "justifications" that in part defend the man, defend the family and blame the woman. Refusal may even involve explicitly taking the side of the violent man himself, in other words complicity. The refusal category also includes less specific responses characterised by incompetence and lack of respect for the woman.

Women who were interviewed in Italy, like those interviewed in Great Britain (Pahl, 1994) or the United States (Bowker & Maurer, 1987), reported that their doctor or social worker suggested they should be "patient", be better wives, be more understanding and try to keep the family together for the sake of their children. Sometimes they were verbally attacked and insulted.

> I went to the Emergency Room full of bruises and the doctor said to me "Don't report him, he's still your husband, the father of your daughter".

Doctor X said, "If a woman is beaten, it means she deserved it".

Even though the results of qualitative studies cannot be generalised, quantitative data confirm that refusals occur frequently. On the basis of the replies of 1000 battered women, Bowker & Maurer (1987) concluded that medical services were used fairly frequently, but that they were seen by the battered women as being less effective than any other group (women's groups, lawyers, the police, the clergy, social service agencies).

Refusal deprives a woman of the services she needs and has a right to receive. Furthermore it makes her feel guilty, sabotages her attempts to evade the violent situation and demoralises her psychologically. These responses represent a form of *de facto* complicity with male violence.

Abusive Psychologisation

The third category, abusive psychologisation or psychiatrisation, works at two levels. First, when confronted with a request for information, financial support, protection or justice, the operator or service provides a response that, whether good or bad, shifts the problem onto hypothetical psychological difficulties of the woman. Second, the experience is labelled by interpretations, such as masochism or co-dependence, of psycho-analytical derivation that create a strong sense of guilt for the woman. At the same time other possible psychological approaches are ignored. In contrast with denial and refusal, health operators do not hide these responses. Indeed, they often claim they are the most appropriate, without realising the consequences for victims of abuse.

An example will help to illustrate this category. It refers to the case of a 50-year-old housewife who had always been abused by her husband. She finally found the strength to think about obtaining a separation and turned to social services for an appointment with a legal counsellor but was instead re-routed to a psychologist who saw her use of her married name as a symptom of her dependence on the affection of her husband. (In Italy, on all official papers, married women have both their maiden and married names, or in some cases only their maiden name. In practice, women with a profession tend to use their maiden name; others, their married name.) Given this "ambivalence", instead of meeting a lawyer, she was advised to have a psychiatric evaluation.

Abusive psychologisation also occurs in the Emergency Room in hospitals. Physicians often sent victims of male violence to the Psychiatric Department in the belief that they could be treated in a more "humanised" way there. In the United States, research by Stark et al. (1983), showed how the mechanism of psychiatrisation works.

Many of the women who came to the Emergency Room with consequences of abuse were redirected to the Psychiatric Department, sometimes even without basic medical attention (tests and treatment) that would have been given had their injuries been caused by a car accident rather than by the fists of their husbands. In the Psychiatric Department, the reason for the women's suffering (violence) was rarely explored. In contrast, they received treatment (sessions and/or psychotropic drugs) focusing on their symptoms of psychological distress. These researchers concluded that certain behaviours of battered women (attempted suicide, alcohol or psychotropic drug abuse) can be traced back equally to the abuses and to the consequent psychiatric conditioning they received when they sought help. Psychologisation also involves other consequences. Because one form of psychological violence perpetrated by the abusive partner is his saying that the woman is crazy and that she is worth nothing, this strategy contributes to assuring the woman that it is she who lies at the heart of the problem and not the husband who maltreated her. Going through psychiatric services may also involve being stigmatised. According to Stark et al. (1983), in certain cases social services have used the fact that the woman in question has been admitted into the psychiatric ward to remove her children.

In addition, many health and social workers use the concepts of masochism and co-dependence in an all too critical manner. Among who were interviewed, some described cases in which the woman did not leave the violent man because she had small children and had neither a house nor a job. In other cases, the husband had threatened to kill her and the children if she left him. Despite the fact that in the months following the interviews three women in the same city were killed by their ex-partners, the obstinately "blind" health and social workers, faced with the difficulties and risks run by the victims of violence, defined their clients as "masochists".

These data are confirmed by research carried out in Bologna (Gonzo, 1997). Among the health workers who were interviewed, 58% believed that it was the psychological problems of the women that set off the violence, 32% believed that the women stayed with the man because they were masochists and 68% were in favour of prescriptions for psychotropic drugs.

The Response of Social Services

Let us now consider the responses of social services to which many women turn when, after separation from a violent man, they are in conflict with him for child custody. My interviews revealed common themes. Often, social services support fathers' requests for greater access to the children and for more convenient conditions in their favour. In one case, the social worker pressured a woman to leave the shelter where she had found refuge and rent a bungalow in a camp site, with her own money, so that the father could visit the children more easily. In other cases, for fear of meeting their partner alone and in an effort to respect the visiting times set to take into account the needs of fathers and not their own, other women end up spending significant sums of money on taxis and baby-sitters. When women resist, the conflict worsens. The courts can order an expert opinion; often the "experts" are psychologists or psychiatrists. Analysis of these reports show surprising results: male violence disappears from the report. The behaviour of women thus becomes unreasonable, symptomatic of inner difficulties and of personal limitations. One example regards a woman who opposed joint custody: even though she recognised the woman as an excellent mother, the psychologist wrote that "This lady is hostile toward her husband and this prevents her from being a just and generous mother". All references to the husband's abuses were omitted from the report. The father obtained custody.

Another case concerned a woman who, after a brief period of cohabitation, left a very violent man who had already seriously injured his ex-wife. He threatened to kill her, their little girl and himself, and thereafter he began to persecute her and her family (car pursuits, insults and assaults) to the point of being convicted three times in 4 years in addition to being the subject of numerous additional complaints to the police. The child witnessed the abuses and the woman feared that the father might abuse the child too. Supported by the Separated Fathers' Movement and on the basis of a favourable report written by social services, the man obtained joint custody. In the psychologist's reports there was no reference to the violence perpetrated by the man, who was justified as being "still in love". The woman was described as having a "persecutionary attitude" and as having "deformed" her ex-partner's image. Once any objective reference to abuse and threats is erased, the reasonable fear held by this woman appears to be paranoia and, in this case, an already convicted man becomes described as merely a stubborn but harmless lover.

In Great Britain we can observe a similar tendency. The 1989 Children's Act emphasised the right to maintainance of the father–children relationship after separation. Thus any conflict was shifted from a legal to a more informal level. Family mediation, with the roots of its theory lying in the systemic approach and in family therapy, became the tool to practise this right. The preliminary condition is that the parents forget their past and their problems as a couple (including abuses), to look to the future and to their roles as parents. This situation is easier for male perpetrators than for those who underwent the abuse. When the women reiterate the need for protection from further abuse, they are labelled as selfish, uncooperative and hostile. For these reasons, in Great Britain as in Italy, a woman can lose custody of her children. To contextualise these service strategies, we must remember that in many countries mediation claims are supported by separated fathers' associations and that many activists of this movement are acknowledged batterers (Walker, 1989; Dufresne, 1998). In Great Britain, a follow-up study was carried out on the arrangements made for children to have contact with the non-resident parent (mostly fathers) following separations that resulted from domestic violence to women. Of the 53 women studied for some years after separation, 50 were assaulted, even seriously, when they met their ex-partners to "exchange" their children. Half of the children were physically or sexually abused during these visits (Radford et al., 1997). An American study found similar results (Shepard, 1992; see also Peled, 1997).

In summary, we find denial of violence, refusal and abusive psychologisation in the responses of social services, albeit in more complex and sophisticated forms than those occurring, for example, in Emergency Rooms.

Adequate Responses

Adequate responses legitimise the experience of a woman and take it seriously. Her rights and needs are recognised and she is provided with the assistance she has a right to receive. The risks she runs are not underestimated and health and social workers treat her with respect and compassion. In some cases, the response is positive because it neutralises abusive psychologisation.

> This psychiatrist said, "You need neither a psychiatrist nor anti-depressants. You need a lawyer".

> The first social worker gave me some tools. It meant telling me: you know you can take out an *ad honouree* loan: a loan with easy terms of repayment which is given to people in certain circumstances. She did not give me any lip-devotion or charity, just information. And once she even asked me "Do you feel any better?"

These positive responses, although infrequent, were also found in other studies (Bowker & Maurer, 1987; Pahl, 1994).

CONCLUSIONS

The responses that social and health services give to female victims of domestic violence are often inadequate, to the point that in some cases they become an objective complicity with the violent man. The violence of these responses is such that, to underline it, the term "secondary victimisation" has been coined to define it.

From a methodological point of view, triangulation reassures us of the validity of these conclusions. In social research, triangulation uses multiple and different sources (e.g. informants), methods, investigators and theories (Denzin, 1988). The fact that the responses can be traced back to denial, refusal and abusive psychologisation emerges from both qualitative and quantitative studies interviewing both women and health/social workers and using very different theory references. Although many studies in this field refer back to a feminist approach, there are others (for example, those done in Emergency Rooms) that reflect back to dominant approaches in the biomedical field and, in particular, to epidemiology. Our conclusions are reinforced by litera-ture describing similar response patterns (denial, refusal and abusive psychologisation) by social, health and educational institutions to child victims of battering and abuse (Frenken & Van Stolk, 1990; Gibbons, 1996; Sundell, 1997) and in the responses which other social institu-tions, such as family and law enforcement bodies give to victims of domestic violence (for the family, see Romito, 1997). Women inter-viewed in Sweden reported that police officers did not worry about protecting them. They belittled and trivialised their abuses, often did not believe them and refused to arrest the violent man (Elman & Eduards, 1991). Police officers interviewed in Great Britain claimed that the victims of violence deserved it, asked for it, enjoyed it, and anyway did nothing to leave their partners (Hanmer, 1990). Police officers I interviewed in Italy described their actions in what they defined as "family conflicts" as mediation and psychological strategies (we listen to them, calm them, we are social workers), without ever mentioning the need to protect the victim nor the possibility of arresting the assailant.

Abusive psychologisation is the "softest", the most sophisticated and perhaps the most pernicious of all inadequate responses. In addition to depriving a woman of "appropriate" responses, it imposes an inter-pretation of the situation that is not just wrong but also considers her to be responsible for the violence she endured (she is paranoid, she is a masochist, etc.). Moreover, social psychologists have shown that psychologisation is a very effective strategy to delegitimise an isolated or deviant individual within a group (Doise et al., 1991).

As we have seen, certain theoretical models are the basis of the responses that social/health workers use to deny the existence or frequency of male violence against women and the destructive role this can have in their lives. The psychoanalytical model not only underes-timates the importance of the current context in a person's suffering, it has also denied the experience of sexual violence (see Masson, 1984; Rush, 1980). Even now patients are told that memories of sexual abuse are Oedipal fantasies rather than memories of actual sexual abuse. Family mediation stems from the systemic approach, which denies the linearity of family violence. In the multi-causal model of family therapy and of mediation, nobody and everybody is responsible for violence and one cannot distinguish between assailant and victim (Bograd, 1984; Dell, 1989). The medical model, on its part, is characterised by a focus on the symptoms, from which follow both reductionism and decontextualisation (Warshaw, 1993). Whether the trauma is caused by a husband's fist or by an accidental fall is irrelevant.

Thus the inadequate responses of social and health services to women who are victims of abuse find their roots partially in widely used theoretical models. After comparing the experiences of several victim types – from family abuse to lagers – psychiatrist Judith Lewis Herman (1992) reminds us of how much easier it is to side with the perpetrator. Those who have been victims of abuse ask us to act, to take sides. All that the perpetrator asks of witnesses is to do nothing. His main strategies are secrecy and silence. When this is not possible, he will do what he can so that nobody listens to the victim or so that the victim is not believed. This is where the strategy of psychologisation enters, with its delegitimising function. If the witness is isolated, the perpetrator's strategy is irresistible. The vision of horror is difficult to tolerate, the stigma associated with the victim seems contagious and, above all, taking sides means commitment and effort and can imply personal and professional costs.

Only in the social context inspired by the feminist movement can there be a political, cultural and material space in which battered women can find a voice, solidarity and hope for the future. In such a context, it is possible to elaborate strategies and initiatives (informational campaigns, education, legal measures and service staff training) aimed at opposing male violence and at preventing secondary victimisation. This will only take place if the level of attention, awareness and political tension regarding this issue is maintained at a high level in society at large.

REFERENCES

Aldarondo, E., & Straus, M. (1994). Screening for physical violence in couple therapy: methodological, practical and ethical considerations. *Family Process*, *33*, 425–439.

Amstrong, L. (1996). In the footsteps of Doctor Freud and down the proverbial garden path. *Feminism and Psychology*, *6(2)*, 298–303.

Andrews, B., & Brown, G. (1988). Marital violence in the community. *British Journal of Psychiatry*, *153*, 303–312.

Bergman, B., & Brismar, B. (1991). Suicide attempts by battered wives. *Acta Psychiatrica Scandinavica*, *83*, 380–384.

Bograd, M. (1984). Family systems approaches to wife battering: a feminist critique. *American Journal of Orthopsychiatry*, *54(4)*, 558–568.

Bowker, L., & Maurer, L. (1987). The medical treatment of battered wives. *Women and Health*, *12(1)*, 25–45.

Campbell, J. (1992). "If I can't have you, no one can": power and control in homicide of female partners. In Radford, J., & Russell, D. (Eds.), pp.99–113. *Femicide. The Politics of Woman Killing*. New York: Twaye.

Campbell, J. (1998). Abuse during pregnancy: progress, policy and potential. *American Journal of Public Health, 88(2)*, 185–186.

Carlson Gielen, A., O'Campo, P., Faden, R., Kass, N., & Xue, X. (1994). Interpersonal conflict and physical violence during the childbearing year. *Social Science and Medicine, 39(6)*, 781–787.

Dell, P. (1989). Violence and the systemic view: The problem of power. *Family Process, 28(1)*, 1–14.

Delphy, C. (1984). *Close to Home: A Materialist Analysis of Women's Oppression*. London: Hutchinson.

Delphy, C., & Leonard, D. (1992). *Familiar Exploitation*. Cambridge: Polity Press.

Denzin, N. (1988). *The Research Act*. Englewood, New York: Prentice-Hall.

Dobash, R., & Dobash, R. (1979). *Violence Against Wives: A Case Against Patriarchy*. New York: Free Press.

Doise, W., Deschamps, J.-C., & Mugny, G. (1991). *Psychologie Sociale Expérimentale*. Paris: Colin.

Dufresne, M. (1998). Masculinisme et criminalité sexiste. *Nouvelles Questions Féministes et Recherches Féministes, 11(2)*, 125–138.

Dye, T., Tolliver, N., Lee, R., & Kenney, C. (1995). Violence, pregnancy and birth outcome in Appalachia. *Paediatric and Perinatal Epidemiology, 9*, 35–47.

Elman, A., & Eduards, M. (1991). Unprotected by the Swedish Welfare State. A survey of battered women and the assistance they received. *Women's Studies International Forum, 14(5)*, 413–421.

Fishbach, R., & Herbert, B. (1997). Domestic violence and mental health: correlates and conundrums within and across cultures. *Social Science and Medicine, 45(8)*, 1161–1176.

Frenken, J., & Van Stolk, B. (1990). Incest victims: inadequate help by professionals. *Child Abuse and Neglect, 14*, 253–263.

Gelles, R. (1997). *Intimate Violence in Families*. London: Sage.

Gibbons, J. (1996). Services for adults who have experienced child sexual assault: improving agency response. *Social Science and Medicine, 43(12)*, 1755–1763.

Gillioz, L., DePuy, J., & Ducret, V. (1997). *Domination et Violence Envers la Femme dans le Couple*. Lausanne: Payot.

Gonzo, L. (1997). *Violenza alle Donne: la Cultura dei Medici e Degli Operatori*. Bologna: City Hall of Bologna.

Grisso, A., Wishner, A.R., Schwarz, D.F., Weene, B.A., Holmes, J.H., & Sutton, R.L. (1991). A population-based study of injuries in inner-city women. *American Journal of Epidemiology, 134(1)*, 59–68.

Hanmer, J. (1990). Men, power and the exploitation of women. *Women's Studies International Forum, 13(5)*, 443–456.

Heise, L., Raikes, A., Watts, C., & Zwi, A. (1994). Violence against women: a neglected public health issue in less developed countries. *Social Sciences and Medicine, 39(9)*, 1165–1179.

Herzberger, S. (1996). *Violence Within the Family. Social Psychological Perspectives*. London: Brown & Benchmark.

HMSO (1993). *The British Crime Survey*. London: HMSO.

Juristat (1994). Résultats d'une enquête nationale sur l'aggression contre la conjointe, K. Rodgers. *Statistique Canada, no. 85, 14(9)*, 1–22.

Kelly, L. (1988). *Surviving Sexual Violence*. Cambridge: Polity Press.

Kelly, L., & Regan, L. (1993). *Abuse of Women and Children. A Feminist Response*. London: University of London Press.

Lewis Herman, J. (1992). *Trauma and Recovery*. New York: Basic Books.

MacLeod, L. (1987). *La Femme Battue au Canada: un Cercle Vicieux*. Ottawa, Ontario: Conseil Consultatif Canadien de la Situation de la Femme.

Masson, J.M. (1984). *The Assault on Truth: Freud's Suppression of the Seduction Theory*. NewYork: Farrar, Straus, Giroux.

McLeer, S., & Anwar, R. (1989). A study of battered women presenting in an emergency department. *American Journal of Public Health, 79(1)*, 65–66.

Mooney, J. (1993). *The Hidden Figure: Domestic Violence in North London. Report*. London: Centre for Criminology, Middlesex University.

Morris, A. (1997). *Women's Safety Survey 1996*. Wellington, New Zealand: Victimisation Survey Committee.

Nazroo, J. (1995). Uncovering gender differences in the use of marital violence: the effect of methodology. *Sociology, 29(3)*, 475–494.

O'Leary, K., & Murphy, C. (1992). Clinical issues in the assessments of spouse abuse. In Ammerman, R.T., & Hersen, M. (Eds.), *Assessment of Family Violence*, (pp.26–46). New York: John Wiley & Sons.

O'Leary, K., Vivian, D., & Malone, J. (1992). Assessment of physical aggression against women in marriage: the need for multimodal assessment. *Behavior Assessment, 14*, 4–14.

Pahl, J. (1994). Health professionals and violence against women. In Kingston, P., & Penhale, B. (Eds.), *Family Violence and the Caring Professions*. Milton Keynes: Open University.

Peled, E. (1997). The battered women's movement response to children of battered women. *Violence Against Women, 3(4)*, 424–446.

Radford, J.E., & Russell, D. (1992). *Femicide. The Politics of Woman Killing*. New York: Twaye.

Radford, L., Hester, M., Humphries, J., & Woodfield, K. (1997). For the sake of the children: the law, domestic violence and child contact in England. *Women's Studies International Forum, 20(4)*, 471–482.

Romito, P. (1997). *Violenza Fisica e Sessuale Contro le Donne e Risposte dei Servizi Socio-sanitari. Research Report*. Trieste: Regione Autonoma Friuli Venezia-Giulia e Commissione Regionale per le Pari Opportunità.

Romito, P. (1999). Dalla padella alla brace. Donne maltrattate, violenza privata e complicità pubbliche. *Polis*, in prep.

Rush, F. (1980). *The Best Kept Secret: Sexual Abuse of Children*. New York: McGraw-Hill.

Rush, F. (1996). The words may change but the melody lingers on. *Feminism and Psychology, 6(2)*, 304–313.

Russell, D. (1990). *Rape in Marriage*. New York: Macmillan.

Shepard, M. (1992). Child-visiting and domestic abuse. *Child Welfare*, *LXXI(4)*, 357–367.

Stark, E., Flitcraft, A., & Frazier, W. (1983). Medicine and patriarchal violence: the social construction of a "private" event. In Fee, E. (Ed.), *Women and Health: The Politics of Sex in Medicine* (pp.177–210). New York: Baywood.

Stewart, D., & Cecutti, A. (1993). Physical abuse in pregnancy. *Canadian Medical Association Journal, 149(9)*, 1257–1263.

Sundell, K. (1997). Child-care personnel's failure to report child maltreatment: some Swedish evidence. *Child Abuse and Neglect, 21(1)*, 93–105.

Tavris, C. (1992). *The Mismeasure of Women*. New York: Simon & Schuster.

United States Department of Justice (1983). *Report to the Nation on Crime and Justice: The Data*. Washington D.C: US Government Printing Office.

Walker, L. (1989). Psychology and violence against women. *American Psychologist, 44(4)*, 695–702.

Warshaw, C. (1993). Limitations of the medical model in the care of battered women. In Bart, P., & Geil Moran, E. (Eds.), *Violence Against Women* (pp.134–146). London: Sage.

Wilson, M., & Daly, M. (1993). Spousal homicide risk and estrangement. *Violence and Victims, 8*, 3–16.

Section 2

WOMEN AND MENTAL HEALTH

Chapter 6

Women and Mental Illness

Jane M. Ussher

University of Western Sydney, Nepean, Australia

Gender differences in the diagnosis and treatment of psychological disorders classified as mental illness are a well-established phenomenon. Prior to puberty, boys are over-represented in significantly greater numbers (by a factor of approximately 4:1) in the whole gamut of psychological or behavioural problems experienced by children. However, after puberty the situation is reversed. Estimates of the ratio of women to men suffering from disorders such as depression, anxiety, and eating disorders range from 6:1 to 5:3. Community surveys, hospital admissions, and statistics on outpatient treatment (both medical and psychological) all concur that women are represented in far greater numbers than men (Bebbington, 1996; Busfield, 1986). The only exceptions are in the diagnosis of schizophrenia, in which there is no clear gender difference, and alcoholism, in which men dominate.

For decades, researchers sought the factors underlying this gender difference, claiming that if we can explain it, we will have the key to understanding mental health problems (e.g. Bebbington, 1996). Numerous competing biological, psychological, and social aetiological theories have been put forward as a result of efforts to understand these gender disparities in mental health diagnoses. The professions of psychiatry, clinical psychology, psychotherapy, and social work dispense expert knowledge and care to ameliorate or prevent such problems. Yet, as we know, their investigations and interventions have not gone unquestioned. A range of critics, including anti-psychiatrists,

Women, Health and the Mind
Edited by L. Sherr and J.S. St Lawrence. © 2000 John Wiley & Sons, Ltd

post-modernists, and feminists from a number of different ideological camps, have subjected expert analyses of women and mental illness to a critical deconstruction. Much of what has for decades (perhaps centuries) been taken for granted has been dissected and discarded as biased, misconceived, or misogynistic in the extreme (Ussher, 1991). However, in mainstream research and clinical practice very little has changed. The categorisation of women's mental health problems as pathology or illness remains unchallenged. Science categorises symptoms into syndromes that are operationally defined and analysed in objective research. Individual women are offered reductionistic explanations and invariably a biomedical cure for the symptoms they experience. Psychological interventions may not blame the body, but they still focus, in the main, on the individual woman (or on her mind). The gap between critical analysis and the institutionalised regulation or treatment of mental health problems seems impossible to bridge.

The question is, why is this the case? And what can be done to effect change? In this chapter I will address these two questions head on, briefly reviewing both mainstream and critical approaches to women and mental illness, as well as the relationship between the two, and arguing that the current positivist/realist, epistemological perspective that underlies mainstream research and clinical interventions should be replaced by a material–discursive–intrapsychic perspective that recognises mental health problems as they are experienced by women, intrapsychic pain, defences, and discursive construction of madness and femininity without privileging one above the others.

EXPLAINING GENDER DIFFERENCES IN MENTAL HEALTH PROBLEMS

There are a number of competing explanations for gender differences in mental health problems. Biomedical accounts have historically dominated the field, providing the basis for widespread use of biomedical interventions, in particular psychotropic drug use. The attribution of symptomatology to "synaptic events", such as noradrenaline, 5-hydroxytryptamine (5-HT) (serotonin), dopamine, and acetycholine neurotransmitters (de Fonseca, 1989) can clearly be applied equally to men and women. The biological key is seen to be "female hormones" (Paykel, 1991), particularly oestrogen and progesterone, which lead to the reproductive syndromes: premenstrual syndrome (PMS), post-natal depression (PND), or menopausal problems. The alternative explanation given is a genetic one. For example, Slater & Cowie (1971) claimed that the gene for depression was located on the X chromosome, and thus women, with two X chromosomes, would be more liable to suffer from it. [Both of these levels of explanation have been subjected to a barrage of critical analysis. It is sufficient to say that there is no evidence for the biological root of reproductive disorders, if indeed such disorders exist (see Bancroft, 1993; Ussher, 1989; Walker, 1997), and the argument for an X-linked genetic hypothesis has been convincingly overturned (Bebbington, 1996, p.319–320).] This focus on the physical body is a direct result of the assumption that it is biomedical factors that can be observed and measured in the most "objective" manner, removing the potentially confounding interface of the woman's subjective interpretation of a symptom. In what is a totally reductionistic viewpoint, the body or biology is conceptualised in terms of physical processes – the action of hormones, neurotransmitters, or ovarian function, considered separately from meaning or from social–cultural contexts.

In recent years, the majority of researchers and clinicians have moved away from a strictly biological model, acknowledging instead the role of psychosocial factors. Social and environmental factors associated with higher reporting of mental health problems include:

- *marital status*, with married women reporting more problems than single women or married men (Bebbington et al., 1988)
- *caring roles*, with women looking after small children (Brown & Harris, 1978) or elderly relatives (Brody & Schoonover, 1986) being at higher risk
- *employment status*, with work generally providing a protective factor, particularly for working class women (Parry, 1986); absence of social support and economic or social power (Chesler, 1995)
- *gender role socialisation*, which leads to depressogenic attributional styles (Wierzbicki & Carver, 1989), a focus on heterosexual relationships as the fulfilment of life (Ussher, 1997a), and an emphasis on affiliation rather than achievement, leading to vulnerability when relationships are under threat (Kessler & MacLeod, 1984)
- *representations of femininity*, which position woman as other, as labile or as Madonna/whore (Ussher, 1997a)
- *multiple role strain and conflict*, as well as devaluation of traditional feminine roles (Bebbington, 1996)
- *sexual violence* or abuse in adulthood or childhood (Browne & Finklehor, 1986; Koss, 1990)

Psychological theories that have been put forward include

- cognitive vulnerability, specifically the greater likelihood of women to attribute problems to internal, stable and global factors (Calicchia & Pardine, 1984);
- coping styles (Sowa & Lustman, 1984);
- perception of control (Martin et al., 1984).

Psychodynamic theories, including object relations theory (Chodorow, 1978; Dinnerstein, 1976), Kleinian theory (Klein, 1984), and Freudian theory (Mitchell, 1975), influential in psychotherapeutic circles as well as in many recent feminist critiques, have had less impact on mainstream research and practice.

A number of suggestions have been offered in an attempt to resolve the apparent contradictions between these different aetiological theories. The adoption of multifactorial models, where biological and psychosocial vulnerability can be addressed within a framework that acknowledges the interaction between the two (e.g. Bancroft, 1993), is one way forward. Alternatively, suggestions of an interaction between cognitive and social vulnerability (i.e. Brown & Harris, 1978), argue that some women are more prone to depression and anxiety as a result of the interaction of environmental factors such as loss or stress and cognitive factors such as overvaluation of one goal at the expense of others.

While these multifactorial models provided a lead in moving away from narrow unidimensional thinking about women's mental health, they only offer a partial answer and arguably operate almost solely at the level of theory, having had little influence on research practice, which continues to be conducted in a unidimensional vein. For example, Paul Bebbington, in acknowledging the aetiological complexity of women's depressions concludes:

> . . . clinical experience suggests that depression arises because of a complex cascade, whereby for instance external circumstances interact with cognitive sets and induce physiological responses that in turn change the way circumstances are appraised. This may then change cognitions and physiological status, leading to a further spiral. If this is actually how depression develops, *it becomes extremely hard to research*, and progress has to fall back on the integration of piecemeal approaches. (Bebbington, 1996, p.299) [*My emphasis*]

It is only "extremely hard to research" within the constraints of methodological naturalism, as practised within a positivist paradigm (Ussher, 1997c). For it is the need to test the influence of antecedent variables within a hypothetico-deductive model that has led to the almost universal adoption of unilinear models in both biomedical and psychosocial research, where the reporting of symptoms is correlated with a single predictive factor. Equally, within this framework, each of the variables that appear in the biomedical, psychosocial, or multifactorial models are clearly operationally defined, reinforcing the assumption that they are discreet antecedent entities which exert independent causal influences in the aetiology of specific syndromes. Thus both mental health problems and the resulting symptoms are positioned as independent variables in research, invariably conceptualised in a dichotomous way as existing or not existing (Walker, 1995).

It is interesting to note that whilst researchers or reviewers are happy to acknowledge the importance of social or psychological aetiological factors (i.e. Bancroft, 1993; Bebbington, 1996; Busfield, 1986), they are less comfortable including any mention of the historical or cultural construction of madness, or of feminist critiques. Because many of the critics of mainstream theories and therapies *rejected* positivism/realism and embraced a social constructionist epistemology, they have had little impact on mainstream research and clinical practice. Social constructionism is seen as being incompatible with positivist/realist research and theory, largely because it contravenes many of the assumptions of this particular model of science. A further reason for these critiques' lack of impact is that, as Mary Parlee commented about feminist research, "very few feminist researchers have over the last few decades gone to the scientific heart of the matter by outlining or carrying out *doable* alternatives in research" (Parlee, 1991, p.29). This, in my view, is the challenge to critical theorists, of whatever persuasion.

SOCIAL CONSTRUCTIONIST AND FEMINIST CRITIQUES: A MOVE AWAY FROM POSITIVISM

Social Constructionism and Feminism

Positivist/realist approaches have been challenged in many areas of health and illness (e.g. Foucault, 1967; Ingleby, 1982; Nicolson, 1986; Stainton-Rogers, 1991; Ussher, 1997c; Yardley, 1997). Alternative models of conceptualising, researching, and, if necessary, treating symptomatology have been developed from within a broadly social constructionist perspective. Social constructionist approaches take a critical stance towards taken-for-granted knowledge; they acknowledge cultural and historical specificity; agree that knowledge is sustained by social practices; and agree that knowledge and social action go together (Burr, 1995). Social constructionists challenge the realist assumptions of traditional biomedical and psychological research, arguing instead that subjectivity, behaviour, and the very definition and meaning of what is "health" and what is "illness" is constructed within social practices and rules, language, relationships, and roles; it is always shaped by culture and history. Science is part of this constructive process, and as a consequence, research or clinical intervention can never be seen as objective or neutral; it is a social practice that partly shapes and constructs knowledge. This does not mean that scientific research is pointless, but merely that reflexivity in theory and practice is an essential part of the scientific enterprise.

Social constructionist critiques (e.g. Foucault, 1989; Ingleby, 1982; Sedgewick, 1987; Tiefer, 1986) have been used to "dethrone" experts in many arenas and to challenge the underlying assumptions of science and scientific practice. But social constructionism has also been used as the epistemological basis of much research and clinical practice (e.g.

McNamee & Gergen, 1992; Shotter & Gergen, 1989), where the gaze of the researcher is on the "social" rather than on the individual and where methodological naturalism is explicitly rejected. For example, there has recently been a move towards the use of discursive theories and methods that focus specifically on the role of language and its relation to cultural practices. From a methodological point of view, this leads to the use of qualitative methods, and again to reflexivity in research practice (for examples see Ussher, 1997b; Wilkinson & Kitzinger, 1995).

Many of the now numerous feminist critiques of women's mental health problems and of the treatment of women within the mental health professions, could also be placed under a broad social constructionist umbrella. Feminist critics have argued that misogynistic assumptions about gender roles and femininity are used to diagnose and treat women who deviate from those assumptions as mad. Assumptions about the proper position of women within the institution of heterosexuality are used to prescribe notions of normality, and the age-old practice of locating distress or deviancy in the womb (or reproductive hormones) reinforces notions of woman as being more animalistic or biologically driven than men. They also dismiss all legitimate anger or discontent as the result of "raging hormones", and ignore social and political inequalities that understandably produce symptoms of distress (see Chesler, 1995; Penfold & Walker, 1984; Ussher, 1991). This has led to critical feminist analyses of mental health research and treatment; to a deconstruction of the very concept of women's madness; and, more recently, to the development of women's centred research and therapy.

Despite the welcome addition of these recent critiques in the field of mental health, there are many issues that remain unaccounted for within a social constructionist epistemological frame. One problem is that adopting a social constructionist perspective or arguing that "mental illness" exists entirely at a discursive level implicitly denies the influence of biology or genetics. Alternatively, we may appear to relegate the body to a passive subsidiary role, which has meaning or interpretation imposed upon it (Turner, 1984; Yardley, 1996). Whilst the emphasis on social and discursive phenomena is understandable as a reaction biological reductionism, positioning the body as irrelevant in the aetiology, interpretation, or meaning of madness or psychological symptomatology is clearly inappropriate. Other material aspects of women's lives may also be negated in a discursive analysis: the influence of age, social class, power, economic factors, ethnicity, sexual identity, personal relationships and social support, or a prior history of sexual abuse, amongst other factors.

Equally, within a social constructionist or discursive approach the "reality" of mental health problems may appear to be denied. "Mental illness" can appear to be conceptualised as merely a social label or category. One of the conundrums facing feminist critics is the contradiction between the social or cultural construction of madness which pathologises and dismisses women and the increasing number of women who seek treatment for mental health problems, as they perceive them to have a significant influence on their lives. As Parlee (1989, p.20) notes, "what is strategically difficult for feminists is that many women now derive genuine benefits in their personal lives from an ideology that functions to explain and obscure social contradictions in their lives and those of other women". Ironically, many women adopt a biological discourse in explaining their psychological symptoms; the body is blamed for what is clearly positioned as "illness". Social constructionist analyses may seem to have little to say to these women. They stand in opposition to what women "know" and may be further rejected for appearing to suggest that madness is a myth. This is a problem facing those who would put forward a radical critique of mental illness; how to reconcile a deconstructive critique at a macro level with the needs of individuals at a micro-level (Ussher, 1991).

In addition, it is not clear how a social constructionist critique that "normalises" madness and denies its status as pathology would impact upon clinical interventions. Whilst social constructionist and feminist therapy *has* been developed in a number of areas, it is notably absent at the level of official discourse – training on mainstream clinical courses, as well as in articles in refereed academic journals. If we are to deconstruct the very notion of madness, how can we offer women treatment for this problem without being accused of reifying its existence? If we are focusing on the social or discursive construction of madness, is the woman an appropriate focus of attention? Does this not reify the notion of madness as an individual illness, to be solved by the woman herself? If we are rejecting realism, does that mean we are embracing relativism, with all the problems that entails?

Moving Forward: A Material–Discursive–Intrapsychic Analysis of Women's Mental Health Problems

In order to understand women's mental health problems, we need an epistemological shift away from a positivist/realist position since so many aspects of the phenomenon categorised as "mental illness" are excluded from the gaze of the researcher by the narrow definition of "science" that this approach implies. However, moving to a hard-line social constructionist position leaves questions unanswered, for the reasons outlined above. I suggest a material–discursive–intrapsychic analysis (Ussher, 1996, 2000), in which material, discursive, and intra-psychic aspects of experience can be examined without privileging one level of analysis above another within an epistemological and methodological framework that does not make *a priori* assumptions about causality, objectivity, or what methods can or should be used. "Material–discursive" approaches have recently been developed in a number of areas of psychology, such as sexuality, reproduction, and mental or physical health (see Ussher, 1997a, 1997b; Yardley, 1997). This is a result of both frustrations with traditional psychology that has tended to adopt a materialist standpoint, thus negating discursive aspects of experience, and dissatisfaction with the negation of the material aspects of life in many discursive accounts. This integrationist material–discursive approach is to be welcomed yet arguably does not always go far enough, as the intrapsychic is often still left out for the reason that it is seen as individualistic or reductionistic, or not easily accessible to empirical investigation. Equally, when intrapsychic factors are considered (for example in psychoanalytical or cognitive theorising) they are invariably conceptualised separately from either material or discursive factors. [There are exceptions. For example, the feminist psychoanalyst Karen Horney (1967) developed theories of sexuality and gender relationships which encapsulated material, discursive and intrapsychic levels of experience.] It is time that all three levels together were incorporated into academic theory and practice, in order to provide a multidimensional analysis of women's lives, of madness as a discursive category, and of the mental health symptoms many women experience. So what is meant by a material–discursive–intrapsychic approach?

The Level of Materiality

To talk of materiality is to talk of factors that exist at a corporeal, a societal, or an institutional level: factors that are traditionally at the centre of biomedical or sociological accounts. This would include biological factors associated with psychological symptomatology; material factors that institutionalise the diagnosis and treatment of mental health problems as "mental illness" or "madness"; gender inequalities and inequalities in heterosexual relationships, legitimating masculine power and control. The latter would encapsulate economic factors that make women dependent on men; presence or absence of the accommodation that allows women in destructive relationships to leave; support for women of a legal, emotional, and structural kind, which allows protection from further harassment or abuse. It would include issues of social class which lead to expectations of "normal" behaviour for women and men that are implicated in educational or employment opportunities available to both, as well as in the way individuals are treated by external institutions such as social services or the mental health professions. The fact of whether children are present in the relationship (or are, in custody battles, withheld) and the material consequences of being married (or not) are also part of this level of analysis. Equally, previous history of abuse or of bereavement is partly a material event, as is family history – the number of siblings, parental relationships, and factors such as parental divorce or separa-

tion from parents in childhood. There are also many material consequences of experiencing or being treated for mental health problems,
in terms of physical or psychological vulnerability, as well as powerlessness at an economic or societal level. The social isolation that can
be a consequence of mental health problems or that can act to exacerbate its effects is also partly a material issue. Sex, ethnicity, and sexuality
are also associated with materiality – with the reproductive body, with
gendered or sexual behaviour, and with physical appearance. Within
a feminist perspective it is recognised that material factors often miti-
gate against women: women are often economically, physically, and
socially disadvantaged in relation to men.

The Level of the Discursive

To focus on the "discursive" is to look to social and linguistic domains
– to talk, to visual representation, to ideology, culture, and power. What
is arguably of most relevance here is the discursive construction of
mental illness or madness, medical or psychological expertise (see
Foucault, 1967, 1979; Ussher, 1991), discursive construction of gender,
and analysis of the relationship between representations of "woman"
and "man" and the social roles adopted by individual women and men.

As many critics have argued, mental illness can be conceptualised
as a social category created by a process of expert definition (Ingelby,
1982; Littlewood & Lipsedge, 1982; Szasz, 1961; Ussher, 1991). In this
view, it is a discursively constructed label, based on value-laden definitions of normality. What is deemed "mental illness" in one context
or at one point in time is deemed normal at another. Parallel arguments
have been made about many other "disorders", both physical and
psychological (Foucault, 1967; Sedgewick, 1987), leading to a deconstruction of expert diagnosis and to a questioning of the existence of
many "syndromes".

Equally, within a discursive account, rather than femininity being seen
as pre-given or innate, here it is seen as something performed or
acquired. In the process of becoming "woman", it is argued that women
follow scripts of femininity taught to them through the family, through
school, and through the myriad representations of "normal" gender
roles in popular and high culture, as well as in science and the law (see
Ussher, 1997a). The taking up of the archetypal feminine position, within
what has been described as a heterosexual matrix (Butler, 1990), has been
seen to put women at risk for mental health problems, as it is a role that
requires self-sacrifice, self-denigration, and a stifling of independence
and desire. The dominance of phallocentric scripts of femininity is one
of the explanations put forward for why women stay in unhappy,
neglectful, or violent relationships (Dobash & Dobash, 1979), and is
arguably one of the explanations for why women internalise marital or
family difficulties as depression (Ussher, 1997d). Women are taught to

gain happiness through relationships, invariably with men. They are also taught that it is their fault if they can't. At the same time, a number of feminist critics have argued that the discursive construction of madness and femininity are closely aligned (Chesler, 1995; Ussher, 1991). Thus, to be "woman" is to be at risk of being positioned as "mad", particularly if one steps out of line – by being violent, sexual or in some other way contravening the feminine role.

The Level of the Intrapsychic

Intrapsychic factors operate at the level of the individual and are the psychological factors that are traditionally the central focus of psychological analyses of women's mental health problems. They include analyses of the way in which women blame themselves for problems in relationships and psychological explanations for why this is so, such as low self-esteem, depression, the impact of previous neglect or abuse, guilt, shame, fear of loss or separation, and the idealisation of both heterosexuality and of men. It would include an analysis of psychological defences, such as repression, denial, projection, or "splitting", as mechanisms for dealing with difficulty or psychological pain. For example, we see evidence of splitting when women see themselves or their man as all good or all bad, with no acknowledgement that everyone can exhibit positive and negative characteristics at the same time, or in the way women blame themselves or their bodies for problems they experience. It would also include women's internalisation of the idealised fantasy of motherhood, and of the expectations of being "woman" in a heterosexual social sphere.

As researchers, clinicians and theorists, we need to move to a position where we can take each of these levels of experience on board, without privileging one above the other. In order to do this, an epistemological shift is required. Critical realism is one example of a material–discursive–intrapsychic approach that can reconcile both the biomedical and psychosocial aspects of experience, as well as acknowledge the cultural and historical context in which individual women and men are positioned, and in which meaning about experience is created. Critical realism (Bhaskar, 1989) affirms the existence of reality, both physical and environmental, as a legitimate field of enquiry, at the same time recognising that its representations are characterised and mediated by culture, language, and political interests rooted in factors such as race, gender, or social class (Pilgrim & Rogers, 1997). Thus the role of hormones, the endocrine system, or physiological arousal, as well as the influence of social stressors, age, or economic factors, can be acknowledged and studied as "real" in analyses of the aetiology of mental health problems. The existence of "real" symptoms would also be acknowledged, whether they are psychological or physical, as would the existence of material factors that might ameliorate symptoms. However, these symptoms or material factors are not conceptualised as independent entities that exist separately from the historical or cultural context in which the woman lives. They are always positioned within discourse, within culture. "Mental illness" is therefore always a product of the symbiotic relationship between material, discursive, and intrapsychic factors; one level of analysis cannot be considered without the other.

SUMMARY

"Mental illness" is a phenomenon experienced by individual women at a material, discursive, and an intrapsychic level; we cannot disentangle one from the other. Its meaning to women, and to the experts who research and treat it, has to be understood in relation to the specific historical and cultural contexts in which they are positioned. It is in the context of dominant cultural discourses associating femininity with madness, infirmity, and reproductive lability that psychological symptoms are interpreted or experienced as "mental illness", by both the women who suffer from these symptoms and by the experts who intervene. It is in the context of the positivist/realist tradition in the biomedical and psychological sciences that madness is positioned as a real entity; as a syndrome or a disease. An epistemological shift to a material–discursive–intrapsychic analysis allows us to incorporate these different layers of women's subjective experience and the different types of expert knowledge about both mental health problems into one framework. What may appear to be contradictions or irrevocable disagreements within a positivist/realist frame, are then transformed into different parts of the complex picture that attempts to understand women's mental health problems; a picture that only makes sense when all the different parts are considered together.

ACKNOWLEDGEMENT

An earlier version of part of this paper has appeared in: Ussher, J.M. (2000), Women's madness: a material–discursive–intrapsychic approach. In Dwight, F. (ed.), *Psychology and the Postmodern: Mental Illness as Discourse and Experience*. London: Sage.

REFERENCES

Bancroft, J. (1993). The premenstrual syndrome – a reappraisal of the concept and the evidence. *Psychological Medicine, monograph supplement 24*. Cambridge: Cambridge University Press.
Bebbington, P. (1996). The origins of sex differences in depression: bridging the gap. *International Review of Psychiatry, 8*, 295–332.

Bebbington, P.E., Brugha, T., MacCarthy, B., Potter, J., Sturt, E., Wykes, T., Katz, R., & McGuffin, P. (1988). The Camberwell Collaborative Depression Study I. Depressed probonds: adversity and the form of depression. *British Journal of Psychiatry, 152*, 754–765.

Bhaskar, R. (1989). *Reclaiming Reality: A Critical Introduction to Contemporary Philosophy*. London: Verso.

Brody, E.M., & Schoonover, C.B. (1986). Patterns of parent care when adult daughters work and when they don't. *The Gerontologist, 26*, 372–382.

Brown, G., & Harris, T. (1978). *Social Origins of Depression*. London: Tavistock.

Browne, A., & Finkelhor, D. (1986). Impact of child sexual abuse: a review of the research. *Psychological Bulletin, 99(1)*, 66–77.

Burr, V. (1995). *An Introduction to Social Constructionism*. London: Routledge.

Busfield, J. (1986). *Men, Women and Madness: Understanding Gender and Mental Disorder*. New York: New York University Press.

Butler, J. (1990). *Gender Trouble: Feminism and the Subversion of Identity*. New York: Routledge.

Calicchia, J.P., & Pardine, P. (1984). Attributional style: degree of depression, respondent's sex, and nature of the attributional event. *Journal of Psychology, 117*, 789–795.

Chesler, P. (1995). *Women and Madness*. New York: Doubleday.

Chodorow, N. (1978). *The Reproduction of Mothering: Psychoanalysis and the Sociology of Gender*. Berkeley: California University Press.

de Fonseca, A.F. (1989). Psychiatry in the 1990s. In Hindmarsh, I., & Stoner, P.D. (Eds.), *Human Psychopharmacy: Measures and Methods*, Vol 2. New York: John Wiley & Sons Ltd.

Dinnerstein, D. (1976). *The Mermaid and the Minotaur: Social Arrangements and the Human Malaise*. New York: Harper.

Dobash, R. E., & Dobash, R. (1979). *Violence Against Wives: A Case Against the Patriarchy*. London: Open Books.

Foucault, M. (1967). *Madness and Civilisation: A History of Insanity in the Age of Reason*. London: Tavistock.

Foucault, M. (1979). *The History of Sexuality, Part 1*. London: Penguin.

Foucault, M. (1989). *Birth of the Clinic*. London: Penguin.

Horney, K. (1967). Premenstrual tension. In Horney, K., *Feminine Psychology*. New York & London: Longman.

Ingleby, D. (Ed.) (1982). *Critical Psychiatry: The Politics of Mental Health*. London: Penguin.

Kessler, R.C., & Macleod, J. (1985). Social support and mental health in community samples. In Cohen, S., & Syme, L. (Eds.), *Social Support and Health*. New York: Academic Press.

Klein, M. (1984). *Envy and Gratitude, and other works 1946–1963*. New York: Free Press.

Koss, M. (1990). The women's mental health research agenda: violence against women. *American Psychologist, 45(3)*, 374–380.

Littlewood, R., & Lipsedge, M. (1982). *Aliens and Alienists: Ethnic Minorities and Psychiatry.* Harmondsworth: Penguin.

Martin, D.J., Abramson, L.Y., & Alby, L.B. (1984). Illusion of control for self and others in depressed and non-depressed college students. *Journal of Personality and Social Psychology, 46,* 125–136.

McNamee, S., & Gergen, K. (Eds.) (1992). *Therapy as Social Construction.* London: Sage.

Mitchell, J. (1975). *Psychoanalysis and Feminism.* London: Allen Lane.

Nicolson, P. (1986). Developing a feminist approach to depression following childbirth. In Wilkinson, S. (Ed.), *Feminist Social Psychology.* Milton Keynes: Open University.

Parlee, M. (1989). The science and politics of PMS research. Paper presented at the annual research conference of the Association for Women in Psychology, Newport, RI, USA.

Parlee, M. (1991). The social construction of PMS: A case study of scientific discourse as cultural contestation. Paper presented to the conference "The Good Body: Asceticism in Contemporary Culture", Institute for the Medical Humanities, Texan University, Galveston, USA, 12–13 April.

Parry, G. (1986). Paid employment, life events, social support and mental health in working class mothers. *Journal of Health and Social Behaviour, 27,* 193–208.

Paykel, E.S. (1991). Depression in women. *British Journal of Psychiatry, 10,* 22–29.

Penfold, S., & Walker, G. (1984). *Women and the Psychiatric Paradox.* Milton Keynes: Open University Press.

Pilgrim, D., & Rogers, A. (1997). Mental Health, critical realism and lay knowledge. In Ussher, J.M. (Ed.), *Body talk: The Material and Discursive Regulation of Sexuality, Madness and Reproduction* (pp.67–82). London: Routledge.

Sedgewick, P. (1987). *Psychopolitics.* London: Pluto Press.

Shotter, J., & Gergen, K.J. (Eds.) (1989). *Texts of Identity.* London: Sage.

Slater, E., & Cowie, V. (1971). *The Genetics of Mental Disorders. Oxford Monographs in Mental Disorders.* Oxford: Oxford University Press.

Sowa, C.J., & Lustman, P.J. (1984). Gender differences in rating stressful events, depression, and depressive cognition. *Journal of Clinical Psychology, 40,* 1334–1337.

Stainton-Rogers, W. (1991). *Explaining Health and Illness.* Hemel Hempstead: Harvester Wheatsheaf.

Szasz, T. (1961). *The Myth of Mental Illness: Foundations of a Theory of Personal Conduct.* London: Secker.

Tiefer, L. (1986). In pursuit of the perfect penis. The medicalization of male sexuality. *American Behavioral Scientist, 29(5),* 579–599.

Turner, B.S. (1984). *The Body and Society.* Oxford: Blackwell.

Ussher, J.M. (1989). *The Psychology of the Female Body.* London: Routledge.

Ussher, J.M. (1991). *Women's Madness – Misogyny or Mental Illness?* Hemel Hempstead: Harvester Wheatsheaf.

Ussher, J.M. (1997a). *Fantasies of Femininity: Reframing the Boundaries of Sex*. London: Penguin.

Ussher, J.M. (1997b). *Body talk: The Material and Discursive Regulation of Sexuality, Madness and Reproduction*. London: Routledge.

Ussher, J.M. (1997c). Premenstrual syndrome: reconciling disciplinary divides through the adoption of a material-discursive epistemological standpoint. *Annual Review of Sex Research, 7,* 218–252.

Ussher, J.M. (1997d). Living with drink from a feminist perspective: a material–discursive–intrapsychic standpoint. In Velleman, R., Copello, A., & Maslin, J. (Eds.), *Living With Drink*, New York & London: Longman. pp. 150–161.

Ussher, J.M. (2000). Women's madness: a material–discursive–intrapsychic approach. In Fee, D. (Ed.), *Mental Illness as Myth and Experience* (pp. 208–230). London: Sage.

Walker, A. (1995). Theory and methodology in premenstrual syndrome research. *Social Science and Medicine, 41(6),* 793–800.

Walker, A. (1997). *The Menstrual Cycle*. London: Routledge.

Wilkinson, S., & Kitzinger, C. (1995). *Gender and Discourse*. London: Sage.

Wierzbicki, M., & Carver, D. (1989). Children's engagement in antidepressive activities. *Journal of Genetic Research, 150,* 163–174.

Yardley, L. (1996). Reconciling discursive and materialist perspectives on health and illness. A reconstruction of the bio-psychosocial approach. *Theory and Psychology, 6(3),* 485–508.

Yardley, L. (1997). *Material Discourses in Health and Illness*. London: Routledge.

Chapter 7

Agoraphobia: Sex-specific Stress or Sex-specific Coping?

Marrie H.J. Bekker

Tilburg University, The Netherlands

In clinical or community samples, agoraphobia is approximately four times more likely to be diagnosed in women than in men. In this chapter, the literature on the relationship between agoraphobia, biological sex, and gender is reviewed. First, explanations referring to the existence of specific sex- or gender-related stressors are discussed. In the second part, perspectives approaching agoraphobia as a sex-specific coping pattern are described. Special attention is paid to the relationship between agoraphobia, dependence, and gender. It is concluded that agoraphobia has sex-specific characteristics at all levels of the syndrome: in underlying, stressful conditions; in stressful aspects of the situations that elicit agoraphobic fear; and in coping with both.

Agoraphobia is generally defined as the inability to be in public situations or alone at home because of the fear of being overwhelmed by panic attacks and/or experiences of depersonalization (Foa et al., 1984; Marks, 1970; de Moor, 1985). The DSM-IV [American Psychiatric Association (APA), 1994] makes a distinction between Panic Disorder With Agoraphobia, Panic Disorder Without Agoraphobia, and Agoraphobia Without History of Panic Disorder. According to Foa et al., it is generally agreed upon that the majority of people suffering from

Women, Health and the Mind
Edited by L. Sherr and J.S. St Lawrence. © 2000 John Wiley & Sons, Ltd

agoraphobia are women, in other words, that agoraphobia is a "women's syndrome" (Foa et al., 1984, p.445). The percentage of women in research populations of at least 25 agoraphobics varies between 63 and 95%. Regardless of whether clinical or community samples are considered, the chance that agoraphobia is diagnosed in women is about four times higher than for men (Chambless & Mason, 1986). Not only are women more likely to have panic with agoraphobia, but they also are more likely to re-experience symptoms after gaining remission (Yonkers et al., 1998). Several sources of bias have been identified that may specifically influence the sex ratio of agoraphobics, all resulting in an underestimation of the total number of male agoraphobics (Bekker, 1996). Future research should determine whether and to what extent the distribution of agoraphobia over the sexes is changing, because data in this area may contribute to insights into the relationship between agoraphobia and demographic, socio-economic, and cultural factors, in particular those relating to employment and the use of anxiety-reducing substances. At this moment, however, it can be concluded that the sex ratios presented in the literature are reasonable starting points (Bekker, 1996).

Agoraphobics usually experience their fears and panic attacks as mysteries. Nevertheless, numerous authors have examined the plausibility of various explanations of the development and/or maintenance of agoraphobic symptoms. Generally, two types of explanations can be distinguished. The first category contains explanations in terms of specific stressors underlying the development and/or maintenance of agoraphobic symptoms. The stressors may vary from basic stressful events or conditions underlying the agoraphobia to stressful features of the situations that elicit the panic attacks or negative emotions. The second category of explanations refers to the way agoraphobics cope with stress. Here, the fact that agoraphobics are predominantly women, is seen as a result of the fact that coping strategies and patterns are highly sex-specific.

The present chapter will review both these types of explanations for the unequal prevalence of agoraphobia in women and men. In particular, the plausibility of explanations referring to the existence of specific, sex- or gender-related stressors is compared with that referring to agoraphobia as a type of sex-specific coping.

AGORAPHOBIA AS AN EXPRESSION OF EXPOSURE TO SEX-SPECIFIC STRESSORS

Why is agoraphobia predominantly occurring in women? One of the answers might be that women are more likely than men to be exposed to specific stressors to which extremely serious agoraphobic fears and, thus, avoidance are intrinsically logical responses. These sex-specific stressors may be fundamental stressful life events or conditions underlying the development and/or mantenance of agoraphobia. Also, these stressors might be more "superficial" stressors, namely features of the situations that elicit the panic attacks or negative emotions, which, in itself, could also be considered the relevant stressors. Like the "fundamental" sex-specific stressors, the stressful characteristics of agoraphobic situations, e.g. being alone in public transport, should be more meaningful for women than for men, in order to be relevant in the context of the unequal sex ratio of agoraphobia's prevalence. The same is true for the stressfulness of experiencing panic or negative emotions.

UNDERLYING, STRESSFUL, SEX-SPECIFIC LIFE-EVENTS AND CONDITIONS

Anxious Attachment Inducing Early Interaction Patterns

Several stressors mentioned in the literature can be categorized in the first subcategory: stressful life events or conditions that form the basis of agoraphobic symptoms. For example, Bowlby (1973) considered agoraphobia as an extreme form of separation anxiety. He postulated several specific, stressful interaction patterns between children and parents, resulting in anxious attachment and agoraphobia in the children when grown-up. One of these interaction patterns implied that the mother, or more rarely, the father, suffered from chronic anxiety regarding attachment figures and retained or still retains her or his child at home to be a companion. From this perspective, anxious attachment is a "logical" psychological condition characterized by lack of trust in the availability and/or responsiveness of the primary attachment person. Anxious attachment can be expressed in several types of behaviors one of them being claiming another person and making sure that he/she will stay close to you. Following the anxious attachment interpretation, it is exactly this way of behaving that is so typical for agoraphobia. A point that must be made is that attachment difficulties are not restricted to agoraphobia; they might set the stage for other types of adult anxiety disorders as well (Lipsitz et al., 1994). Furthermore, not all persons suffering from anxious attachment develop psychological symptoms. An important point in the context of this chapter is that Bowlby did not differentiate between boys' and girls' experiences. The retrospective research on agoraphobia that was inspired by Bowlby's ideas has focused on separation anxiety in childhood, stressful life events, and/or parental rearing practices (for overviews, see: Barlow, 1988; Dijkman-Caes, 1993) without explicitly taking into account that these might have sex-specific aspects and implications. Kerig et al. (1993), for instance, demonstrated in their microanalytical study of family interaction that marital quality was related to gender differences in both parent and child behavior. More

research has to be done in the area of parent–child attachment and the
development of agoraphobia that is prospective in nature, focusing not
only on early childhood but also on adolescence, and taking into account
that parent–child interaction patterns and childhood experiences in
general may be sex-specific. In particular the feminist theorizing about
mother–daughter relationships (e.g. Chodorow, 1978) might be helpful
in understanding why daughters (compared with sons) may be more
at risk for developing anxious attachment in the case of psychological
problems in the mother; due to a more enduring and more intense
symbiosis between mothers (still most often the primary attachment
person) and daughters, daughters would more easily become an object
of mothers' projections.

Sexual Violence

Second, sexual violence can be mentioned as a sex-specific stressor of
etiological importance to agoraphobia. Of course, sexual violence experiences might overlap with the first mentioned stressor: growing up
under unfavorable conditions regarding the availability and responsiveness of the primary caretaker(s). In several studies, the threat of
sexual harassment turned out to be an important variable in the perception of, attitude towards, and emotions about situations that
agoraphobics usually avoid, such as public transport, streets, and being
alone at home. It should be noted that the role of actual and feared
sexual violence in phobias has not been systematically investigated.
Chambless (1989) suggested that women's higher levels of anxiety
leading to their more easily acquiring fears could be rooted in sexual
abuse of girls, domestic violence against women, rape, and poverty of
women. From a screening of women over 18 years of age regarding
sexual assault histories during childhood, childhood rape victims
appeared to be more likely than non-victims to have ever met the DSM-
III diagnostic criteria for agoraphobia and other mental disorders
(Saunders et al. 1992). A comparison of the report frequency of childhood physical or sexual abuse between a sample of patients suffering
from anxiety disorders (panic disorder with or without agoraphobia,
social phobia, or obsessive–compulsive disorder) and a matched
community sample revealed a higher frequency of physical abuse in
both men and women of the first group (Stein et al., 1996). Childhood
sexual abuse was higher among women with anxiety disorders than
among comparison women, and highest among women with panic
disorder. Unfortunately, a control group of women with other mental
disorders was lacking. Consequently, it remains unknown whether
sexual abuse as a stressor of etiological significance is specific for anxiety
disorders, or can result in other kinds of symptom behavior as well.
Moreover, it should be noted that avoidance behavior resulting from
sexual violence (rape) in public places is best interpreted as post-

traumatic stress syndrome (PTDS; see APA, 1994), whereas agoraphobia involves the fear of panic.

Conflicts in Intimate Relationships

Third, marital problems have been considered a stressful source of agoraphobic symptoms. In the system-theoretical perspective, the focus is on the interaction within the (marriage-)system of the help-seeking, agoraphobic woman and her protecting, latently anxious husband. Following this perspective, the prototypical agoraphobic woman is married, and feels more able to go outside if accompanied by her partner (Marks, 1970; Thorpe & Burns, 1983). The husband's protectiveness can go to great lengths. Fry (1962), for instance, describes a husband who refrained completely from any activity without his wife and spent every possible minute with her. System-theoretically speaking, these observations have been interpreted as indicating a certain psychological interest of the partner in the development and/or maintenance of his wife's phobia. As long as the interpersonal system focuses on her symptoms and, as the authors in this tradition call it, her excessive dependence on her husband, his anxieties and his other psychological problems can remain latent. In addition to protectiveness, extreme jealousy (Barendregt & Bleeker, 1973; Hafner, 1979) and obstructing behavior with respect to the wife's therapeutic recovery (Haley, 1963; Holmes, 1982) have been described as partners' behaviors indicating a similar function of *her* agoraphobia. Authors such as Symonds (1971) and Holmes (1982) localized the dependence problems primarily in the agoraphobic woman (in particular in her childhood experiences), but also considered marriage as the trigger that activates repressed dependence needs. The agoraphobia is seen as a symptom that "protects the protector" (Deutsch, 1929) or masks the couple's problems (Holmes, 1982; Shafar, 1976; Webster, 1953). As Holmes (1982) has postulated in the same vein as Bowlby (1973), both partners may suffer from a similar psychological condition, i.e. anxious attachment, while their coping style is completely different.

de Swaan (1981; see also Dijkman & de Vries, 1987) extended this system-theoretical interpretation of agoraphobia by situating the "agoraphobic couple" in its cultural–historical context. de Swaan mentions the first case histories about agoraphobia, presented by Westphal in 1871 (and which, paradoxically, all referred to agoraphobic *men*!). A specific cultural code prohibited nineteenth-century well-to-do women from leaving their houses without husbands, brothers, or fathers acting as "chaperons". This "going out restriction" existed until the end of the last century in the province of Holland, and the cities of Brussels and London, and was imposed upon women in order to prevent them from having dangerous, rough, offensive, and seductive contacts with the "mob", the great unnumbered. From de Swaan's point of view, the prevalence of agoraphobia arose when these and other socio-economic limitations upon women disappeared at the end of the nineteenth century. While in the previous century interpersonal relationships between men and women were characterized by the existence of a clear hierarchy, according to de Swaan, the sexes now relate to each other in compliance with a model of symmetrical negotiation. Within this process of socio-relational changes, the restrictive code was replaced by the phenomenon of agoraphobia, although the agoraphobia still enables a woman to impose her dependence upon her husband who, in turn, can keep his wife under constant surveillance.

To what extent does the system-theoretical interpretation of agoraphobia fit into the reality of agoraphobics and their partners (and/or other relevant people; cf. Vandereycken, 1983)? Most interpretations originating in this approach are based on relatively small numbers of striking cases (Arrindell, 1987; Vandereycken, 1983). First, are agoraphobias (still) more prevalent among (married) women who live together with a male partner? Bourdon et al. (1988) report a "lack of an association between being married and the [agoraphobic] disorder" (p.237) and, furthermore, for the majority of agoraphobics, an onset of the disorder that *pre-dated* marriage. Thus, the *development* of agoraphobic symptoms seems to be largely independent of marriage.

Second, how representative is the image of the protective or extremely jealous husband for partners of agoraphobics in general? A study by Arrindell and Emmelkamp (see Arrindell, 1987) using self-report measures, showed that partners of agoraphobics as a group did not appear to be more defensive or psychologically more disturbed than their control counterparts. From a system-theoretical perspective, however, it can be argued that the agoraphobic's partner will not reveal psychopathological problems while the couple is still focusing upon *her* agoraphobia.

Third, and more importantly, how valid is the assumption that marital problems underly the symptoms of (married) agoraphobics? Kleiner & Marshall (1985) concluded in their review that relational conflict is more common among agoraphobics (in approximately 45% of the cases) than among patients from other clinical groups. "The interaction . . . between interpersonal difficulties and agoraphobics' personal characteristics (e.g., dependence, lack of assertiveness, etc.) might . . . be important in the development and, particularly, the maintenance of the phobia" (p.593). However, several later studies did not support the importance of marital satisfaction for the maintenance of agoraphobia in general. A study by Arrindell (1987) revealed that neither agoraphobic women nor their partners rated their marriages as more maladjusted or unpleasant than non-phobic psychiatric patients or their partner controls. In a study by Fisher & Wilson (1985) no differences appeared between agoraphobics and non-agoraphobic controls in reported marital satisfaction. However, if one takes the system-theoretical perspective (the agoraphobia masks the couple's and/or the husband's troubles), it can be deemed unlikely that the couple will report marriage problems, while the wife's agoraphobia is fully present and enduring. Therefore, an important contribution has been made by studies in which marital satisfaction of agoraphobics was investigated as a predictor for treatment outcome. These studies (Craske et al., 1989; Emmelkamp, 1980; Himadi, 1986; Jansson et al., 1987) failed to confirm any relation between marital satisfaction before treatment and treatment outcome in agoraphobics. This suggests very strongly that interpersonal *difficulties* are *not* relevant in maintaining agoraphobia in general. The phenomenon that marital satisfaction generally improves with treatment-produced improvements in phobic behavior (Cerny et al., 1987; Himadi, Cerny, Barlow, Cohen & O'Brien 1986) provides further support for this conclusion. This does not necessarily mean that other marital factors never can play a role, such as a sex-stereotypical exchange of anxious helplessness and self-confident helpfulness by wife and husband, respectively.

It can be concluded that, *in general*, marriage problems are not relevant to the development of agoraphobia nor its maintenance. Nevertheless, the empirical data available do not exclude the possibility that marital dissatisfaction may play a role in isolated cases of agoraphobia, or that other interpersonal factors may contribute to its development and/or maintenance.

In summary, stressful events or conditions that have been studied so far because of their presupposed role in the development and/or maintenance of agoraphobia, are specific interaction patterns in childhood resulting in anxious attachment, sexual violence experiences, and (unconscious) conflicts in intimate relationships. Of course, these three possible stressful sources of agoraphobic symptoms do not exclude each other; they can overlap. For example, sexual violence experiences can be a specific type of experiences occurring in a context of anxious attachment inducing interaction patterns, and these interaction patterns might contribute to later marital conflicts. Although empirical evidence supports the hypothesis that both first mentioned stressors can be etiologically relevant for agoraphobia, they do not seem to be *specifically* relevant. Both can also result in other syndromes, e.g. other anxiety disorders; moreover, they do not necessarily result in syndromes. Although the role of actual interactional factors cannot be ruled out, empirical evidence indicates that marital conflicts should not be considered stressors with relevance for the majority of agoraphobic complaints. This review shows the difficulty of distinguishing the relative relevance of stressors and coping in explaining agoraphobia. Particularly when agoraphobia is considered a way of dealing with anxious attachment, both – stress (early and/or actual, e.g. marital, interactional stress) and coping (seeking support and closeness) – seem equally important.

STRESSFUL CHARACTERISTICS OF AGORAPHOBIC SITUATIONS

Although there is a tendency in the literature to consider (agoraphobic) anxieties to be irrational, that is, not to be explained from the characteristics of the situations in which they arise, some attempts have been made to relate both agoraphobic fears and stressful situational characteristics to each other. In most of these studies and theories, the fact that most agoraphobics are women is taken into account, whether by examining aspects or meanings of the situations that are specifically stressful for women and/or by postulating characteristics of women that cause coping problems in such situations. We use the term *gendered* meanings to express possible differences in meanings of situations due to gender.

As is well known, agoraphobics avoid a range of situations such as supermarkets, public transport, streets, etc. In many cases, the aversion is proportional to the physical distance between the specific public situation outside and the agoraphobic's house. Also, many agoraphobics avoid being alone. Summing up the criteria for agoraphobia, DSM-IV (APA, 1994, p.396) described the relevant places or situations as those "from which escape might be difficult (or embarrassing) or in which help may not be available in the event of having an unexpected or situationally predisposed panic attack or panic-like symptoms". Marks (1970) characterized the significant situations for agoraphobics outside the house as *public* situations. In some cases, agoraphobia has been defined as *fear of open spaces*, probably due to an erroneous translation of the Greek word *agora* meaning *meeting point of people outside* (Arrindell, 1987; Barlow, 1988). In fact, closed spaces such as public transport and elevators also belong to the relevant situations. In their large community sample, Bourdon et al. (1988) found that, compared with agoraphobic men, agoraphobic women scored higher on the two agoraphobia items dealing with fear of *being alone* and *going out of the house alone*. The authors consider this sex difference as meaningful and to be explored in future research. Several authors examined the cultural meanings of the situations that are feared and avoided by agoraphobics, and, in some cases, related them to gender.

No Affirmation of One's Personal Identity

Situations relevant to agoraphobics were characterized by Van Zuuren (1982) as *anonymous* (public) and *solitary* situations. Van Zuuren distinguishes both types of situations from two other types: *intimate* and *social* situations. From her perspective, the crucial aspect of the situations that agoraphobics fear and avoid is the absence of affirmation of one's personal identity by significant others (Van Zuuren, 1982; see also Dijkman

& de Vries, 1987). Van Zuuren found some empirical support for her typology, although the results were contaminated by classification criteria: compared with social phobics, agoraphobics reacted extremely strongly to solitary and anonymous situations using such reasons as *feeling lost, not oneself*, etc. According to Van Zuuren, individuals with a weak sense of identity have coping problems in anonymous and solitary situations. She postulated that being a housewife – housewives form the larger part of the agoraphobic population – is a risk factor in developing agoraphobic symptoms, because a housewife's identity is based upon the small world of the home and the family.

In a pilot study by Bekker (1987) agoraphobics and (non-phobic, non-neurotic) controls rated their aversion to and avoidance of 17 situations and were asked for reasons in a subsequent interview. The impersonal formal atmosphere of public anonymous situations, in which showing emotions is not appropriate behavior, emerged as the main reason for aversion and avoidance. Especially women reported having problems with this specific aspect, possibly because they had been socialized towards functioning in the emotionality and intimacy of the private area. Gelfond (1991) compared, among other variables, the interiors of houses of highly independent women, averagely independent women, and agoraphobic women. She found *highly personalized* interiors in the houses of the latter group, that is, many objects referring to the personal lives and experiences of the agoraphobic residents, whereas the houses of highly independent women were used more as places for short stays. Of course, the interpretation of all these data is problematic because the direction of causality is unclear. Is agoraphobia preceded by a preference for the more feminine, personal, and emotional inside world with intimate others and an aversion to the more masculine, impersonal, and non-emotional outside world? Or are both, preference and aversion, consequences of being agoraphobic?

Going Out as "Not Done"

In the past, the possibility of seduction and the threat of sexual harassment formed, in particular for women, the specific characteristics of those public or anonymous situations that are nowadays relevant for agoraphobics (de Swaan, 1981; see also p. 95). It could be hypothesized that public anonymous situations are still associated with residues of the restricting norms from the previous century. (The situation of being alone at home is neglected in de Swaan's theory.) Some support can be found in the results of the research carried out by Sinnott et al. (1981). They demonstrated that being unaccompanied (in de Swaan's terms *without chaperon*) versus being with a beloved person was a relevant dimension in provoking agoraphobic anxiety. However, the same results are also supportive of the assumption that agoraphobics may have a strong need for intimacy and personal affirmation.

Going Out as Not Learnt

In general, it can be argued that specific skills are acquired for functioning both in solitary and in public, anonymous situations (as well as for functioning in the intimacy of the private area!). It has been described how girls are encouraged to avoid public places and how sex differences develop in adolescence with respect to participation in solitary and instrumental activities, and with respect to functioning in the absence of intimates: girls spend more time interacting with family members and friends, and are more likely to function in a dyadic relationship with an intimate friend, a *soul mate*. The mobility of girls compared to that of boys is restricted in space (only *street girls* hang around), in time (not after sunset), as regards company, and as regards activities (de Waal, 1989; Dijkman-Caes, 1993). It would be worth investigating in a longitudinal study to what extent adolescent girls and boys who become agoraphobics, and those who remain free from these restricting symptoms, differ in their freedom to *explore* the *world outside* and in the acquisition of skills to enter this world and to function in solitary situations (cf. Bourdon et al., 1988; Dijkman-Caes, 1993; Gelfond, 1991).

Sexuality

Also other meanings of public anonymous and solitary situations could be mentioned that have specific relevance to certain groups of women. Like the role of sexual harassment (see above), that of seduction or sexual taboos is also rather unknown. From the classical psychoanalytic point of view, agoraphobic fears are considered to be fears of punishment following the release of sexual impulses with unknown people (Freud, 1926). Fenichel (1945) explained how streets are seen as areas in which seduction occurs frequently, adding that also solitary situations may confront a person with her or his sexual desires. No research has been done on the sexual desires of agoraphobics in specific situations. Studies on sexual (dis)satisfaction of agoraphobics differ with respect to results. Earlier studies (Roberts, 1964; Webster, 1953) reported low sexual satisfaction in agoraphobic women; in later studies (Buglass et al., 1977; Marks & Herst, 1970), the frequency of sexual problems of agoraphobics and normals did not differ (Foa et al., 1984).

In summary, it seems plausible that several characteristics of public, anonymous situations in our culture are more stressful for women than for men, in particular for certain subgroups of women, e.g. those who are in a strong need of personal affirmation and/or those who are relatively untrained in the world outside.

PANIC AND NEGATIVE EMOTIONS AS SEX-SPECIFIC STRESSORS?

Agoraphobia has often been considered a fear of fear. Experiencing fear and managing one's anxious body might also be more stressful for women than for men. The research on agoraphobia has emphasized cognitive factors, in particular selective attention to and misinterpretation of bodily sensations that result in panic (Beck, 1988; Clark, 1988). According to Beck (1988), panic patients are particularly sensitive to internal sensations and tend to fix their attention on bodily or mental experiences that can be interpreted as signs of danger (see also Clark, 1988). It seems that panic patients with agoraphobia report more fear of bodily sensations than panic patients without agoraphobia (Chambless & Graceley, 1989; de Ruiter & Garssen, 1989). When these results are linked to the high incidence of agoraphobia in women, several questions can be raised. Do women in general experience more bodily sensations than men and/or are they more sensitive to them? Do they produce other cognitive responses resulting more frequently in the experience of lack of control over their bodies? Remember here that bulimics too experience their binge eating as overwhelming them (and note that the prevalence of bulimia nervosa is also much higher in women than in men). Is the experience of panic more stressful for women than it is for men; does it trigger more negative emotions? Clum & Knowles (1991) suggest that fear of negative social consequences of panic may be directly related to the disproportional frequency of women with avoidance.

Future research should take into account the relevance of demographic, daily-life differences among women, such as the amount of time spent alone in the house, the amount and quality of external stimuli because of job characteristics, the presence of children, etc. For instance, do housewives (or, more in general, home-makers) focus more on bodily sensations owing to the fact that their specific circumstances lead them to fix their attention more inside than outside themselves? In other words, there could be relevant differences *within* the female sex, specified by demographic characteristics and to be linked to experiences in daily life, that are relevant to the specific cognitive responses of agoraphobic women to bodily sensations (cf. Pennebaker, 1982).

AGORAPHOBIA AS A SEX-SPECIFIC COPING PATTERN

In the previous section, I examined the possibility that agoraphobia might be a reflection of exposure to specific stressors, operative as etiological factors or as momentary triggers, respectively, and having more impact on women than on men. Another interpretation of agoraphobia underlines its function in dealing with stressful conflicts rather irrespective of what these underlying or triggering stressors may be. From this point of view, agoraphobia is primarily a way of sex-specific coping. There is reason to believe that factors other than anxiety and panic determine avoidance behavior (cf. McNally, 1990) and that avoidance behavior is correlated with biological sex (cf. Barlow, 1988). By taking into consideration the sex ratios of Panic Disorder Without Agoraphobia, Panic Disorder With Agoraphobia, and Agoraphobia Without History of Panic Disorder, all mentioned in DSM-IV, it can be seen that they are diagnosed twice as often, three times as often, and far more often, respectively, in women than in men (APA, 1994). Clum & Knowles (1991) report a "clear sex difference between panic disorder with avoidance and panic disorder without avoidance" (p.308), the difference between proportions of females being 82 and 59%, respectively.

The coping pattern that is generally considered typical for agora-phobia, is characterized by *dependence*, referring primarily to the behaviorally manifested excessive reliance by agoraphobics upon signif-icant others. Precise ideas about the nature of agoraphobics' dependence vary with the theoretical perspectives of the various authors. One frame-work is a *system-theoretical* perspective, which was elaborated above. In this perspective, the focus is on the interaction within the (marriage-) system of the help-seeking, agoraphobic woman and her protecting, latently anxious husband. *Her* dependence emerges here primarily as an interpersonal product. A second approach combines the high percentage of female agoraphobics with dependence considered a char-acteristic of traditional femininity in general, and conceptualizes dependence as a part of *sex roles*. Other authors focus on dependence as a *personality characteristic* of agoraphobics. Thus, one approach focuses on interpersonal factors, while the second approach is socio- and cultural-psychological, and the third is primarily (personality-)psycho-logical and psychodynamic. These three approaches to dependency are not mutually exclusive and do, in fact, overlap considerably. The first approach has already been examined in the part of this chapter that focused on underlying stressors, in this case marital problems; the second and third approaches will be discussed below.

DEPENDENCE AS A PART OF FEMININITY IN AGORAPHOBIA

From the sex role perspective, agoraphobia is an inevitable product of Western culture, in which the traditional feminine sex role discourages assertiveness and self-supportive behavior in women and prescribes for them a reaction to stress via dependence and helplessness (Al Issa, 1980; Chambless & Goldstein, 1982; Fodor, 1974; Gelfond, 1991; Symonds, 1971; Wolfe, 1984). As a consequence, agoraphobias in women are expected to decrease in frequency the more Western culture demands employment outside the house and self-reliant, assertive behavior on the part of women (Chambless, 1988). In recent decades, the participation of West European and American women in the labor force has increased greatly. While the female participation rates in 1973 were 35, 53, 51, and 62% for The Netherlands, the United Kingdom, the United States, and Sweden, respectively, in 1991 these rates were 53, 63, 69, and 81%. Recent epidemiological studies (Bourdon et al., 1988; Eaton et al., 1994; Lindal & Stefansson, 1993) do offer some empirical support for Chambless' assertion by consistently presenting the ratio of agoraphobic women to agoraphobic men as approximately 2.7:1, instead of the ratio 4:1 that was usually reported in earlier years (Chambless & Mason, 1986). This seems to suggest that male and female proportions of agoraphobics are growing more equal. One difficulty is, however, that epidemiological data in different studies since the first study by Agras et al. (1969) are not based on uniform diagnostic criteria and methods; it is therefore not possible to determine whether the prevalence of agoraphobia among women and men has changed in time.

Two studies, in particular, investigated the relationship between agoraphobia and sex-role stereotyping. In both studies, sex-role stereo-typing was measured by self-ratings on adjectives that were *a priori* determined as being masculine, feminine, or neutral [Bem's Sex Role Inventory (BSRI), Bem, 1974; and Personal Attributes Questionnaire (PAQ), Spence & Helmreich, 1978]. In these studies, femininity and masculinity were no longer seen as two extremes of one dimension, but rather as two distinct, independent dimensions. Hafner & Minge (1989) found no differences in masculinity and femininity between agoraphobic and non-agoraphobic women, nor between the two groups of male partners. However, it appeared that the more masculine and autonomous the agoraphobic women rated themselves, the less serious they considered their agoraphobia to be. A similar result was found by Chambless & Mason (1986) who studied masculinity and femininity in relation to measures of psychopathology for agoraphobic men and women separately and compared them with normative samples. Here masculinity was found to be negatively correlated, for both sexes, in most measures of psychopathology (such as severity of avoidance behavior, trait anxiety, and depression). Furthermore, agoraphobic women tended to be more avoidant when alone than agoraphobic men. This sex difference was accounted for by their lower scores on the masculinity sex-role stereotyping scale. Both studies suggest that sex-role stereotyping plays a role in agoraphobia and, more precisely, that the absence of masculine traits such as assertiveness, instrumentality and active approach behavior, is a relevant variable for agoraphobia, and not femininity. In particular, the finding by Chambless & Mason (1986) that low masculinity in female agoraphobics played a substantial role in their relatively high levels of avoidance behavior, supported Fodor's assertion that fearful behavior is culturally more acceptable for women (Fodor, 1974). However, the nature of the explanatory power of sex roles in agoraphobia is still quite unclear. Due to their correlational nature, the data do not allow definitive conclusions regarding the assumption that a society which does not teach women to be instrumental, competent, and assertive, rather than nurturant and expressive, breeds phobic women (Chambless & Mason, 1986). The relationship found between (lack of) masculinity and psychopathology could be primarily a reflection of the effects of being agoraphobic on an individual's sense of competence. It also allows a more far-reaching, tautological interpretation: a culture that defines psychopathology in terms of low masculinity such as fearful and avoidant behavior produces a lack of masculinity in the self-concepts of agoraphobic women (cf. Cadbury, 1991; Kaplan, 1983).

Several conceptual questions arise when the sex-role approach is looked at more closely. First, the assumption that agoraphobia is a product of sex roles suggests that its symptoms are likely to develop in many subjects belonging to one sex. How could the sex-role approach explain that not the majority but only a very small minority of Western women suffers from agoraphobia? Second, other psychological symptoms have also been explained from the traditional female sex role, for instance eating disorders (Orbach, 1978) and depression (Gove, 1972; Gove & Tudor, 1973). But how can we learn from a sex role perspective that women develop such different syndromes?

A third problem concerns the fact that men also develop agoraphobia. Should we hypothesize from the sex-role approach that male agoraphobics are high in traditional femininity or low in masculinity? More generally, what is the relationship between biological sex, sex roles, and sex-specific syndromes, in this case, agoraphobia?

Like the system-theoretical approach, the sex-role approach of agoraphobia also focuses primarily on two of its aspects: fearfulness and dependence. But fearfulness or dependence *per se* cannot explain why agoraphobics avoid very specific situations. At the same time, the specific situations being avoided by agoraphobics form a very crucial aspect of the syndrome. Additionally, focusing on fearfulness and dependence (what is mentioned is, in fact, focusing on avoidance and reliance on company) the sex-role approach neglected possible sex differences in the experience and interpretation of panic. Besides, no thorough research has been done on the question of whether all agoraphobics use the same coping style, i.e. rely heavily on other people in the case of (the anticipation of) fear of going outside or staying at home alone. In summary, the relationship between sex roles and agoraphobia deserves more research and more theorizing, especially with regard to questions of *specificity*, viz. the specificity of the symptoms of agoraphobia. Also the fact that only a small proportion of Western women (*and* an even smaller proportion of Western men) develop these symptoms needs to be researched.

DEPENDENCE AS A PERSONALITY CHARACTERISTIC OF AGORAPHOBICS

In many reviews on agoraphobia, a personality profile of agoraphobics is presented, in most cases separated from aspects such as sex ratio and demographic characteristics. The agoraphobic is usually described as a timid, dependent, anxious, and subassertive personality, attributes for which, as will be made clear in the next section, some studies offer empirical support, whereas others do not. As was pointed out above, both the system-theoretical approach and the sex-role approach of agoraphobia rely heavily on the assumption that agoraphobics as a group are dependent persons. For this reason too, a further examination of the studies in this area is worthwhile.

Buglass et al. (1977) compared agoraphobic women with normal women, and concluded that they feel more dependent on their mothers. In a study by Harper & Roth (1962), agoraphobics appeared to be more dependent than epileptics. Roth (1959) compared agoraphobics with normals and with other neurotics, and found a higher dependence. Hafner & Minge (1989) reported lower autonomy scores of agoraphobic women compared with normal women. All the women (agoraphobic and non-agoraphobic) and men in their study rated not only themselves but also their partners. It was remarkable that the partners of the agoraphobic women attributed more autonomy to them than the control women's partners did. Subjects in the study by Reich et al. (1987) were panic disorder patients with varying degrees of phobic avoidance. The authors specifically reported more dependent personality disorder and a larger number of third-cluster personality disorders (dependent, avoidant, compulsive, passive, aggressive) in patients with more avoidance. Reich et al. (1987) found that people who had recovered from panic disorder (with or without agoraphobia) were more dependent and had less *emotional strength* than control subjects. Arrindell & Emmelkamp (1987) compared agoraphobic women with normal controls and with non-phobic female psychiatric patients. No difference in affective dependence was found among the three groups; the only difference that emerged was that the agoraphobic women scored higher on situational dependence, discomfort, and uncertainty in new situations. A similar design was conducted by van der Molen et al. (1988), who compared the scores on locus of control (Rotter, 1954) of agoraphobics (both sexes), non-phobic controls, and non-phobic neurotic controls. The hypothesis that particularly agoraphobics are characterized by a more external orientation was not confirmed; instead, more external locus of control was found in *both* neurotic groups. Bekker (1991) obtained similar results when the autonomy scores of agoraphobics (both sexes) were compared with those of bulimic women, normals, and, as will be explained below, wheelchair users. The agoraphobics and the bulimics were *both* found to be lower in autonomy.

In summary, studies that have compared agoraphobics with non-phobic, non-neurotic controls have revealed higher dependence in agoraphobics. From the comparative studies in which agoraphobics, normals, *and* non-phobic, neurotic controls participated, except for the study by Roth (1959), it appeared that *both* neurotic groups are higher in dependence than the normal group. Thus, it seems to make a difference whether a non-phobic neurotic control group participates in the study. From this perspective, dependence is not a characteristic of agoraphobia only. Another reason why the results of these studies are partly contradictory may be the variety in designs and methodology (Arrindell & Emmelkamp, 1987; Bekker, 1991; Foa et al., 1984). Furthermore, different concepts and operationalizations of dependence (or analog terms) were used. This has to be taken into account when the results are compared; for example, Hafner & Minge (1989) used the concept *autonomy*, the study by Arrindell & Emmelkamp (1987) was about *dependence*, van der Molen et al. (1988) examined *locus of control*, and Bekker (1991; 1993) used an autonomy concept based on recent insights into gender identity.

An interesting question, touching the core of agoraphobic problems and its relationship with dependence, is the following: If agoraphobia and/or other neurotic disorders are characterized by dependence, should we consider the latter as an antecedent or a predisposition? In other words, if we assume that agoraphobia is primarily a sex-specific coping pattern characterized by dependence, should we consider this as *emotional* (Rossmann, 1984) or *affective* (Birtchnell, 1984) dependence, deeply rooted in (passive–dependent; Millon, 1969) personality? Or is *instrumental* (Rossmann, 1984) or *situational* dependence (Arrindell & Emmelkamp, 1987) a more adequate interpretation, reflecting the fact that a person has to live with the symptom (Arrindell & Emmelkamp, 1987; Barlow, 1988; Thorpe & Burns, 1983)? The association, reported by Mavissakalian & Hamann (1987), between recovery from agoraphobia and reductions in dependent personality disorder symptoms does not resolve this question; recovery from agoraphobia could have implied changes in (pre-agoraphobia) personality characteristics and/or dependence could have diminished because coping with panic and anxiety was no longer necessary. The study by Bekker (1991) was primarily aimed at the question whether a low degree of autonomy is an effect of living as an agoraphobic. Agoraphobics were compared with a third control group with a similarly constricted range of action and a daily life rather similar to that of agoraphobics: wheelchair users whose physical handicap (caused by accidents or physical illnesses) had begun in early adulthood. Agoraphobics and non-phobic neurotics (bulimics), compared with normals *and* with wheelchair users, appeared to be less autonomous. The similarity in the constricted range of action between agoraphobics and wheelchair users suggests that the lower autonomy of agoraphobics (and bulimics as well) may not be considered an effect of living as an agoraphobic, and may indicate the presence of an antecedent or predisposing factor. Nevertheless, this study still does not resolve the question of whether dependence antedates agoraphobic behavior; dependence may simply be a concomitant of agoraphobia (and bulimia). Further prospective research is needed to obtain more insight into the nature of the relationship between agoraphobia and dependence.

A further point that has to be discussed is the question of biological sex in relation to agoraphobics' (and other neurotics') dependence. Most studies described above only focused on women. In the study by van der Molen et al. (1988), in which also men participated, no sex effects were found. In other words, the higher scores on external locus of control reported in agoraphobics and in neurotic controls apply to the women in these groups as well as to the men. Similarly, Bekker (1991) found that male and female agoraphobics and female bulimic controls were, compared with control groups of normals and wheelchair users, all lower in autonomy. However, one sex difference appeared: compared with men, women were higher in sensitivity for others, which was one of the three aspects of autonomy distinguished. This higher sensitivity for others in women was confirmed in other, non-clinical samples (Bekker, 1993). It seems that this aspect of autonomy has to be regarded as a gender-related variable that at least plays a role in agoraphobia and bulimia nervosa.

In summary, it has to be concluded that high (emotional) dependence or low (psychological) autonomy plays a significant role in agoraphobia; probably as a preceding factor, but in any case as a factor that does not play a role *specifically* in agoraphobia. So, it is relevant, but fails to explain the *specificity* of the symptom agoraphobia.

The implication of this conclusion for perspectives on agoraphobia, which, like the system-theoretical and the sex-role approach, mainly focuses upon (feminine or non-masculine) low autonomy, is clear and consistent with the objections mentioned above. First, the *low autonomy* perspectives neglect the fact that dependence or low autonomy does not exclusively characterize people (in particular women) suffering from agoraphobia. Second, because not *all* agoraphobics are low in autonomy, agoraphobia in subjects with normal or high autonomy need further explanation. Third, the specificity of agoraphobia, in particular its characteristic that specific situations are feared and avoided, is still to be explained.

CONCLUSIONS

The aim of this chapter was to discuss theories of agoraphobia referring to specific, sex- or gender-related stressors and those considering agoraphobia as a sex-specific coping pattern. The first category contained explanations in terms of specific stressors underlying the development and/or maintenance of agoraphobic symptoms. The stressors varied from stressful events or conditions underlying the agoraphobia, to stressful characteristics of panic (or other aversive feelings) situations or panic itself.

Two stressors were identified as probably etiologically relevant for agoraphobia. These were stressful interaction patterns resulting in anxious attachment, and sexual violence. However, neither seemed to be *specifically* relevant; that is, they can also result in other syndromes, e.g. other anxiety disorders, or in no syndromes at all. It appeared difficult to determine what is more essential for agoraphobia: (early, interactional) stress, or coping (with anxious attachment, by seeking support and closeness). Furthermore, it seemed plausible that certain characteristics of public, anonymous situations in our culture are more stressful for (certain subgroups of) women than for men; the same is true for experiencing aversive, bodily sensations. Regarding agoraphobia as a coping pattern, it can be concluded that high (emotional) dependence or low (psychological) autonomy is a characteristic that probably precedes the syndrome but, again, does not *exclusively* characterize agoraphobia.

Several suggestions have been made for further research. It seems to be worth examining, prospectively, *sex-specific* childhood and adolescence experiences that result in agoraphobia in later life, taking into account that agoraphobia occurs more frequently in women. In research on agoraphobia, attention has been paid to parent–child interactions, but not specifically with respect to the types of activities and skills that were trained, and not with a special focus upon *sex-specific* parent–child interactions. In particular, exploratory activities and the acquisition of skills necessary for functioning in the world outside as well as in solitary situations may be relevant. Furthermore, sex differences with respect to the experience of and coping with bodily sensations and cognitions should be explored more systematically in the context of agoraphobia, also from a developmental perspective. What different cultural meanings are attributed by boys and girls, and by men and women, to their bodies and bodily functionings? A special issue in this field is the role of sexual violence in agoraphobia, which is rather an unknown hitherto. In future studies of agoraphobia in relation to the meanings of the situations feared and avoided, as well as in agoraphobia research focusing upon the interaction between bodily sensations and cognitive factors, attention should be paid to the fact that until now the majority of agoraphobics seem to form a specific demographic group, namely housewives. What specific meanings are given to anonymous and solitary situations by housewives compared with other groups? What is the role of situational factors in the specific ways in which agoraphobics experience bodily sensations or develop cognitions?

Several authors (e.g. Barlow, 1988; Gorman et al., 1989) developed models of the etiology of panic disorder, especially agoraphobia. In these models a distinction is made between the panic attack (conceptualized as originating from biological vulnerability, stress, and a focus

on interoceptive cues), anticipatory anxiety or learned alarm (the interaction between bodily sensations and cognitive responses), and phobic
avoidance. The high incidence of agoraphobia in women has, until now,
partly been localized in the first part of the model: the panic attack.
However, a hormonal approach is not able to explain the sex ratio suffi-
ciently; one of the reasons is that panic disorder without agoraphobia
occurs only twice as often, but agoraphobia without panic "far more
often", in women than in men (Bekker, 1996). Most of the explanations
that have so far been offered for agoraphobia as a women's syndrome
refer to the last part of the model, i.e. the phobic avoidance, but mainly
in as far as coping by dependence and reliance on another person is
concerned. Future research should also focus upon the gendered meanings of the situations that are feared and avoided, and should relate
these to their significance for specific demographic differences between
women. The gender-sensitive approach for future research on agoraphobia that I would propose covers the complete model: the sex-specific
stressors, the panic, the phobic avoidance (including its interpersonal
functions, the fact that it is developed by specific, sex-related, demographic groups, the gendered meanings of the situations being avoided),
and what Gorman et al. (1989) postulated in between: the again sex-
specific interaction between bodily sensations and cognitive responses.

ACKNOWLEDGEMENTS

Parts of this chapter are reprinted from Bekker, M.H.J., Agoraphobia
and gender; a review, *Clinical Psychology Review, 16 (2)*, 129–146, copy-
right 1996, with permission from Elsevier Science.

REFERENCES

Agras, S., Sylvester, D., & Oliveau, D. (1969). The epidemiology of
    common fears and phobia. *Comprehensive Psychiatry, 10*, 151–156.
Al Issa, I. (1980). *The Psychopathology of Women*. New Jersey: Prentice Hall.
American Psychiatric Association (APA) (1994). *Diagnostic and Statistic
    Manual of Mental Disorders*, 4th Edition. Washington DC: APA.
Arrindell, W.A. (1987). *Marital Conflict and Agoraphobia: Fact or Fantasy?*
    Doctoral Dissertation, Eburon: Delft.
Arrindell, W.A., & Emmelkamp, P.M.G. (1987). Psychological states and
    traits in female agoraphobics: a controlled study. *Journal of Psycho-
    pathology and Behavioral Assessment, 9*, 237–253.
Barendregt, J.T., & Bleeker, A.A.M. (1973). Een geval van een agorafobie
    bij een esoferie [A case of agoraphobia along with esophoria]. *De
    Psycholoog, 8*, 43–49.
Barlow, D.H. (1988). *Anxiety and its Disorders. The Nature and Treatment
    of Anxiety and Panic*. New York/London: The Guilford Press.

Beck, A.T. (1988). Cognitive approaches to panic disorder: Theory and therapy. In Rachman, S., & Maser, J.D. (Eds.), *Panic: Psychological Perspectives*. Hillsdale, NJ: Erlbaum.

Bekker, M.H.J. (1991). *De bewegelijke grenzen van het vrouwelijk ego. De relatie tussen autonomie, sekse en welbevinden* [Moving boundaries of the female ego. The relation between autonomy, gender, and well-being]. Doctoral Dissertation, Eburon: Delft.

Bekker, M.H.J. (1993). The development of a new autonomy-scale based on recent insights into gender identity. *European Journal of Personality, 7*, 177–194.

Bekker, M.H.J. (1996). Agoraphobia and gender: a review. *Clinical Psychology Review, 16*, 129–146.

Bem, S.L. (1974). The measurement of psychological androgyny. *Journal of Consulting and Clinical Psychology, 42*, 155–162.

Birtchnell, J. (1984). Dependence and its relation to depression. *British Journal of Medical Psychology, 57*, 215–225.

Bourdon, K.H., Boyd, J.H., Rae, D.S., Burns, B.J., Thompson, J.W., & Locke, B.Z. (1988). Gender differences in phobias: results of the ECA Community Survey. *Journal of Anxiety Disorders, 2*, 227–241.

Bowlby, J. (1973). *Attachment and Loss. Vol. 2: Separation: Anxiety as Anger*. London: The Hogarth Press.

Buglass, D., Clarke, J., Henderson, A.S., Kreitman, N., & Presley, A.S. (1977). A study of agoraphobic housewives. *Psychological Medicine, 7*, 73–86.

Cadbury, S. (1991). The concept of dependence as developed by Birtchnell: a critical evaluation. *British Journal of Medical Psychology, 64*, 253–261.

Cerny, A.J., Barlow, D.H., Craske, M.G., & Himadi, W.G. (1987). Couple treatment of agoraphobia: a two-year follow-up. *Behavior Therapy, 18*, 401–415.

Chambless, D.L. (1988). Sekse en fobie [Sex and phobia]. *Gedragstherapie, 21*, 283–293.

Chambless, D.L. (1989). Gender and phobias. In Emmelkamp, P.M.G., Everaerd, W.T.A.M., Kraaimaat, F., & van Son, M.J.M. (Eds.), *Fresh Perspectives on Anxiety Disorders*. Amsterdam/Lisse: Swets & Zeitlinger.

Chambless, D.L., & Goldstein, A.J. (1982). *Agoraphobia. Multiple Perspectives on Theory and Treatment*. New York: John Wiley & Sons Ltd.

Chambless, D.L., & Graceley, E.J. (1989). Fear of fear and the anxiety disorders. *Cognitive Therapy and Research, 13*, 9–20.

Chambless, D.L., & Mason, J. (1986). Sex, sex-role stereotyping and agoraphobia. *Behaviour Research and Therapy, 24*, 231–235.

Chodorow N. (1978). *The Reproduction of Mothering*. Berkeley: University of California Press.

Chodorow, N. (1989). *Feminism and Psychoanalytic Theory*. Cambridge: Polity Press.

Clark, D.M. (1988). A cognitive model of panic attacks. In Rachman, S., & Maser, J.D. (Eds.), *Panic: Psychological Perspectives* (pp.71–89). New Jersey: Erlbaum.

Clum, G.A., & Knowles, S.L. (1991). Why do some people with panic disorders become avoidant? A review. *Clinical Psychology Review, 11,* 295–313.

Craske, M.G., Burton, T., & Barlow, D.H. (1989). Relationships among measures of communication, marital satisfaction and exposure during couples treatment of agoraphobia. *Behaviour Research and Therapy, 27,* 131–140.

Deutsch, H. (1929). The genesis of agoraphobia. *International Journal of Psychoanalysis, 10,* 51–69.

Dijkman, C.I.M., & de Vries, M.W. (1987). The social ecology of anxiety. *Journal of Nervous and Mental Disease, 175,* 550–557.

Dijkman-Caes, C.I.M. (1993). *Panic Disorder and Agoraphobia in Daily Life.* Doctoral Dissertation, University of Maastricht.

Eaton, W.W., Kessler, R.C., Wittchen, H.U., & Magee, W.J. (1994). Panic and panic disorder in the United States. *American Journal of Psychiatry, 151,* 413–420.

Emmelkamp, P.M. (1980). Agoraphobics' interpersonal problems: their role in the effects of exposure in vivo therapy. *Archives of General Psychiatry, 37,* 1303–1306.

Fenichel, O. (1945). *The Psychoanalytical Theory of Neurosis.* New York: Norton.

Fisher, L.M., & Wilson, G.T. (1985). A study of the psychology of agoraphobia. *Behaviour Research and Therapy, 23,* 97–107.

Foa, E.B., Steketee, G., & Young, M.C. (1984). Agoraphobia: Phenomenological aspects, associated characteristics, and theoretical considerations. *Clinical Psychology Review, 4,* 431–457.

Fodor, I.G. (1974). The phobic syndrome in women. In Franks, V., & Burtle, V. (Eds.), *Women in Therapy.* New York: Brunner/Mazel.

Freud, S. (1926). *Hemmung, Symptom und Angst* [Inhibition, symptom, and anxiety]. Frankfurt am Main: Fischer.

Fry, W.F. (1962). The marital context of an anxiety syndrome. *Family Process, I,* 245–252.

Gelfond, M. (1991). Reconceptualizing agoraphobia: a case study of epistemological bias in clinical research. *Feminism and Psychology, 1,* 247–262.

Gorman, J.M., Liebowitz, M.R., Fyer, A.J., & Stein, J. (1989). A neuroanatomical hypothesis for panic disorder. *American Journal of Psychiatry, 146,* 148–161.

Gove, W.R. (1972). The relationship between sex roles, marital status and mental illness. *Social Forces, 51,* 34–44.

Gove, W.R., & Tudor, J.F. (1973). Adult sex roles and mental illness. *American Journal of Sociology, 78,* 812–835.

Hafner, R.J. (1979). Agoraphobic women married to abnormally jealous men. *British Journal of Medical Psychology, 52,* 99–104.

Hafner, R.J., & Minge, P.J. (1989). Sex-role stereotyping in women with agoraphobia and their husbands. *Sex Roles, 20,* 705–711.

Haley, J. (1963). *Strategies of Psychotherapy.* New York: Grune & Stratton.

Harper, M., & Roth, M. (1962). Temporal lobe epilepsy and the phobic anxiety–depersonalization syndrome. *Comprehensive Psychiatry, 3,* 129–151.

Himadi, W.G. (1986). The relationship of marital adjustment to agoraphobia treatment outcome. *Behaviour Research and Therapy, 24,* 107–115.

Holmes, J. (1982). Phobia and counterphobia: family aspects of agoraphobia. *Journal of Family Therapy, 4,* 133–152.

Jansson, L., Ost, L.G., & Jerremalm, A. (1987). Prognostic factors in the behavioral treatment of agoraphobia. *Behavioural Psychotherapy, 15,* 31–44.

Kaplan, M. (1983). A woman's view of DSM-III. *American Psychologist, 29,* 786–792.

Kerig, P.K., Cowan, P.A., & Cowan, C.P. (1993). Marital quality and gender differences in parent–child interaction. *Developmental Psychology, 29,* 931–939.

Kleiner, L., & Marshall, W.L. (1985). Relationship difficulties and agoraphobia. *Clinical Psychology Review, 5,* 581–595.

Lindal, E., & Stefansson, J.G. (1993). The lifetime prevalence of anxiety disorders in Iceland as estimated by the US National Institute of Mental Health Diagnostic Interview Schedule. *Acta Psychiatrica Scandinavica, 88,* 29–34.

Lipsitz, J.D., Martin, L.Y., Mannuzza, S., Chapman, T.F., Liebowitz, M.R., Klein, D.F., & Fyer, A.J. (1994). Childhood separation anxiety disorder in patients with adult anxiety disorders. *American Journal of Psychiatry, 151,* 927–929.

Marks, I.M. (1970). The agoraphobic syndrome. *Archives of General Psychiatry, 23,* 538–553.

Marks, I.M., & Herst, E.R. (1970). A survey of 1200 agoraphobics in Britain. *Social Psychiatry, 5,* 16–24.

Mavissakalian, M., & Hamann, M.S. (1987). DSM-III personality disorder in agoraphobia. II. Changes with treatment. *Comprehensive Psychiatry, 28,* 356–361.

McNally, R.J. (1990). Psychological approaches to panic disorder: a review. *Psychological Bulletin, 108,* 403–419.

Millon, T. (1969). *Modern Psychopathology; A Biosocial Approach to Maladaptive Learning and Functioning.* London: W.B. Saunders.

de Moor, W. (1985). The topography of agoraphobia. *American Journal of Psychotherapy, 36,* 371–388.

Nathanson, C.A. (1980). Social roles and health status among women: the significance of employment. *Social Science and Medicine, 14 A,* 463–471.

Orbach, S. (1978). *Fat is a Feminist Issue. The Anti-diet Guide to Permanent Weight Loss.* New York: Paddington Press, Ltd.

Pennebaker, J.W. (1982). *The Psychology of Physical Symptoms.* New York: Springer Verlag.

Reich, J., Noyes, R. Jr., & Throughton, E. (1987). Dependent personality disorder associated with phobic avoidance in patients with panic disorder. *American Journal of Psychiatry, 144(3),* 323–326.

Roberts, A.H. (1964). Housebound housewives: a follow-up study of a phobic anxiety state. *British Journal of Psychiatry, 110*, 191–197.

Rossmann, P. (1984). Assessing different aspects of psychosocial dependence: a new scale and some empirical results. *Studia Psychologica, 26*, 317–321.

Roth, M. (1959). The phobic anxiety–depersonalization syndrome. *Proceedings of the Royal Society of Medicine, 52*, 587–595.

Rotter, J.B. (1954). *Social Learning and Clinical Psychology*. Englewood Cliffs, NJ: Prentice Hall.

de Ruiter, C., & Garssen, B. (1989). Social anxiety and fear of bodily sensations in panic disorder and agoraphobia: a matched comparison. *Journal of Psychopathology and Behavioral Assessment, 11*, 175–184.

Saunders, B.E., Villeponteaux, L.A., Lorenz, B.A., Lipovsky, J.A., & Kilpatrick, D.G. (1992). Child sexual assault as a risk factor for mental disorders among women: a community survey. *Journal of Interpersonal Violence, 7*, 189–204.

Shafar, S. (1976). Aspects of phobic illness: a study of 90 personal cases. *British Journal of Medical Psychology, 49*, 221–236.

Sinnott, A., Jones, B., & Fordham, A.S. (1981). Agoraphobia: a situational analysis. *Journal of Clinical Psychology, 37*, 123–127.

Spence, J.T., & Helmreich, R.L. (1978). *Masculinity and Femininity. Their Psychological Dimensions, Correlates, and Antecedents*. Austin: University of Texas Press.

Stein, M.B., Walker, J.R., Anderson, G., Hazen, A.L., Ross, C.A., Eldridge, G., & Forde, D.R. (1996). Childhood physical and sexual abuse in patients with anxiety disorders and in a community sample. *American Journal of Psychiatry, 153*, 275–277.

de Swaan, A. (1981). The politics of agoraphobia: on changes in emotional and relational management. *Theory and Society, 10*, 359–385.

Symonds, A. (1971). Phobias after marriage. Women's declaration of dependence. *American Journal of Psychoanalysis, 31*, 144–152.

Thorpe, G.L., & Burns, L.E. (1983). *The Agoraphobic Syndrome*. Chichester: John Wiley & Sons Ltd.

van der Molen, G.M., Merckelbach, H., & van den Hout, M.A. (1988). The possible relation of the menstrual cycle to susceptibility to fear acquisition. *Journal of Behavior Therapy and Experimental Psychiatry, 19*, 127–133.

Van Zuuren, F.J. (1982). *Fobie, Situatie en Identiteit* [Phobia, situation, and identity]. Doctoral Dissertation. Lisse: Swets & Zeitlinger.

Vandereycken, W. (1983). Agoraphobia and marital relationship: theory, treatment, and research. *Clinical Psychology Review, 3*, 317–338.

de Waal, M. (1989). *Meisjes, een Wereld Apart: een Etnografie van Meisjes op de Middelbare School* [Girls, A World Apart: Ethnographics of High-School Girls]. Amsterdam, Meppel: Boom.

Webster, A.S. (1953). The development of phobias in married women. *Psychological Monographs, 67*, 1–18.

Westphal, C. (1871). Die Agoraphobia. Eine neuropathische Erscheinung [Agoraphobia. A neuropathic phenomenon]. *Archives für Psychiatrie und Nervenkrankheiten*, *3*, 384–412.

Wolfe, B.E. (1984). Gender ideology and phobias in women. In Spatz Widom, C. (Ed.), *Sex Roles and Psychopathology* (pp.51–72). New York: Plenum Press.

Yonkers, K.A., Zlotnick, C., Allsworth, J., Warshaw, M., Shea, T., & Keller, M.B. (1998). Is the course of panic disorder the same in women and men? *American Journal of Psychiatry*, *155*, 596–602.

Chapter 8

Gender, Stress and Coping: Do Women Handle Stressful Situations Differently from Men?

Denise T.D. de Ridder

Utrecht University, The Netherlands

Stereotypical beliefs about gender and the way stress is handled lead to the belief that women primarily cope with adversity in an emotional fashion while men confront it in an instrumental, problem-oriented way. Such a viewpoint parallels cultural beliefs in our society that depict men as oriented towards autonomy and attempting to control the environment and women as nurturing and dependent on others (Bem, 1974). Such gender-related differences in coping responses are often proposed as an explanation for the documented differences between women and men in health and health-related behaviour (Verbrugge, 1985, 1989).

In general, it has been reported that women suffer more from psychological distress, depression, and minor somatic disorders, whereas men seem to be especially vulnerable to life-threatening diseases such as myocardial infarction and cancer (Verbrugge, 1989). Also, throughout most of life men report healthier states than women, although their health advantage decreases with age, perhaps due to unhealthier

Women, Health and the Mind
Edited by L. Sherr and J.S. St Lawrence. © 2000 John Wiley & Sons, Ltd

life-styles (Ross & Bird, 1994). Although the assumption that this variation may be explained by gender-related differences in stress and coping
is attractive, gender-related differences in health may also be associated
with genetic differences or differences in activities and health habits. In
addition, the stress and coping perspective on the association between
gender and health is not the straightforward explanation it appears at
first glance. Complex explanations exist, such as the extent to which men
and women are exposed to stress in our society, the biological and cultural determinants of the way men and women perceive stress, appraise
their options to deal with it, the availability of coping resources, and,
ultimately, the behavioural strategies they have at their disposal to deal
with adversity. Therefore, whenever the "stress coping" perspective is
invoked to understand gender-related differences in health, one must
carefully examine these different explanations.

Notwithstanding the complexity of these issues, the stress and coping
framework is considered one of the most powerful psychological paradigms to explain gender differences in health and health-related
behaviour and may contribute to their understanding in at least three
ways (cf. Thoits, 1991):

1. The methodological artifact explanation, suggesting that women are
   socialized to be more expressive and therefore will admit more stress
   than men in response to standard distress scales.
2. The stress-exposure argument, suggesting that women face more
   stressors in general or more severe and persistent stressors.
3. The vulnerability argument, suggesting that women lack coping
   resources or appropriate coping strategies for handling the stressors
   to which they are exposed.

In the recent literature the third explanation seems to be favoured, since
either greater expressiveness or greater exposure alone have proved
insufficient to understand the observed differences in health. Nevertheless, elements of both approaches have been incorporated in the
third explanation, highlighting gender-related behavioural and cognitive differences in response style.

The third explanation needs critical examination as it leaves many
questions open to debate. One of the major questions relates to the
issue whether differences between men and women in the way they
perceive and handle stress are primarily *socialized* (Pearlin & Schooler,
1978), that is caused by enduring differences in the way boys and girls
are raised, or whether they are associated with the *social constraints*
imposed upon men and women as they take up their social roles and
encounter different kinds of stressful situations (Rosario et al., 1988).
Although the socialization perspective and the social constraints
approach are often presented as competing, a more plausible account
of their relationship is that they are complementary as they each highlight different aspects of the way coping behaviour is determined.

Therefore, this chapter will not focus on the value of either explanation but instead will address them in the context of an account of the different elements of the stress coping process. The issue of gender, stress, and coping will be addressed by taking the different stages of the stress coping process as a line of reasoning, including research that has included both women and men. A perspective dictated by the most authoritative account of the stress coping perspective, provided by the transactional theory of Lazarus & Folkman (1984), will be adopted. Despite its shortcomings (De Ridder, 1997), this theory provides the most detailed account of what happens during a stressful encounter and as such offers different but coherent angles to understand the way men and women experience stress and do things to minimalize the health effects of stress. In addition, this perspective also parallels the historical development of research on gender, stress, and coping, as many of the earlier attempts to understand their relationship were dominated by a sociological perspective on differential exposure to stressful events, followed by a more psychologically oriented line of research on differential coping responses. The most recent developments in the stress and coping field focus on the appraisal stage of coping and relate to such issues as differential sensitivity of men and women for stressful cues in their environment and the way that these cues are interpreted. This latter line of research will be discussed in the fourth section of this chapter. The discussion of each of these stages will examine psychological as well as biological and social aspects of gender in order to provide a full account of the association between gender, stress, and coping. Finally, the major issues brought up in this chapter will be summarized and some promising lines for future research will be discussed.

EXPOSURE TO STRESSFUL LIFE CONDITIONS

Early research on gender-related stress and stress responses has been predominantly sociological–epidemiological in nature, attempting to highlight differential exposure to stressful conditions for men and women. These sociological studies were inspired by the societal changes in the position of women, many of whom had entered the labour market by the 1970s. Statistical data, showing that in the United States about 75% of women including those with pre-school and school-age children had moved into paid employment, raised concern about the "double role" of these women combining domestic roles and employment obligations (Crosby, 1988). Beginning with Walter Gove's initial formulation of the *role strain hypothesis* (Gove, 1972), a considerable body of research has accumulated which focused on the role that various work-related strains played in contributing to higher levels of symptoms of ill health among women in general, and married women in particular. Interestingly, Gove found a similar distress profile of single men and women in contrast to the discrepancies among the married, which would reflect the disadvantaged social situation of married women (Gove & Tudor, 1973). Also more recent research has demonstrated sex differences in distress among the married and the greater emotional costs of parenthood for women, especially in those with dependent children when parental role demands are greatest (e.g. Bolger et al., 1990; Simon, 1992). The evidence is not conclusive. Data have been reported that fail to find a significant difference in the distress of employed, married men and women. Paradoxically, married women in the labour force, precisely those women one would expect to be most overloaded, have been found to be healthier than married women who do not work (Gore & Mangione, 1983). This discrepancy can only be understood by assuming that women's health is improved by paid labour work because they are in better health than non-employed women, but that employment also involve costs for their health because they are in poorer health than employed men.

In an attempt to understand the impact of differential social roles of men and women a more proximal approach to exposure has been undertaken by studying critical life events associated with social roles. This approach corresponds with the central idea of classical stress research that stress is caused by breaches in the continuity of previous routines, imposed by life changes and other forces outside the individual. The work of Brown & Harris (1978), especially, has been seminal in this domain as it demonstrated the significance of sets of life events that were typical for women, e.g. absence of a spouse, social isolation, and chronic poverty, and played a role in the development of depression. Some of these studies have shown that women are indeed exposed to more life stressors than men, but few have been able to demonstrate that the greater exposure of women to life events explains their higher symptom levels (Mirowsky & Ross, 1989). Other studies call into question the assumption that women's lives are fraught with more stressors and strains. Martocchio & O'Leary (1980), for example, concluded on the basis of a critical examination of 15 studies on gender differences in occupational stress, that there was no evidence that working women encountered more work stressors than working men did. However, the appropriateness of life event inventories to study women's exposure to stress has been called into question as critical stressors in the lives of women, such as being victim of sexual abuse, discrimination, and violence, have been omitted (Belle, 1982).

More generally, the life event approach has been criticized for its lack of attention to the interrelatedness of exposure to stress and the availability of coping resources, indicating a differential *vulnerability* of men and women to stressors. A model of greater female vulnerability to the effects of stress predicts an interaction between sex and exposure, suggesting that women are more highly affected by the stressful situations to which they and men are similarly exposed. In contrast to the differential exposure explanation which proposes that women's greater distress is the result of higher exposure alone, the differential vulnerability hypothesis suggests that although men and women may be exposed to similar levels of stress, differences in response to these stressors result in women experiencing the same environmental cues as being more stressful. Several studies suggest that men and women are indeed differentially vulnerable as they dispose of less resources to cope with stress or use other ways to cope with stress (e.g. Roxburgh, 1996). Turner, Wheaton & Lloyd (1995) have reported that vulnerability differences account for over 50% of the total gap in men's and women's distress – although it has been questioned whether a generalized female vulnerability exists which relates to all kinds of stressors. It is argued instead that women are particularly reactive only to certain types of stressors, especially undesirable events that occur within their network of family and friends (Conger et al., 1993; Kessler & McLeod, 1984; Thoits, 1982; Wethington et al., 1987) – an issue to be dealt with in the section on appraisal of stress. A major problem in determining their relative vulnerability relates to the difficulty in comparing men and women due to the likelihood of differential selection effects. To determine the extent to which women in the same (mostly, working) conditions may be more vulnerable than men to the harmful effects of stress, more should be known about the effects of selection on women who succeed in occupying the same jobs as men.

In conclusion, the assumption that women are exposed to more stressors or more persistent stressors than men is not corroborated by empirical evidence. Indeed, in the past 20 years the exposure approach has been broadened by research in which differences in the way men and women adapt cognitively, emotionally, and behaviourally to stressful life conditions are studied. In this type of research, the way individuals respond to stress is considered a key factor in understanding the assumed greater vulnerability of women to stress. This leads us to another major issue in research on gender, stress, and coping: to what extent do women and men use differential strategies to handle stress?

COPING STRATEGIES

Cultural imagery portrays men as rational problem solvers and women as emotional and depending on others when faced with adversity. This conventional wisdom is corroborated by a large number of empirical studies, showing indeed that men engage more in problem-focused ways of coping (Billings & Moos, 1981; Diehl et al., 1996; Lazarus & Folkman, 1984; Stone & Neale, 1984) or individualistic, sometimes aggressive behaviour, such as turning against others (Hobfoll et al., 1994; Frank et al., 1984). Women, in contrast, appear to engage more in emotion-focused coping (Brems & Johnson, 1989; Carver et al., 1989; Endler & Parker, 1990; Folkman & Lazarus, 1980; Stone & Neale, 1984), or seek more social support (Carver et al., 1989; Jung, 1995; Rosario et al., 1988; Stone & Neale, 1984). Stone & Neale (1984), for example, studied longitudinally seven coping strategies in a sample of 60 middle-aged married couples and found that men used direct action more often whereas women endorsed more emotion-focused strategies such as distraction, catharsis, tension release, and prayer.

A less cited gender stereotype relates to another major distinction in coping efforts and concerns the difference between avoidant and approach strategies (cf. Roth & Cohen, 1986). Although some authors are inclined to treat avoidant and emotion-focused coping as strategies of a similar type and as such assume that women engage more than men in avoidant coping, evidence regarding this aspect is mixed. Some authors have reported data showing that women endorse avoidant strategies more than men (Endler & Parker, 1990; Long, 1990; Pearlin & Schooler, 1978: Stone & Neale, 1984). Others, however, have reported the opposite. Veroff et al. (1981) asked a large national sample of adult respondents how they handled worries and periods of unhappiness. Men were significantly more likely than women to report "doing nothing" or "not thinking about it". Men are also more likely than women to report having used drugs and alcohol (Carver et al., 1989; Sigmon et al., 1995) – which in fact may be classified as an avoidant strategy. These findings correspond with Nolen-Hoeksema's (1987) theory on differential response style stating that men are more likely to engage in distracting behaviours when distressed, while women are more likely to ruminate about it, thus amplifying and prolonging their negative mood states. However, avoidant coping may be a form of dealing with the emotional aspects of stress, since avoiding may also represent problem-oriented handling. Hobfoll et al. (1994) found that women avoiding an interpersonal conflict may actually enact actively and instrumentally upon their environment because they value harmony.

A number of considerations limit the univocality of these findings.

Adaptiveness of Emotion-oriented Coping

Many researchers simply assume that emotion-oriented coping (and also avoidant coping) is a less adaptive way of dealing with stress. The widely held belief that emotion-oriented coping results in poorer health outcome is questioned, both theoretically and empirically. The effec-tiveness of coping is said to be determined by examining it in relation to the demands of the situation (Lazarus & Folkman, 1984). That is, it is plausible to state that situations that are controllable call for more problem-focused efforts because the individual is in a position to control the situation. In contrast, situations that do not allow for control require adequate management of the emotions evoked by such a situation (Folkman, 1984). Effectiveness must also take into account the duration of stressors. Research concludes that with short-term stressors avoidant strategies are preferred, while long-term stressors require attentional strategies (Suls & Fletcher, 1985). This implies that men would be better at coping with short-term events because of their predominant use of avoidant coping but that women adjust better to less frequent but more severe events (e.g. death of a spouse; cf. Stroebe, 1998) because of their more frequent use of attentional strategies, which provides them with timely warning signs to take action (Weidner & Collins, 1993). Futhermore, although many studies report that women engage more frequently in emotion-focused ways of coping than men, the majority of female coping efforts is characterized by a problem-oriented focus (e.g. Ptacek & Dodge, 1994). The observation that women are emotion-oriented copers is a relative one and does not correspond to the stereotype of all women as emotional copers.

In general, the studies show that women more than men engage in emotion-focused ways of coping. Methodological problems must be considered relating to the validity of conventional coping question-naires responses (De Ridder, 1997). These questionnaires may elicit preferences in response to a general stressor instead of actual behaviour adopted in specific situations (cf. Ptacek & Dodge, 1994; Rosario et al., 1988; Sigmon et al., 1995). It has been demonstrated that the presenta-tion of more specific situations elicit less stereotypical answers and also produce less gender differences. Gender differences may be most likely to occur when subjects are simply asked to indicate how they coped with the most stressful event of the recent past, and coping compar-isons are then made without regard to the nature of the recalled event (Vitaliano et al., 1987). Studies that have not used traditional indices of coping based on the reported extent to which each coping method was employed, also provide a different picture. Ptacek et al. (1992) examined the order in which coping methods were used and found that although men and women did not differ in the extent to which they applied problem-focused coping, men more often than women reported using it first in their coping sequence. Also, using an index developed by Vitaliano et al. (1987) indicating the relative coping effort defined as the proportion of the total coping effort, Ptacek found that men engaged more in problem-focused coping than women, even though no differences appeared when the traditional extent-used scoring method was used. Although these results corroborate the tradi-tional findings that women engage emotion-focused coping more than men, they also show that a more sophisticated measurement of coping results in a more balanced picture of female coping efforts. Similarly, Thoits (1991) was able to demonstrate that women engage in *more* coping efforts than men (cf. de Vries et al., 1997; Long, 1990) – possibly indicating a higher sensitivity for stress; an issue discussed later.

To summarize, it has proved important to reflect on what qualities of coping behaviour are relevant for use in research on gender differ-ences in coping. Studies that move beyond the conventional coping scales (which elicit the extent to which one or more particular coping strategies were employed), and instead focus on qualities such as the order or the relative amount of specific coping efforts, lead thus to surprising results.

Classification of Coping Efforts

A second consideration lies in the classification of coping efforts. First, it must be pointed out that there is no general consensus about which particular behaviours should be classified as either emotion-focused or problem-focused, as these broad categories may involve very different behaviours. This lack of clarity has led to dubious classifications possibly producing a biased picture of gender differences in coping. Vingerhoets & Van Heck (1990), for example, categorized behaviours that are often believed to represent emotional ways of dealing with stress, such as positive thinking and daydreaming, as problem-focused strategies and concluded that males had a tendency to prefer problem-focused strategies. Aggregating different coping behaviours into particular strategies may produce a distorted picture because apparently univocal behaviours may serve different goals and should therefore be classified according to their objective. This is especially apparent in the strategy of social support seeking, which may either correspond to problem-solving efforts (as in seeking advice) or correspond to emotion-focused coping (as in venting emotions to a friend). Nevertheless, regardless of which type of social support is involved, social support seeking is often classified as an emotion-focused strategy.

Recently, the very concept of emotion-focused coping has been questioned by Stanton et al. (1994) as it incorporates such different behaviours as taking responsibility ("blame myself"), cognitive avoidance and adaptive outcomes ("become very tense", "get upset"), and omit behaviours that reflect working through emotions (disclosure and rumination). In a study on the effectiveness of Emotional Approach Coping, a scale developed by Stanton et al., which they claim to be "uncontaminated", they were able to demonstrate that women more frequently worked through their emotions than men and that this greater attempt to understand and express one's emotions was also more adaptive for them – either because women have developed greater skill in using this strategy or because such strategies are more congruent with women's values, while men are more likely to perceive emotional expression as irrational and immature. Similarly, Stroebe (1998) has suggested that widowers may be more vulnerable to physical illness and depression than widows because widowers find it easier to avoid confrontation with feelings and deal with the problems that are concurrent with bereavement rather than the emotions that it evokes, while widows can access their emotions and express them more easily. Disentangling these various forms of emotion-focused coping in the future may help to clarify to what extent women are indeed emotion-focused copers. Also, taking into account that the issue of emotion versus problem-focused coping is closely connected to issues relating to the effectiveness of coping (and the role of coping with stress as a determinant of health outcomes), this promises to be an important line of research.

Relevance of the Emotion- Versus Problem-focused Classification

A third issue is related to this as some researchers have questioned the relevance of the emotion-focused versus problem-focused classification as the most important distinction to understand differential coping behaviour of men and women. Hobfoll et al. (1994) have proposed a different approach, highlighting two other aspects of coping, namely active versus passive and prosocial versus antisocial behaviour. Although evidence for the approach is mixed, Hobfoll was able to demonstrate that women acted more prosocially than men when confronted with stress. Men, on the other hand, were more likely to use antisocial and aggressive strategies, but also less assertive coping strategies than women. Although these gender-differences were evident, they were constrained by gender-role orientation. Men and women with more traditional opinions about sex roles differed more distinctly in their coping behaviour. Interestingly, active coping was related to lower distress for both men and women, while prosocial coping was beneficial for women but not for men – neither was antisocial coping for men. Hobfoll concludes that men may have a narrower band of beneficial coping strategies.

Although uncorroborated, these findings are especially interesting since one of the more robust differences reported in the coping behaviour of men and women relates to the issue of social support seeking. Although social support seeking is often classified as a form of emotion-focused coping, such a categorization is questionable since, as stated earlier, the mobilization of social support can involve both problem-solving objectives and emotional relief. In an extensive review of gender-related variations in social support, Vaux (1985) concluded that differences in support seeking typically favour women and that such differences are most likely to emerge with respect to emotional support. Also, other studies demonstrate that women appear much more likely than men to seek out social support (e.g., Billings & Moos, 1981; Defares et al., 1985; Ptacek et al., 1992; Stone & Neale, 1984). The finding that women rely more on their social networks as a coping strategy is also consistent with other research that women have larger, more inter-dependent social networks (Kessler et al., 1985) and generally higher needs for affiliation (Wong & Csikszentmihalyi, 1991). Nevertheless, it must be kept in mind that social involvement can not only increase the availability of social support, but also create more stress. Women with low levels of personal resources appear to be more distressed by stressful conditions in the lives of significant others (Riley & Eckenrode, 1986).

Role of Different Types of Stressful Situation

Finally, a fourth consideration pertains to the role of the different types of stressful situations that men and women are involved in as a factor in explaining gender differences in coping, and as such it relates directly to the issue of socialization versus social constraint introduced in the first section of this chapter. As stated earlier, the socialization approach predicts that gender differences are fairly stable and will manifest themselves across a wide variety of different situations. Cantor & Kihlstrom (1987), for example, have suggested that gender-related differences in social knowledge caused by differential upbringing have a profound effect on the development and the selection of problem-solving strategies in life-tasks. In contrast, the social constraint perspective states that situational constraints are powerful determinants of stress responses and will limit the number of possibilities either men or women have at their disposal for reaction to the stressful encounters they engage in. This perspective predicts that, when confronted with similar stressful situations, men and women will react in a similar way. As such, this approach corresponds with the transactional approach to stress and coping advocated by Lazarus & Folkman (1984), who stated that the experience of stress is the result of a "transaction" between person and situation, in which the personal relevance of a stressful situation is determined by the extent to which it threatens or challenges the values and goals cherished by the person. As such, situational demands are believed to shape and constraint coping responses (Lazarus & Folkman, 1984).

There appears to be some evidence for the social constraint view. A number of studies report no sex differences in coping when men and women are faced with similar stressful conditions, for example college life (Hamilton & Fagot, 1988; Ptacek et al., 1992), working conditions (Long, 1990; Rosario et al., 1988), or other particular stressful conditions (Folkman & Lazarus, 1980; Porter & Stone, 1995; Ptacek et al., 1992). However, it remains to be determined to what extent these results really do support the social constraint view, as it is unclear whether the key issue is about different or similar situations. A more detailed test of the social constraint view is provided by Folkman & Lazarus (1980) who studied the coping reactions of middle-aged men and women in specific situations. They found that there were no gender differences at an aggregated level (across situations) but, on closer examination, men were more likely to use problem-focused strategies than women in response to work problems, whereas women were more likely to use problem-solving strategies within marriage and parenting contexts. Similar observations have been made by Billings & Moos (1981) and Pearlin & Schooler (1978).

Perhaps problem-solving efforts are more likely to be used when individuals are more familiar with a situation and perceive more control, power, or responsibility in a particular role domain (women in the family arena, men in the occupational arena). In that respect, the findings also allow for a socialization view in which socialized values determine in what particular way specific sets of stressful situations are evaluated. Gore & Colten (1991), for example, have emphasized the profoundly interpersonal nature of stress for women because losses, disruptions, and conflicts with significant others threaten their self-esteem. It is difficult to evaluate the impact of socialization, however, since very little research has been concerned with evaluating the impact of socialization on actual coping behaviour (Kliewer et al., 1996). One would assume that, if socialization of typical male and female behaviour patterns played a role in stress and coping, the effects of socialization should be visible in traditional attitudes towards gender-appropriate behaviour (e.g. gender-role orientation). Unfortunately, most studies on gender differences in coping rely on biological sex only as the basis for comparisons. The few available studies incorporating gender-role orientation demonstrate a moderating role of gender-role orientation on the effects of biological sex on coping behaviour, but also show that biological sex continues to have a large main effect (Conway et al., 1990; Levit, 1991; Nezu & Nezu, 1987; Ptacek & Dodge, 1994). One study reports that gender-role stereotypes hinder women in the employment of "masculine" coping strategies (Abraham & Hansson, 1996). These findings point to the relevance of situational appraisals as an important stage of the stress coping process which may account for differential reactions of men and women.

Differences in Coping Strategies of Men and Women

Despite methodological constraints associated with the assessment and the classification of coping behaviours it appears that there is a significant difference in the way men and women handle stress. This difference may be small and constrained by either the typical stressful situations men and women encounter in their daily lives or by their gender-role orientations. Nevertheless the trends are evident. It remains to be determined, however, to what extent these differences are able to explain gender differences in health, as the observed differences appear to relate to some functionality, with problem-focused coping efforts employed in situations with which one is familiar. Also, some kinds of emotion-focused coping may be more adaptive than is generally believed. To the extent that emotion-focused coping is not adaptive, it must be kept in mind that also women primarily engage in problem-focused ways of coping.

DETERMINANTS OF DIFFERENCES IN COPING BEHAVIOUR: APPRAISAL AND RESOURCES

The previous section made clear that gender differences in the use of coping strategies exist and can partly be explained by the different types of situations men and women confront. When controlling for situational constraints, however, differential use of coping strategies by men and women remain (Long, 1990; Ptacek & Dodge, 1994). To account for these observations, it must be assumed that additional factors are involved that can help to explain the observed gender differences in coping behaviour. These factors can be classified as being related either to the appraisal stage of coping or to the availability of and access to such coping resources as social support, personal dispositions, and material conditions.

To begin with the role of appraisal as a determinant of differential coping behaviour, unfortunately few empirical studies are available; this, in part, may reflect the methodological difficulties associated with measuring the inherent evanescence of such cognitions (De Ridder, 1997). Some research exists that suggests that women, relative to men, are more affected by life events and obtain higher ratings of how "upsetting" an event is or how much adjustment would be required to deal with it (Bradley, 1980; De Ridder & TeVaarwerk, 1995; Sigmon et al., 1995; Wethington et al., 1987), which may be interpreted as an indication of the *primary appraisal* of the event in which its "stressfulness" (harm, threat, or challenge – Lazarus & Folkman, 1984) is evaluated. Women also appraise a set of life events as likely to produce more stress and tension and as requiring more recovery time than men (Jorgensen & Johnson, 1990), and they are more inclined to label the experience of stress as "emotion" (instead of mere "stress") which may, in turn, lead to less anticipation of problem solving strategies (Robinson & Johnson, 1997). These findings are consistent with the notion that women as a group (relative to men) appraise potentially threatening events as more stressful (Miller & Kirsch, 1987). Nevertheless, as was reported earlier with respect to coping strategies, one must be careful of stereotypical answering tendencies when gender differences in primary appraisal are evaluated. That is, when more specific events are presented to men and women, gender differences become less pronounced. Ptacek & Dodge (1994), for example, observed that men and women responding to the same event (a college achievement situation) under controlled laboratory conditions reported similar amounts of stress (cf. Porter & Stone, 1995; Sigmon et al., 1995). In contrast, De Ridder & TeVaarwerk (1995) demonstrated striking differences in the appraisal of the same stressors (presented by vignette), with women reporting significantly higher scores on a primary appraisal scale. Also, studies of partners sharing the same event have shown remarkable differences between men and women, men being more inclined to ignore the stressful situation (McGreal et al., 1997; Schilling et al., 1985).

In a more general sense, these results may be taken as evidence of a general (psychological or physiological) reactivity of women regarding their evaluation of potentially harmful events. In correspondence with research on avoidance and approach as coping strategies (see above), research on appraisal strategies shows that women are more inclined to highlight potential dangers brought up by the situation while men have been found to make more use of such strategies as denial and avoidance (see 1993 for a review, Weidner & Collins). Such an appraisal strategy may set men at a disadvantage in comparison to women, especially when controllable stressors are concerned (cf. Suls & Fletcher, 1985). That is, men's initial avoidance reactions may not allow them to perceive and act upon early warning signs and, as a result, leaves them overwhelmed by the problem once they realize it is of long-term consequence and indeed requires attention. In contrast, women may be disadvantaged employing attentional strategies when it concerns uncontrollable stressors of short duration. It appears that women are better adjusted than men when exposed to stressful events of extended duration (more than 1 week) while men are advantaged when transient stressors are involved.

At present, it is unclear to what extent these differential appraisal strategies are of either a social or a biological origin or both. There is some evidence of a physiological reactivity in women (Polefrone & Manuck, 1987; Stoney et al., 1987). On the other hand, there is also research suggesting that differential cognitive strategies may be socialized, since they relate to different attitudes regarding stress. Lower rates of primary appraisal are associated with an attitude in which stressful situations are considered being a part of daily life and will dissolve without any real efforts to control them – an attitude which is found more frequently in men (De Ridder & TeVaarwerk, 1995). However, despite its intuitive appeal, evidence of consistent socialized gender differences in sensitivity to stressful events, as for example demonstrated in learned helplessness or other attitudinal features, is not conclusive (Kliewer et al., 1996; Miller & Kirsch, 1987). Indeed, one must be careful to conclude that a generalized reactivity in women exists, because a number of studies show that women are more reactive to particular classes of events, depending on the extent to which these events threaten the values they cherish. Thoits (1991; cf. Wethington et al., 1987), for example, has suggested that women's greater responsiveness to family role strains may reflect the salience that women attach to these roles relative to men. In itself, such greater responsiveness to particular events does not need to be dysfunctional. When, for example, network events are involved, women are more able to make a realistic appraisal of what is at stake (Belle, 1987). A striking example of this phenomenon is provided by Ben-Zur & Zeidner (1996), who demonstrated that during the Gulf War Israeli women unexpectedly showed more problem-oriented coping efforts than men, which can only be accounted for because most of the coping options that could be exercised were related to family and home (e.g. such as buying provision and taking care of children); men, in contrast, had fewer tasks to accomplish because it was impossible to protect their country in the traditional sex-appropriate way (via military service).

The second set of factors that may determine gender-related differences in coping behaviour concerns coping resources. Studies on coping resources show that women have less access to social resources (e.g. income or education) due to their disadvantaged social situation (for a review see Belle, 1987). While the social gains made by recent generations of women have broadened their roles and the coping resources to which they have access, women's social position in general remains lower than that of men – an issue we have discussed to some extent in the second section of this chapter. Regarding more specific coping resources, such as the availability of social support, research shows that women, in comparison with men, have more access to emotional and informative help from their social networks (Belle, 1987; Riley & Eckenrode, 1986). Help from the network may have a price, though. Women's greater involvement in the network of family and friends provides them with their opportunity to turn to these network members for help, but it also confronts them with more requests for help when these network members, in their turn, are confronted with stressful situations. Men, on the other hand, are more inclined to use their social networks in an instrumental way; the network provides them with support when they ask for it but they do not feel obliged to do something in return (Jorgenson & Johnson, 1990).

Other coping resources involve such personal characteristics as a positive orientation, personal control, or extraversion. Although research on systematic gender differences in these personal characteristics is scarce, some studies show that these characteristics may have a moderating effect on the use of particular coping strategies (Kobasa, 1987; Rim, 1986). Studies by Houtman (1990) and Jung (1995) also demonstrate that men and women make differential use of particular personal characteristics, although a systematic pattern remains unclear. One coping resource that has been studied more extensively is personal control. Although some studies have reported a lower sense of personal control in women (e.g. De Ridder & TeVaarwerk, 1995; Wheaton, 1980), others have failed to do so (Thoits, 1991). More striking is the finding that a low level of personal control has a differential effect on the use of coping strategies in men and women: while women do not appear to be bothered much by low levels of personal control, for men a low level of personal control interferes with their attempts to deal with the stressful situation (Jorgensen & Johnson, 1990). In addition, it must be stated that although it is often assumed that a high level of personal control promotes the adoption of problem-oriented ways of coping, some authors have suggested that only when subjective control of the situation matches objective control may one actually benefit from a high level of control (Folkman, 1984).

In conclusion, research on the appraisal stage of the coping process shows that women are somewhat more reactive to stressful situations than men but that whether higher reactivity leads to less adequate coping is dependent on the type of stressful situations involved. Higher reactivity may disadvantage women when transient stressors are concerned but may be useful in the interpretation of signs that the situation calls for action. Higher reactivity appears also to be protective in familiar situations in which one knows what to do, which promotes problem-oriented coping.

FURTHER QUESTIONS

In general, the studies reported in this chapter show that women, relative to men, react in a more emotion-oriented fashion when confronted with stress. It remains to be determined, however, to what extent these preferences of women make them disadvantaged insofar as their health outcomes are at stake. Depending on the duration and the controllability of the kind of stressful situations, emotion-oriented coping may be adequate. Unfortunately, duration and controllability of specific events have rarely been assessed in the literature that discusses gender differences in coping. To arrive at a more profound understanding of gender differences coping, more attention should be paid to the objective characteristics of stressful situations. In addition, it appears that on top of these objective situational demands, subjective demands as perceived by the individual are also relevant to determine. There is some evidence suggesting that women, relative to men, are more inclined to pay attention to the potential upsetting aspects of stressful situations (ruminate), while men are inclined to ignore them. Women's tendency to use attentional strategies when encountering short-term stressors of no particular consequence may be maladaptive because emotional energy is spent on transient events that are beyond their control. Compared with women, the typical male avoider benefits from not being upset by uncontrollable events of short duration. On the other hand, not paying attention to early warning signs may result in feeling overwhelmed and helpless when encountering a severe threat of prolonged duration, such as divorce or another loss event.

In addition to paying more attention to both situational and appraisal aspects of the coping process and broadening the perspective from simply coping strategies to a more complete account of the coping process, we need to pay more attention to the conceptualization of gender. Most studies have taken biological sex as their point of departure, ignoring its physiological, psychological, and social concomitants. Regarding psychological and social aspects, it is remarkable that few studies on gender differences in coping strategies have paid respect to such relevant characteristics as gender role or gender-role orientation, or life-roles associated with the social position of women in our society. As such, it is also remarkable that the sociological–epidemiological research, discussed in the second section of this chapter, has not merged with the psychological stress and coping research discussed in the third section – although some sociological researchers have broadened their view with research on psychological variables such as role identity (cf. Thoits, 1991). Theoretical reflections on the nature of gender differences and its impact on stress and coping are rare. Incorporating theoretical notions of what level gender differences in reaction to adversiveness would manifest themselves could also help to clarify the heuristic value of the socialization versus social constraint opposition that has dominated coping research on gender differences over the past 10 years. The available research, although not conclusive, strongly suggests that gender differences in coping are present during several stages of the coping process. In order to explain and understand the nature of these differences it is necessary to study both social and biological as well as psychological aspects of these differences. The sometimes unexpected findings that women, in particular circumstances, engage more in problem-oriented strategies than men may be interpreted as a sign that the "classic" socialization hypothesis must take account of recent social changes in which women are also socialized to be more assertive, instrumental, and independent.

Finally, it must be stressed that stress coping research on gender differences could benefit from using more detailed measures of health outcomes because it is often assumed that gender differences in coping can account for gender differences in health, though empirical validation of this assumption is lacking. Prospective designs incorporating proximal indicators of health status are obligatory to substantiate this claim.

REFERENCES

Abraham, J.D., & Hansson, R.O. (1996). Gender differences in the usefulness of goal-directed coping for middle-aged and older workers. *Journal of Applied Social Psychology, 26,* 657–669.

Belle, D. (1982). The stress of caring: women as providers of social support. In Goldberger, L., & Breznitz, S. (Eds.), *Handbook of Stress: Theoretical and Clinical Aspects.* New York: Free Press.

Belle, D. (1987). Gender differences in the social moderators of stress. In Barnett, R.C., Biener, L., & Baruch, G.K. (Eds.), *Gender and Stress* (pp.257–277). New York: Free Press.

Bem, S.L. (1974). The measurement of psychological androgyny. *Journal of Consulting and Clinical Psychology, 42,* 155–162.

Ben-Zur, H., & Zeidner, M. (1996). Gender differences in coping reactions under community crisis and daily routine conditions. *Personality and Individual Differences, 20,* 331–340.

Billings, A.G., & Moos, R.H. (1981). The role of coping responses and social resources in attenuating the stress of life events. *Journal of Behavioral Medicine*, *4*, 139–157.

Bolger, N., de Longis, A., Kessler, R.D., & Wethington, E. (1990). The microstructure of daily role related stress in married couples. In Eckenrode, J., & Gore, S. (Eds.), *Stress Between Work and Family* (pp.95–105). New York: Plenum.

Bradley, C. (1980). Sex differences in reporting and rating of life events: a comparison of diabetic and healthy subjects. *Journal of Psychosomatic Research*, *24*, 35–37.

Brems, C., & Johnson, M.E. (1989). Problem-solving appraisal and coping style: the influence of sex-role orientation and gender. *Journal of Personality*, *123*, 187–194.

Brown, G.W. and Harris, T. (1978). *Social Origins of Depression A Study of Psychiatric Disorder in Women*. New York: Free Press.

Brown, G.W., & Harris, T. (1987). *Social Origins of Depression: A Study of Psychiatric Disorders in Women*. London: Tavistock.

Cantor, N., & Kihlstrom, J.F. (1987). *Personality and Social Intelligence*. Englewood Cliff, NJ: Prentice Hall.

Carver, C.S., Scheier, M.F., & Weintraub, J.K. (1989). Assessing coping strategies: a theoretically based approach. *Journal of Personality and Social Psychology*, *59*, 267–283.

Conger, R.D., Lorenz, F.O., Edler, G.H., Simons, R.L., & Ge, X. (1993). Husband and wife differences in response to undesirable life events. *Journal of Health and Social Behaviour*, *34*, 71–88.

Conway, M., Giannopoulos, C., & Stiefenhofer, K. (1990). Response styles to sadness are related to sex and sex-role orientation. *Sex Roles*, *22*, 579–587.

Crosby, F. (1988). *Spouse, Parent, Worker: On Gender and Multiple Roles*. New Haven, CT: Yale University Press.

Defares, P.B., Brandjes, M., Nass, C., & Van den Ploeg, J.D. (1985). Coping styles, social support and sex differences. In Sarason, I., & Sarason, B. (Eds.), *Social Support: Theory, Research and Applications* (pp.173–186). Dordrecht: Nijhoff.

De Ridder, D.T.D. (1997). What is wrong with coping assessment? A review of conceptual and methodological issues. *Psychology and Health*, *12*, 417–431.

De Ridder, D.T.D., & TeVaarwerk, M. (1995). Het belang van de omstandigheden. Over de invloed van stresserende situaties op het copingproces. In Sanderman, R., van den Heuvel, W.J.A., & Krol, B. (Eds.), *Interveniëren in de determinanten van gezondheidheid: resultaten van een onderzoeksprogramma* [Situational Determinants of Coping Processes] (pp.27–47). Assen: Van Gorcum.

De Vries, H.M., Hamilton, D.W., Lovett, S., & Gallagher-Thompson, D. (1997). Patterns of coping preferences for male and female caregivers of frail older adults. *Psychology and Aging*, *12*, 263–267.

Diehl, M., Coyle, N., & Labouvie-Bief, G. (1996). Age and sex differences in strategies of coping and defense across the life span.
Psychology and Aging, 11, 127–139.

Endler, N.S., & Parker, J.D.A. (1990). Multidimensional assessment of
coping: a critical evaluation. *Journal of Personality and Social Psychology,
58,* 844–854.

Folkman, S. (1984). Personal control and stress and coping processes:
a theoretical analysis. *Journal of Personality and Social Psychology, 46,*
839–852.

Folkman, S. & Lazarus, R.S. (1980). An analysis of coping in a middle-
aged community sample. *Journal of Health and Social Behaviour, 21,*
219–239.

Frank, S.J., McLaughlin, A.M., & Crusco, A. (1984). Sex role attributes,
symptom distress, and defensive style among college men and
women. *Journal of Personality and Social Psychology, 47,* 182–192.

Gore, S., & Colten, M.E. (1991). Gender, stress, and distress. In Eckenrode,
J., (Ed.), *The Social Context of Coping* (pp.139–163). New York: Plenum.

Gore, S., & Mangione, T. (1983). Social roles, sex roles and psychological distress: additive and interactive models of sex differences. *Journal
of Health and Social Behaviour, 24,* 49–53.

Gove, W.R. (1972). The relationship between sex roles, marital status,
and mental illness. *Social Forces, 51,* 34–44.

Gove, W.R., & Tudor, J.F. (1973). Adult sex roles and mental illness.
American Journal of Sociology, 26, 64–78.

Hamilton, S., & Fagot, B.I. (1988). Chronic stress and coping styles: a
comparison of male and female undergraduates. *Journal of Personality
and Social Psychology, 55,* 819–823.

Hobfoll, S.E., Dunahoo, C.L., BenPorath, Y., & Monnier, J. (1994). Gender
and coping: the dual-axis model of coping. *American Journal of
Community Psychology, 22,* 49–79.

Houtman, I.D. (1990). Personal coping resources and sex differences.
Personality and Individual Differences, 11, 53–63.

Jorgensen, R.S., & Johnson, J.H. (1990). Contributors to the appraisal of
major life changes: gender, perceived controllability, sensation
seeking, strain, and social support. *Journal of Applied Social Psychology,
20,* 1123–1138.

Jung, J. (1995). Ethnic group and gender differences in the relationship
between personality and coping. *Anxiety, Stress and Coping, 8,* 113–126.

Kessler, R.C., & McLeod, J.D. (1984). Sex differences in vulnerability to
undesirable life events. *American Sociological Review, 49,* 620–631.

Kessler, R.C., McLeod, J.D., & Wethington, E. (1985). The costs of caring:
a perspective on the relationship between sex and psychological
distress. In Sarason, I.G., & Sarason, B.R. (Eds.), *Social Support: Theory,
Research and Applications* (pp.491–506). The Hague: Nijhof.

Kliewer, W., Fearnow, M.D., & Miller, P.A. (1996). Coping socialization in middle childhood: tests of maternal and paternal influences.
Child Development, 67, 2339–2357.

Kobasa, S.C.Q. (1987). Stress responses and personality. In Barnett, R.C., Biener, L., & Baruch, G.K. (Eds.), *Gender and Stress* (pp.308–329). New York: Free Press.

Lazarus, R.S., & Folkman, S. (1984). *Stress, Appraisal, and Coping.* New York: Springer Verlag.

Levit, D. (1991). Gender differences in ego defenses in adolescence: sex roles as one way to understand the differences. *Journal of Personality and Social Psychology, 61,* 992–999.

Long, B.C. (1990). Relation between coping strategies, sex-typed traits, and environmental characteristics: a comparison of male and female managers. *Journal of Counseling Psychology, 37,* 185–194.

McGreal, D., Evans, B.J., & Burrows, G.D. (1997). Gender differences in coping following loss of a child through miscarriage or stillbirth: a pilot study. *Stress Medicine, 13,* 159–165.

Martocchio, J.J., & O'Leary, A.M. (1980). Sex differences in occupational stress: A meta-analytic review. *Journal of Applied Psychology, 74,* 495–501.

Miller, S.M., & Kirsch, N. (1987). Sex differences in cognitive coping with distress. In Barnett, R.C., Biener, L., & Baruch, G.K. (Eds.), *Gender and Stress* (pp.278–307). New York: Free Press.

Mirowsky, J., & Ross, C.E. (1989). *Social Causes of Psychological Distress.* New York: Aldine.

Nezu, A.M., & Nezu, C.M. (1987). Psychological distress, problem solving, and coping reactions: sex role differences. *Sex Roles, 16,* 205–214.

Nolen-Hoeksema, S. (1987). Sex differences in unipolar depression: Evidence and theory. *Psychological Bulletin, 101,* 259–282.

Pearlin, L.I., & Schooler, C. (1978). The structure of coping. *Journal of Health and Social Behaviour, 19,* 2–21.

Polefrone, J.M., & Manuck, S.B. (1987). Gender differences in cardiovascular and neuroendocrine response to stressors. In Barnett, R.C., Biener, L., & Baruch, G.K. (Eds.), *Gender and Stress* (pp.13–38). New York: Free Press.

Porter, L.S., & Stone, A.S. (1995). Are there really gender differences in coping? A reconsideration of previous data and results from a daily study. *Journal of Social and Clinical Psychology, 14,* 184–202.

Ptacek, J.T., & Dodge, K.L. (1994). Gender differences in coping with stress: when stressor and appraisals do not differ. *Personality and Social Psychology Bulletin, 20,* 421–430.

Ptacek, J.T., Smith, R.E., & Zanas, J. (1992). Gender, appraisal, and coping: a longitudinal analysis. *Journal of Personality, 60,* 747–770.

Riley, C., & Eckenrode, J. (1986). Social ties: subgroup differences in costs and benefits. *Journal of Personality and Social Psychology, 51,* 770–778.

Rim, Y. (1986). Ways of coping, personality, age, sex and family structural variables. *Personality and Individual Differences, 7,* 113–116.

Robinson, M.D., & Johnson, J.T. (1997). Is it emotion or is it stress? Gender stereotypes and the perception of subjective experience. *Sex Roles, 36,* 235–258.

Rosario, M., Shinn, M., Morch, H., & Huckabee, C. (1988). Gender differences in coping and social supports: testing socialization and role constraints theories. *Journal of Community Psychology, 16,* 55–69.

Ross, C.E., & Bird, C.E. (1994). Sex stratification and health lifestyle: consequences for men's and women's perceived health. *Journal of Health and Social Behaviour, 35,* 161–178.

Roth, S., & Cohen, L.J. (1986). Approach, avoidance, and coping with stress. *American Psychologist, 41,* 813–819.

Roxburgh, S. (1996). Gender differences in work and well-being: effects of exposure and vulnerability. *Journal of Health and Social Behaviour, 37,* 265–277.

Schilling, R.F., Schinke, S.P., & Kirkham, M.A. (1985). Coping with a handicapped child: differences between mothers and fathers. *Social Science and Medicine, 21,* 857–863.

Sigmon, S.T., Stanton, A.L., & Snyder, C.R. (1995). Gender differences in coping: A further test of socialization and role constraint theories. *Sex Roles, 33,* 565–587.

Simon, R.W. (1992). Parental role strains, salience of parental identity and gender differences in psychological distress. *Journal of Health and Social Behaviour, 33,* 25–35.

Stanton, A.L., Danoff-Burg, S., Cameron, C.L., & Ellis, A.P. (1994). Coping through emotional approach: problems of conceptualization and confounding. *Journal of Personality and Social Psychology, 66,* 350–362.

Stone, A.A., & Neale, J.M. (1984). New measure of daily coping: developments and preliminary results. *Journal of Personality and Social Psychology, 46,* 892–906.

Stoney, C.M., Davis, M.C., & Matthews, K.A. (1987). Sex differences in physiological responses to stress and in coronary heart disease: a causal link? *Psychophysiology, 24,* 127–131.

Stroebe, M.S. (1998). New directions in bereavement research: explorations of gender differences. *Palliative Medicine, 12,* 5–12.

Suls, J., & Fletcher, B. (1985). The relative efficacy of avoidant and nonavoidant coping strategies: a meta-analysis. *Health Psychology, 4,* 249–288.

Thoits, P.A. (1982). Life stress, social support, and psychological vulnerability: epidemiological considerations. *Journal of Community Psychology, 10,* 341–363.

Thoits, P.A. (1991). Gender differences in coping with emotional distress. In Eckenrode, J. (Ed.), *The social context of coping* (pp.107–138). New York: Plenum.

Turner, R.J., Wheaton, B., & Lloyd, D.A. (1995). The epidemiology of social stress. *American Sociological Review, 60,* 104–125.

Vaux, A. (1985). Variations in social support associated with gender, ethnicity, and age. *Journal of Social Issues, 41,* 89–110.

Verbrugge, L. (1985). Gender and health: an update on hypotheses and evidence. *Journal of Health and Social Behaviour*, *26*, 156–182.

Verbrugge, L. (1989). The twain meet: empirical explanations of sex differences in health and mortality. *Journal of Health and Social Behaviour*, *30*, 282–304.

Veroff, J., Kulka, R.A., & Douvan, E. (1981). *Mental Health in America: Patterns of Help-seeking from 1957 to 1976*. New York: Basic.

Vingerhoets, A.J.J.M., & Van Heck, G.L. (1990). Gender, coping and psychosomatic symptoms. *Psychological Medicine*, *20*, 125–135.

Vitaliano, P.P., Maiuro, R.D., Russo, J., & Becker, J. (1987). Raw versus relative scores in the assessment of coping strategies. *Journal of Behavioral Medicine*, *10*, 1–18.

Weidner, G., & Collins, R.L. (1993). Gender, coping, and health. In Krohne, H.W. (Ed.), *Attention and Avoidance. Strategies in Coping with Aversiveness* (pp.241–265). Seattle: Hogrefe & Huber.

Wethington, E., McLeod, J.D., & Kessler, R.C. (1987). The importance of life events for explaining sex differences in mental health. In Barnett, R.C., Biener, L., & Baruch, G.K. (Eds.), *Gender and Stress* (pp.144–155). New York: Free Press.

Wheaton, B. (1980). The sociogenesis of psychological disorder: an attributional theory. *Journal of Health and Social Behaviour*, *24*, 208–229.

Wong, M.M., & Csikszentmihalyi, M. (1991). Affiliation motivation and daily experience: Some issues on gender differences. *Journal of Personality and Social Psychology*, *60*, 154–164.

Chapter 9

Leading the Troops or Just Entertaining? Women, Humour and Stand-up

Bathsheba Doran

London, UK

MOIRA:	Now this is Victoria – she's a comedienne! On telly! Yes!
CHARLES:	Well, call me old-fashioned but I don't like to see a woman telling jokes.
HILLARY:	Charles thinks women aren't funny.
GERALD:	Well I'm sorry; I agree.
HILLARY:	But there are hundreds of funny women. There's the woman who does the column in *The Sunday Telegraph* for a kick off.
CHARLES:	Well you name me a funny woman who's attractive with it.
DULCIE:	Attractive narrows it down.

Victoria Wood, "Staying In", Chunkey

For feminist academics looking at the relatively new field of women and humour there is one key problem which they need to confront before attempting serious, coherent, critical analysis. Its name is Joan Rivers. There is an entirely appropriate feminist instinct to applaud her success in the male-dominated field of stand-up. Joan Rivers grasped

Women, Health and the Mind
Edited by L. Sherr and J.S. St Lawrence. © 2000 John Wiley & Sons, Ltd

the phallic microphone when there were few female precedents. Her fame is a beacon to any aspiring comediennes, as well as a rebuke to the recurring patriarchal suspicion that women just aren't funny. However, lurking between the claps there is also the nagging suspicion that whilst Joan Rivers has contributed to the feminist fight, she won't be invited to entertain the feminist troops. After all, Rivers is a comedienne who freely acknowledges that "daring to admit that Elizabeth Taylor was a blimp ... skyrocket[ed] ... [her] ... career" (Rivers, 1992). Her material is frequently about her own "unattractiveness" and that of other women in the public eye. At the feminist victory party where we all eat cake without worrying about weight and drink beer without worrying about propriety, Joan Rivers will be left slinking behind some performance artistes from New Mexico who brought the house down earlier with their latest "My Body is a Yam" number.

Considering where Joan Rivers will stand at a feminist victory party is necessary because for the feminist critics who have written on the subject, women in comedy have revolutionary potential. According to such critics, women's humour is potentially "transformative and violent" (Wilt, 1980), marked by "revolt and inversion" (Little, 1983) and most frequently about claiming "autonomy and power" (Walker, 1988). "When women's laughter is directed towards authority," writes one author, "it can bring the house down" (Barreca, 1994).

The logic behind such pronouncements provides a key framework from which to begin any consideration of women and comedy. There are three recurring themes in the existing feminist analysis which relate to women as both professional and social comedians.

The first is that laughter and power are interconnected. As Frances Gray puts it, "to define a joke, to be the class that decides *what is funny*, is to make a massive assumption of power" (Gray, 1994). Such an "assumption of power" works on a variety of levels. Socially it defines the leader of the group – the joker with enough confidence to decide who is to be excluded from the circle (the object of laughter) and who is invited inside (those expected to laugh with the joker). On a general level this paradigm is far more dangerous. Conceptions of "the norm" and "the incongruous", which are the basis for most comic perception, are coloured by prejudice. Comedy is an "ideological construct" which exploits existing ideological constructs. Frequently it is traditional "others" who are the object of laughter (Barreca, 1988). However, the pervasive conception of laughter as involuntary and harmless relief makes objection difficult. "To object to a specific joke, in a specific context," Gray observes, "is to be perceived as an enemy of laughter in general"; indeed sociological studies imply that "both men and women prefer the butt of the joke to be female, regardless of the theme of the joke" (Palmer, 1994).

The second point that feminist critics have made is that it is far harder for women to access comedy's power than it is for men. In many cases there are real prejudices for women to overcome every time they make a joke. There is an ancient insistence that women are not very funny; or if they are funny, it is to compensate for physical flaws. Regina Barreca observes that "'she's got a terrific sense of humour' has become a kind of shorthand for 'physically unattractive'" (Barreca, 1991). If it is meant as a compliment, she points out, "it typically means that she gets the joke, not that she makes any of her own" (Barreca, 1991). In addition, comediennes are disabled by notions of female propriety. A degree of confidence is required for a successful joke, but assertive women run the risk of alienating a male audience. The power that feminists have identified as fundamental to the structure of joke telling is not meant to be accessed by the "second sex". Furthermore, women are rarely encouraged to be aggressive and thus frequently lack the assurance to carry a joke off. Stand-up comedian Jerry Seinfeld describes what he sees to be the essential relationship between an audience and a comic: "to laugh is to be dominated" (Auslander, 1992). Women are inevitably not used to taking such a stance.

The problem of propriety is intensified when it comes to the subject matter of the joke. Women particularly cause raised eyebrows if they make "dirty" jokes, or simply jokes about their body. As late as the 1960s most Shakespeare critics refused to acknowledge Cleopatra's bawdy, on the grounds that it was too inappropriate for a woman to wield such metaphors (Fitz, 1994). Popular British comediennes, such as Jo Brand and Jenny Eclair, are described in the press as "brash" and "bawdy" far more regularly than male counterparts who swear and use "smutty" material to an equal or greater extent. According to *The Times* journalist Brian Appleyard, for example, the smut by old school comics like Benny Hill and Bernard Manning is "inspired filth" which "celebrate[s] our common humanity". Such dirty jokes "seem to spring directly from a tradition from Chaucer". Jo Brand, Jenny Eclair and Joan Rivers, by contrast, are "outrageous" and "grotesque" (Appleyard, 1996).

Another fundamental difficulty that women face when they make jokes is that frequently men will not have experienced what the women comics are describing. "Tell him, just tell him, it's quicker", Victoria Wood, the British stand-up, calls out if she makes a joke the men in the audience clearly do not understand. She comments that it is at private functions that she feels most aware of sexual difference: "if you say 'privatisation' they think you're the funniest thing on earth. If you say 'tampon' it would be little blank faces all round" (Rosenguard & Ward, 1989). The gulf between men and women's knowledge of each other is perhaps indicated by this section from the American comedienne Kate Clinton's material:

> *Tootsie* would have been a very different film if once, just once, Dustin Hoffman could have known what it was like to sneeze and blow out a Tampax. (Quoted in Kader, 1990)

Annie Beatts, a writer on the American comedy show *Saturday Night Live*, had to find another women writer to work with because her male colleagues on the show were baffled by some of her material. For her, the question of a different comic understanding between men and women goes beyond knowing discreet information about women's bodies. "There's a woman's *culture* that men just don't know about," she explains. "So when they say, 'hey, that joke's not funny,' it's sometimes because they don't understand the vocabulary" (Barreca, 1991; my emphasis).

Beatts' analysis anticipates the third feminist point about women and humour, a point which is the logical conclusion from the first two. A number of critics have argued that there is a distinctly female sense of humour. Whether or not this difference is materially or essentially located is seldom made clear. Arguments based upon psychological and sociological studies usually do affirm that women tend to laugh at those in power and are thus subversive; men tend to laugh at inferiors. This information is not surprising given the existing feminist analysis: comedy tends to define the teller against the told – therefore the patriarchal binary guarantees the sociological equation. Feminists often give the information more of an essentialist slant, however, and implicit in their analysis is that women have the moral high ground when it comes to humour. Regina Barreca, for example, categorically states that women do not find Norman Mailer or *The Three Stooges* funny. Instead "women's humour is about power and it's systematic misappropriation . . . [it] . . . allows us to gain perspective by ridiculing the implicit insanities of a patriarchal culture" (Barreca, 1991). Emily Toth similarly argues that whereas men's humour uses comic "types", women's humour "involves an attack on types" (Toth, 1981).

These three considerations, power, access and difference, should begin to give substance to the feminist claim that women's humour has revolutionary potential. Nonetheless there are a number of difficulties with the feminist position. The argument that women are unable to access aggression and comic power has little resonance in the lives of individual comediennes, most of whom became comics because telling jokes came naturally to them; and among these comediennes, there is not really enough common ground for there to be obvious examples of a distinctly female sense of humour, suggesting that behind the feminist notion of a "woman's laugh" is a prescriptivism, implying that women should be laughing at some things and not others. Countering that instinct is the need to claim as many female comics as possible; consequently the selections in the anthologies of women's humour are so catholic that the whole notion of a specific women's laugh – especially a feminist laugh – is undermined. In a recent anthology, the rather dismal joke "a man in the house is worth two in the street" is on the same page as Gloria Steinem's comment that "some of us are becoming the men we wanted to marry" (Morgan, 1995).

Not only does comediennes' material vary so much as to make the possibility of a clear common ground between every female comic suspect, but there are also male comics who don't use humour in the aggressive manner that the feminist analysis implies. Feminist critics make no mention, for example, of the "alternative" circuit that has been current in England and America for the last 20 years. Alternative comedy professes to be "politically committed" comedy "which avoids the easy but offensive laugh" and has for the most part been true to its word (Rosenguard & Ward, 1989). One of its early stars, Jim Barclay, used to open his act with "Good evening ladies and gentlemen. My name's Jim Barclay and I'm the wacky and zany Marxist Leninist comedian, and it's my job to come here and tell you jokes which precipitate the downfall of capitalism and bring an end to tyranny and injustice wherever it rears it's ugly head, so 'ere we go with a starter for ten." (Rosenguard & Ward, 1989).

There is also comic material, from puns to *Monty Python* sketches, that does not contain the exploitative power structure that feminist critics emphasise. There is extremely sophisticated neutral humour (Eddy Izzard's absurd material about cats drilling behind sofas, for example) and material that draws attention to the nature of existing power structures and deconstructs them. *Fawlty Towers*, for example, is an (often painful) critique of both class and gender pretension. It portrays the power relations between the served and the servers, between the husband and the wife, between employer and employees, but it is an exploration of the social relationships, and one that, overall, tends to debunk the logic of social hierarchy. Polly, the waitress, is the most competent of the hotel staff whilst Basil Fawlty, the manager, is the least.

Equally essentialist are the claims about what women do and do not find funny as they fail to consider the effect that race, class and sexuality might have on each individual female in the audience. Susan J. Wolfe comments that "some women's comedy is so heterosexist that lesbians find it offensive" (Walker and Dresner, 1988). The reception of comedy is dependent on a degree of "psychical accord", to use Freud's term, and feminist critics have been right to use that to explain divisions between men and women in comic appreciation. However, psychical accord depends on a variety of frames of reference, which extend beyond sex and gender to other factors such as class and culture.

The biggest rebuff to the possibility of women and comedy's revolutionary potential comes from three interconnected arenas which none of the feminist analyses have considered in depth: post-modern, television and comedy culture. The absence of these considerations is a serious omission if comediennes are to be considered in their professional and artistic context. Women have become noticeably prominent in comedy specifically over the last 20 years, in other words within the period roughly described as post-modern. Post-modern culture is frequently accused of political apathy, as is the television industry, on which stand-up comics particularly rely for promotion. Comedy culture insists on the primacy of laughter above politics. Consequently the immediate surroundings of comediennes estrange them from any complicity with revolutionary agendas.

Television is one of the most inappropriate forums for political debate. Feminist debate is generally unwelcome, which is not surprising considering the male-dominated hierarchy. There is an obsession with ratings that makes the possibility of subversive programmes slight. As Michael Morgan explains, to ensure maximum profit "programme producers *have* to create programmes with the broadest possible appeal." Consequently it has become doctrine that making good television involves "avoiding perceived extremes" and "striving for a safe, respectable, 'middle-of-the-road' balance" so that "all presentations appear 'objective', 'moderate', 'non-ideological', and otherwise suitable for mass-marketing" (Morgan, 1989). If a programme is broadcast that does risk offence, the viewer can change the channel. Television encourages spectators to "prospect for images that astonish" rather than challenge; it is a "continually recording meter for desire" (Twitchell, 1992). For feminists challenging the status quo, television arguably offers the least attentive or responsive audience. This is particularly depressing with regard to comedy, as comics come from a tradition of live shows in which audience interruption is the norm.

The availability of images via mass media is a microcosmic example of the plurality that is a fundamental tenet of post-modern thought and culture. There is an emphasis on multiplicity rather than a "master discourse", on truth as contingent and local rather than fixed. Whilst this approach is invaluable inasmuch as it deconstructs the power bases and prejudices inherent in single-minded perspectives, it also leaves post-modernism potentially guilty of relativism or indifference. There is an awkward relationship between the desire for political activism and the knowledge that we cannot transcend the terms of our cultural and epistemological context. This political inertia has influenced both post-modern culture and its audience. The style of post-modern work, as Todd Gitlin has characterised it, "calls attention to its constructedness ... Instead of a single center there is pastiche, cultural recombination ... Not only has the master voice disappeared but any sense of loss is rendered deadpan" (Gitlin, 1989). These works draw and encourage an audience for whom "commitment dissolves into irony". It is also primarily the market for a specific post-modern class and generation: "Yuppies – urban professional products of the late baby boom ... [who] ... cannot remember a time before television, suburbs, shopping malls. They are accustomed therefore, to rapid cuts, discontinuities, breaches of attention, culture to be indulged and disdained at the same time". Post-modernism has given rise to neither an audience nor a culture prepared to accommodate a political method.

The plurality of post-modern culture and the potential indifference that it fosters is not limited to television comedy culture. The same sort of variety is available at club nights. The organisers expect the audience to laugh at material that reveals a large variety of political standpoints. As the comedian Jeremy Hardy wrote of one of his appearances at the London Comedy Store:

> There was a traditional club comic who got up at the comedy store and was racist and sexist and he just stormed. The audience might like me as well but they would be quite happy to see Jim Davidson or Bernard Manning. (Quoted in Rosenguard & Ward, 1989)

This political indifference of the comedy audience, whilst encouraged by the relativism of post-modern culture that Gitlin identifies, is also perpetrated by the ethos surrounding comedy in general. Most comics insist on a clear distinction between the comic and the political, and inevitably, given the imposed binary, give priority to the former. For example, in *Didn't You Kill My Mother-In-Law: The Story of Alternative Comedy in Britain From the Comedy Store to Saturday Night Live*, by the founder (Peter Rosenguard) and manager (Don Ward) of the London Comedy Store, the writers are at pains to establish their liberal credentials whilst equally anxious to point out that comedy is about making people laugh, not making "a point". Thus, whilst alternative comedy "avoids the easy but offensive laugh", this is because it is like the "best comics in any tradition". On Alexi Sayle they write "he did make politically flavoured jokes but he did not make the political message the *raison d'être* of his act." On feminist comedians they write "there is still a tendency to do very old fashioned anti-men material, but the best of them are now making their points with more subtlety" (Rosenguard & Ward, 1989).

The apolitical affectations of comedy culture affect female comics' perception of their political situation. Whereas there are fragments within most artistic circles that are informed by certain political debates (frequently feminist ones), comics are seldom divided by abstract ideas. In an essay on feminism and artistic strategies, Rozsika Parker and Griselda Pollock discuss some of the issues female artists consciously address (Parker & Pollock, 1987). They include whether or not to attempt mainstream success, how to encourage more women to become artistes, how to retrace female artistes who have not been recognised and what particular subjects and techniques are most suitable to feminist artistic practices. Similar discussions are also circulating amongst women dramatists (Forte, 1996). Amongst female comics, however, there is a sense that such issues are irrelevant. According to stand-up comic Jenny Lecoat "if you really want to change the world, you don't go into comedy. You learn to fire a gun and you go to El Salvador" (Rosenguard & Ward, 1989). The point is taken, but within the world of comedy and within the larger society that contains it there are a number of battles to be fought. With regards to feminism, activism seems to be muted not only out of the feeling that comedy is an inappropriate forum, but also a pronounced sense of professional competition. "My idea of hell is ten young women my age who are just absolutely brilliant", the comic Jenny Éclair once said. Similar sentiments have been voiced surprisingly often by female comics, each one sounding playful in isolation, but taken collectively indicating a possible reason why feminist strategies are not discussed among comediennes. There is a sense that there is only room for a few on the circuit.

There are of course exceptions to television and comedy's avoidance of the political. Critics in the 1970s were complaining that situation comedy projected myths that hide the fact that most women do jobs that "are normally unproductive and often socially useless" and that "most of them pay minimal wages" and that America is presented as a "country where almost everyone is middle class" (Kaplan, 1992).

Now the mass popularity of the television show *Roseanne*, which centres around a working class family, marks an almost isolated but significant indication that the old structure can be successfully attacked. The attack is endorsed by ratings rather than Utopian ideals, but none the less the journey from fighting to air what would have originally been considered subversive and revolutionary within the world of television comedy to the establishment of a programme like *Roseanne* as official, endorsed, (popular) culture, indicates that there is room both in comedy and television for the subversive to gain access to the mainstream.

There is a school of thought that would argue that any female comic, regardless of the content and delivery of her material, is a revolutionary performer.

> All women's performances are derived from the relationship of women to the dominant system of representation, situating them within a feminist critique. Their disruption of the dominant system constitutes a subversive and radical strategy of intervention *vis à vis* patriarchal culture. (Forte, 1990)

Forte's comment above is from an article about women's performance art – a form of performance which can sometimes resemble stand-up comedy so closely that the generic category into which some performers fit is unclear. The most significant common ground between performance art and stand-up comedy is that in both the artiste has complete control over how to represent the body that performs. This accounts for the prominence of women in performance art, the overtly political nature of many women's performances and the wealth of feminist analysis of the genre. Stand-up comedy by women has received less critical attention, and is embraced by less self-consciously political artistes. This is partly because performance art is considered to be a form of "high art" with polemical potential, whereas stand-up is associated with general entertainment with any political commitment dampened by the constraints of the media and mass popularity. None the less, there are a number of ways in which stand-up comedy by women can and does work towards some of the same feminist goals that women's performance art has been associated with. As an appendage to previous studies of the revolutionary potential of women's humour, I would like to suggest some of the ways in which stand-up comedy, as an art form, is particularly well suited to strategic feminist artistic practices.

As Lesley Ferris has argued, since the beginning of theatre women have been represented reductively. When women were excluded from performing on the stage, theatre "created the notion of women as sign, a symbolic object manipulated and controlled artistically by male playwrights and male actors". These "women" were broad caricatures – the speechless heroine, the wilful woman, the golden girl (Ferris, 1990). Once women were allowed on the stage "they merely played themselves", wearing their own clothes, and were encouraged to impose their own persona upon each role. They were thus "removed from any possibility of cultural creativity". The effect was the same both before and after women were allowed onto the stage: "the individual woman herself stood for the role." Any woman could signify the sign.

Stand-up comedy provides a departure from this condition as public and pervasive as the legacy theatrical misogyny has left. Stand-up is dependent not only on strong material but also on the strong and distinctive personality of the performer. Women write themselves, and although there is inevitably a distinction between the nuances of the comic's true personality and the persona that she projects on stage, stand-up is quite distinct from the traditional role of women on the stage.

This is equally true of women performance artists. Forte connects the strategies used by women performance artists in representing themselves with the emphasis that Luce Irigaray and especially Hélène Cixous place on using the female body as a base for female empowerment. She makes the thought-provoking suggestion that Cixous' and Irigaray's promotion of the female body and sexuality as the inspirational sites for a new, marked women's writing outside the phallocentric system of representation is a strategy "much more vividly realised in the context of women's performance than in writing".

> The very placement of the female body in the context of performance art positions a woman and her sexuality as speaking subject, an action which cuts across numerous sign-systems, not just the discourse of language. (Forte, 1990)

Forte's assumption here is that the performance artiste is able to control how her body is perceived by the gestural or verbal text that she inscribes upon it. In practice, however, a lot of women's performance art attracts audience and critical attention by the strong element of interest on the explicit and "obscene" presentation of the (often naked) female body. This practical consideration reflects some of the more abstract criticisms of the work of Irigaray and Cixous: they, like the voyeurs in the audience, arguably reduce the woman to no more than the physical. Furthermore, "if language, as they claim, is phallocentric, then female drives are by definition incapable of representation within it" (Bowlby, 1983). Even if the performance artiste considers her representation as seeing beyond the world of the symbolic, the female body in performance art cannot be freed from the patriarchal signs already inscribed on it because the audience, contaminated by phallocentrism, can re-code the symbols back into their own reductive terms.

Whilst performance artistes have worked on strategies to prevent voyeuristic reception, the very nature of stand-up comedy helps to bypass this problem, whilst still leaving space for Forte's (and Irigaray's and Cixous') "woman and her sexuality as speaking subject". Comedy is one of the very few instances that an audience is paying to hear and respond to women's words. Whilst a female comic who is not well established may be reduced to a sexual sign by her audience (as in "get your tits out"), there is little space for voyeurism. Yet this does not in any way neutralise the impact of the female body and its presence on the stage. The female body in performance is empowered by the audience's interest but not reduced to a sexual symbol. "Comedy," according to Elaine Boostler, "is very very sexy when it's done right" (Barreca, 1996), but the sexual attractiveness and indeed "otherness" of the performer involves her wit rather than her tits.

Whilst women in stand-up comedy may be attacking the patriarchal order, comedy protects them against the accusation levelled at Cixous and Irigaray about being unable to escape the confines of phallocentrism. Rather than an attempt at escape, a staple in most stand-up sets is parody and pastiche. This can range from observational comedy about fairly neutral issues which once articulated sound absurd ("I could *see* the ring road, couldn't get at it . . .") to more directly political and aggressive mimicry:

> When this judge let a rapist go because the woman had been wearing a miniskirt and so was "asking for it" I thought, ladies, what we all should do is this: next time we see an ugly guy on the street shoot him. After all, he knew he was ugly when he left the house. He was asking for it. (Quoted in Barreca, 1996)

Ellen Cleghorn, quoted above, deconstructs through an imitation that highlights the absurdity of the original model. This sort of comedy, it is worth noting, effectively responds to the post-modern concern that as critics we are unable to transcend our own subjectivity and limited viewpoint. As well as being a strategy that responds to post-modern anxieties, it is also connected to the concerns that feminists have about the nature of artistic practices. Elin Diamond, amongst others, has suggested that the concept of "mimesis" and "realism" are problematic for feminists and feminist artistic practices. "Mimesis" implies a truthful relation between the world and its representation, a concept that feminists, and post-modernist discourses in general, have done much to undermine. For feminists, she points out, this "truth" is inseparable from gender-biased epistemologies. However, she continues, feminists do have a stake in the concept of objective truth: "the critique of patriarchy carries with it a commitment to the truth value of one's own position, however complex and nuanced that position might be" (Diamond, 1993). She concludes by suggesting that although mimesis is suspect when used unself-consciously, it "can be retheorised as a site of, and means of, feminist intervention". Comic parody is part of this process.

Stand-up comedy also addresses feminist concerns with regard to realism from another perspective. As Catherine Belsey puts it, "classic realism is dominated by 'illusionism', a narrative which leads to 'closure,' and a 'hierarchy of discourses' which establishes the 'truth' of the story." She goes on:

> . . . the story moves inevitably towards closure which is also disclosure, the dissolution of enigma through the re-establishment of order, recognisable as a re-instatement or a development of the order which is understood to have proceeded the events of the story itself. (Quoted in Forte, 1996)

Belsey's description of realism is remarkably similar to conventional descriptions of comedy as a literary genre. Northrop Frye, as a representative example, writes in the "Argument of comedy" that comedy's closure is marked by "a renewed sense of social integration" (Frye, 1984). Riddles are unravelled, lovers make up and marry, and the disruptive holiday is replaced by the re-establishment of welcome order and maturity. This sort of understanding of the comic structure ("the *laws* of comic form", he calls it) is unsatisfactory to feminists. It imposes reintegration into a society within which disruption may well have been a welcome release for women. Thus in Shakespeare's comedies, for example, the freedom permitted heroines such as Rosalind and Viola when disguised as men in the middle of *As You Like It* and *Twelfth Night* is cancelled at the end of each play when they return to their dresses and "social integration" in both cases through wedlock. A feminist "happy ending" is not met by the closure that inflexible definitions impose on the genre of comedy.

Thus, suitably, in her study of comedy in Virginia Woolf and Murial Spark, Judy Little argues that a "lack of closure, this lack of resolution, characterises the feminist comedy" (Little, 1983). Whilst a lack of closure is a technique that these writers consciously imitate, it is the essence of the form of stand-up comedy. The stand-up's set is always inconclusive.

It is abruptly terminated with a "thank you and good night" and then picked up again the next time the comic does a set. Rather than a temporary disruption that is resolved, the stand-up comedienne remains constantly disruptive in the audience's imagination: time removes her from the stage but her disruptive presence is not reintegrated into the social order by common consensus.

The potential and problems relating to women and stand-up comedy would justify a much longer analysis. This is an overview of issues that could be explored in more detail, and it has barely touched on questions about class, race and sexuality, all of which complicate and invigorate analysis and indeed closure. By way of conclusion here, suffice to say that the scope for parody, the fusion of realism with the absurd and the anti-closure that stand-up comedy allows, together with the space it can give the female subject to articulate her concerns and present herself and her body as she chooses, mark it as a genre that, regardless of content, has inherent and potential space for feminist strategies. Which is all a very long-winded justification of the fact that I find Joan Rivers funny.

REFERENCES

Appleyard, B. (1996). Why smut is no laughing matter. *The Times*, 1 December 1996.

Auslander, P. (1992). *Presence and Resistance: Postmodernism and Cultural Politics in Contemporary American Performance*. Ann Arbor: University of Michigan Press.

Barreca, R. (1988). *Last Laughs: Perspectives on Women and Comedy*, Vol. 1. Philadelphia: Gordon and Breach.

Barreca, R. (1991). *They Used to Call Me Snow White But I Drifted: Women's Strategic Use of Humor*. New York: Penguin.

Barreca, R. (1994). *Untamed and Unabashed: Essays on Humor in British Literature*. Detroit: Wayne State University Press.

Bowlby, R. (1983). The feminine female. *Social Text*, Spring/Summer 1983, 54–61.

Diamond, E. (1993). Mimesis, mimicry, and the 'True–Real'. In Hart, L., & Phelan, P. (Eds.), *Acting Out: Feminist Performances* (pp.363–379). Ann Arbor: University of Michigan Press.

Ferris, L. (1990). *Acting Women: Images of Women in Theatre*. London: Basingstoke: Macmillan.

Fitz, L.T. (1994). Egyptian queens and male reviewers: sexist attitudes in *Antony and Cleopatra*: criticism. In Drakakis, J. (Ed.), *New Casebook: Antony and Cleopatra* (pp.180–192). Basingstoke: Macmillan.

Forte, J. (1990). Women's performance art: feminism and postmodernism. In Case, S.E. (Ed.), *Performing Feminisms: Feminist Critical Theory and Theatre* (pp.251–261). Baltimore: Johns Hopkins University Press.

Forte, J. (1996). Realism, narrative and the feminist playwright. In Keysser, H. (Ed.), *Feminist Theatre and Theory* (pp.19–30). Baltimore: Johns Hopkins University Press.

Frye, N. (1984). The argument of comedy. In Palmer, D.J. (Ed.), *Comedy: Developments in Criticism, A Casebook* (pp.74–85). London: Macmillan.

Gitlin, T. (1989). Postmodernism: roots and politics. In Angus, I., & Jhally, S. (Eds.), *Cultural Politics in Contemporary America* (pp.347–361). London: Routledge.

Gray, F. (1994). *Women and Laughter*. Basingstoke: Macmillan.

Kader, C. (1990). Kate Clinton: the production and reception of feminist humour. In Raymond, D. (Ed.), *Sexual Politics and Popular Culture* (pp.49–55). Bowling Green, Ohio: Bowling Green State University Press.

Kaplan, C.A. (1992). Feminist criticism and television. In Allen, R. (Ed.), *Channels of Discourse: Television and Contemporary Criticism* (pp.247–283). London: Routledge.

Little, J. (1983). *Comedy and the Woman Writer: Woolf, Spark, and Feminism*. Nebraska: Lincoln, Nebraska: University of Nebraska Press.

Morgan, M. (1989). Television and democracy. In Angus, J., & Jhally, S. (Eds.), *Cultural Politics in Contemporary America* (pp.240–253). London: Routledge.

Palmer, J. (1994). *Taking Humour Seriously*. London: Routledge.

Parker, R., & Pollock, G. (1987). Fifteen years of feminist action: from practical strategies to strategic practices. In Parker, R., & Pollock, G. (Eds.), *Framing Feminism: Art and the Women's Movement 1970–1985* (pp.3–79). London: Pandora.

Rivers, J. with Merryman, R. (1992). *Still Talking*. London: Arrow.

Rosenguard, P., & Ward, D. (1989). *Didn't You Kill My Mother-In-Law: The Story of Alternative Comedy in Britain From the Comedy Store to Saturday Night Live*. London: Methuen.

Toth, E. (1981). Female wits. *The Massachusetts Review*, Winter 1981, 783–794.

Twitchell, J.B. (1992). *Carnival Culture: The Trashing of Taste in America*. New York: Columbia University Press.

Walker, J. (1988). *A Very Serious Thing: Women's Humor and American Culture*. Minneapolis: University of Minnesota Press.

Walker, N., & Dresner, Z. (Eds.) (1988). *Redressing the Balance: American Women's Literary Humor from Colonial Time to the 1980s*. Jackson: University Press of Mississippi.

Wilt, J. (1980). The laughter of the maidens and the cackles of the matriarchs. In Todd, J. (Ed.), *Women and Literature* (pp.171–182). New York: Holmes and Meier.

Wood, V. (1996). *Chunky*. London: Methuen.

Chapter 10

Psychological, Social, and Economic Implications of Bereavement Among Older Women

Christine L. McKibbin,[1,2,4,5] **Darrelle Koonce-Volwiler,**[1,2,4,5]
Ruth C. Cronkite,[3–5] **and Dolores Gallagher-Thompson**[1–5]

Older Adult and Family Research and Resource Center,[1] *Geriatric Research and Clinical Center,*[2] *Department of Health Services Research and Development,*[3] *Veterans Affairs Palo Alto Health Care System,*[4] *and Stanford University School of Medicine*[5]

CURRENT AND EXPECTED INCIDENCE OF BEREAVEMENT

The number of bereaved women in the United States will dramatically increase by the middle of the next century. This projected growth is largely due to the fact that life expectancy has increased and baby-boomers are now reaching geriatric age. Currently, there are about 12 million widowed men and women in the United States, with approximately 800 000 new widows and widowers annually. Strikingly, it has been estimated that by the age of 65 years, 35% of all women have been widowed at least once and this rate of widowhood rises to 59% at age 75 and 79% at age 85 and over (United States Bureau of the

Women, Health and the Mind
Edited by L. Sherr and J.S. St Lawrence. © 2000 John Wiley & Sons, Ltd

Census, 1993). These rates may be considerably higher if one were to take into account other common types of bereavement (e.g. death of an adult child, aging parent, or sibling). Given these bereavement rates and the fact that the number of elderly in the population is on the rise, it stands to reason that there will be many more bereaved older women in the United States by the middle of the next century than there are today. Because women of the baby-boom generation are more likely to enjoy a longer life expectancy, many may be bereaved later and may experience more years of being bereaved than do the women of today (Hobbs & Damon, 1996).

These future scores of bereaved older women are expected to differ from today's older women in several ways especially in their social, demographic, and health characteristics (Hobbs & Damon, 1996). Because each of these factors are believed to be related to the bereavement experience and recovery process, continued attention to both mental and physical health implications of bereavement, as well as intervention strategies to ameliorate negative effects of bereavement, is critical. Therefore, the purpose of this chapter is to provide a brief overview of well-known bereavement literature widely presented in chapters and journals that pertain to stages of grief, pathological grief reactions, the grief experiences of today's older women, and factors that impact their adjustment process. Finally, there will be a section highlighting areas in need of future research.

OVERVIEW OF THE BEREAVEMENT PROCESS

Before discussing what is understood as the normal and pathological bereavement processes, it is important to differentiate grief from mourning, for which it is often interchanged. Bereavement is differentiated from grief in that bereavement is the objective situation of having lost someone significant in life, while grief is the actual emotional response to that loss. Mourning, on the other hand, reflects the manner of expressing grief that often reflects cultural practices (Stroebe et al., 1988). Although bereavement, grief, and mourning are distinct, we will use the term bereavement process to encompass the bereavement event, process of mourning, and experience of grief.

The modern conceptualisation of bereavement originated with Freud's (1917) definition of mourning in which he described mourning as the process by which "each single one of the memories and situations of expectancy which demonstrate the libido's attachment to the lost object is met by the verdict of reality that the object no longer exists." Later theorists such as Kubler-Ross (1968), Bowlby (1971, 1980), Glick et al., (1974), and Pollock (1987) delineated stage models of the bereavement process that take either a sequential or non-sequential course. The general consensus among these theorists is that the bereavement process is comprised of an initial state of shock, disbelief, and denial, followed by pining and yearning, then despair, and finally acceptance and return to normal functioning (Bowlby, 1971; Parkes, 1965; Parkes & Brown, 1972). Although these stage models are attractive for understanding the bereavement process and its chronological course, one must be cautious in the application of these stages to bereaved persons. Specifically, research has shown that grief reactions do not tend to follow distinct stages and bereaved persons may not pass through stages in the same order or in the same time frame and some may skip a particular stage entirely. Further, there is little agreement about the time-course of normal bereavement. Depressive symptoms associated with normal bereavement vary, lasting from 6 months (Prigerson et al., 1996) up to 2½ years after the loss or longer (Farberow et al., 1992; Zisook et al., 1987).

Although the grief experience associated with bereavement typically declines with time for most women, the process of recovery can be more difficult and long lasting for others. The point at which normal grief actually becomes pathological has only recently become better understood. According to Rosenzweig et al. (1997), symptoms of pathological grief, taken together, are more likely to represent a major depressive episode and include:

- feelings of guilt other than regarding actions taken or not taken by the survivor at the time of death
- thoughts of death other than the survivor feeling that he or she would be better off dead or should have died with the deceased person
- morbid preoccupation with worthlessness
- marked psychomotor retardation
- prolonged and marked functional impairment
- hallucinatory experiences other than thinking that he or she hears the voice of, or transiently sees the image of the deceased person

Others have addressed criteria from additional disorders which may mark a pathological reaction to grief, including the anxiety disorders and post-traumatic stress disorder (Stroebe et al., 1993).

Prigerson et al. (1995) argued that symptoms of complicated grief are distinct from bereavement-related depression (i.e. sad mood, apathy, guilt) and anxiety (i.e. irritability, nervousness, tenseness, and restlessness). In fact, they developed a scale titled the Inventory of Complicated Grief in order to accurately assess and identify maladaptive grief reactions in widowed elderly populations. They found that complicated grief includes, but is not limited to, thinking about the person so much that it creates disruptions in daily routines, being drawn to places associated with the deceased person, feeling lonely or bitter, avoiding reminders of the person, being upset by memories of the person who died, or angry about the person's death. Symptoms such as these signify a complicated grief process when they are experienced frequently over time and tend to disrupt an individual's capacity to carry out daily activities.

Scrutton (1995) conceptualised pathological grief in a similar way. However, he differentiated between several types of complicated grief reactions that encompass many of the symptoms described by Rosenzweig et al. (1997), including complicated, exaggerated, chronic, delayed, and masked grief. Those experiencing "complicated" grief believe that they cannot recover from their loss. This response is characteristic of "exaggerated" grief when the grief is an excessively intense feeling which frequently disables the individual. "Chronic" grief occurs when the reaction to loss is unremitting and continues for months or even years. On the other hand, grief may also be "delayed" and the individual appears to be acting quite normally by diverting initial pain. Finally, the grief may become "masked" when intense emotions manifest in physical and medical symptoms for which the surviving individual seeks medical attention.

REACTION TO DIFFERENT TYPES OF BEREAVEMENT

It is generally accepted that the type of relationship lost due to death influences the grief reaction and bereavement process of the survivor. The relationship to the deceased has such an influence because the needs, hopes, and expectations differ with each type of relationship as do the personal meaning and social implications of the loss (Osterweis et al., 1984). The influence of relationship on the bereavement process will be very briefly described with a review of the literature based on two types of bereavement common to older women: loss of a spouse and loss of an adult child. Because bereavement experiences of older women are the focus of this chapter, women's reactions to prenatal and infant deaths as well as deaths of young children will not be reviewed. However, there are several substantial overviews of bereavement theory and reactions among younger women (Klass, 1996; Osterweis et al., 1984; Rubin, 1993).

A woman's loss of her spouse is widely accepted as being one of the most stressful of all possible losses (Holmes & Rahe, 1967). This loss is particularly stressful because death of a spouse really encompasses many important losses including the loss of her household and financial co-manager, her companion, and her social and sexual partner. As a result, a woman is left to either make many task, emotional, and identity transitions or face tolerating a more difficult and lonelier life. In terms of expression of grief, widows tend to be more emotionally expressive and tend to cry more than do widowers. Widows also tend not to reinvest in new intimate relationships for a year or more after their husband's death (Glick et al., 1975). Among physically frail elderly women, the process of redefining their social identities and social and intimate relationships may be further impeded.

Although some believe that loss of a spouse is one of the most stressful events, others believe that loss of an adult child in later life is even more painful (Moss et al., 1984). In spite of this view, little empirical research (Cacace & Williamson, 1996; Goodman et al., 1991; Leshner & Bergey, 1988) has addressed this latter type of bereavement. Attention to losses of children among elderly women is important because this untimely death may generate many losses, including loss of identity as a life-long parent (Hocker, 1988; Schatz, 1986), loss of love, companionship, decision-making loss pertaining to treatment and burial (Rando, 1986a), and loss of financial security. These many losses may engender fears of isolation, particularly if she has already lost her spouse or other members of her social support network (Karlan, 1988; Rando, 1986a); insecurity; guilt (Miles & Demi, 1986); and anxiety (Schatz, 1986; Stevenson, 1988). According to a recent study conducted by Cacace & Williamson (1996), most elderly parents were able to overcome some of their initial devastation and resume regular activities within a few weeks of their child's death. A few strategies seemed to help the elderly bereaved parents in this study with their coping. Those who were able to help with direct care and emotional support of their dying children and their families reported feeling less guilt and regret. In addition, parents stressed the benefits of helping grandchildren cope with the loss of their parents and benefits of seeking support from friends, extended family, support groups, and counseling (Cacace & Williamson, 1996).

IMPLICATIONS OF CONJUGAL BEREAVEMENT AMONG OLDER WOMEN

When a woman in today's era loses her spouse, there are a number of gender specific issues that surface. This is especially true when the woman is elderly, as she was probably raised in a time of clear, specific roles for women. Some of the issues that pertain to today's elderly woman who loses a spouse or partner have been outlined by previous authors including Anderson & Dimond (1995), Cline (1995), and Scrutton (1995). Some of the general conclusions of these authors are outlined below.

Generally speaking, we can discuss the change in an older woman's role in the context of our current time. Older women of future generations, such as the baby-boomers, will probably not experience the same role changes, because of the current differences in male/female roles. Rather, these women will likely be more independent and have their own sources of income separate from their partners (Hobbs & Damon, 1996). Therefore, the issues related to older women of today will be discussed, keeping in mind that these issues will change over time as the baby-boom generation ages.

Role Loss

A significant issue faced by today's older bereaved woman is that of a role change. The vast majority of the women over age 65 were raised to be dependent on their husbands for financial well-being and also for important decision-making. Women have not only assumed the role of the passive spouse who carries out the requests of her husband, but also may not see themselves as whole people without their husbands (Scrutton, 1995). Cline (1995) has described the older widow as stigmatised as not having a role in our society, in addition to being subjected to agism. She wrote that widows are often treated as being "touched by death", and therefore avoided. People in our culture don't like to talk about death or be reminded of it. This puts the widow in a difficult position. The widower, on the other hand, is usually the subject of great concern and is not avoided but sought out to nurture, primarily by women. The older widow may also lack the skills to complete tasks formerly handled by her husband. Such difficulties have been reported in a study on responses to bereavement (Anderson & Dimond, 1995) and include yard work, home maintenance, and car repairs.

Impact on Social Life

Many bereaved older women find themselves without the skills to initiate and maintain new social relationships following the loss of their spouse. They may struggle with beliefs that they are dishonoring their lost husband if they date other men and may not know how to go about meeting new people. Many social functions for older adults are geared towards couples, making it uncomfortable and difficult to find male companionship. Often they may not be invited or feel awkward at functions previously attended with a spouse, due to an overall feeling of low social worth (Cline, 1995). Due to previous roles, older women may also lack assertiveness skills necessary to pursuing new relationships. If family members live nearby, they often become an important focal point of the bereaved older woman's socialisation (Anderson & Dimond, 1995).

Financial Implications

Often, due to previous roles and limited skills, the bereaved older woman is less practiced at handling financial matters and less knowledgeable as well. She may have fears and experience hesitation in making important financial decisions (Scrutton, 1995). A particularly special financial concern that has received more attention recently is that of the partnered women who is cohabiting but is either unmarried to her male partner or is lesbian. This cohabitation status often leaves women with no legal right to inheritance. Unless these women have totally independent sources of income, they may be left financially drained by the loss of their partners.

Sexual Issues

The older bereaved woman is more likely than younger widows to adhere to traditional sexual roles and to be hesitant to date, spend an evening alone in public with a man, or become sexually involved with another person (Scrutton, 1995). This may make it more likely that a bereaved older woman remarries as opposed to having a long dating history following the loss of a husband.

Cline (1995) presents a different view on sexuality of widows. She believes that our culture assumes that all women want to be sexually involved, and that celibacy constitutes failure. Friends and family of the widow may persist in trying to "set her up" with some eligible bachelor, without first consulting with her to determine her needs and desires. In some cases the elderly widow is interested in pursuing a sexual relationship but may want to do it at her own pace. Other women are content with their celibacy and may even wish to remain partnerless.

With all of these potential areas of difficulty for the older bereaved woman, there is good news. Zisook et al. (1993) found in their report on aging and bereavement, that older widows and widowers had more positive perceptions of their ability to adjust to loss than younger ones, and the oldest had more consistent improvement over time. We can conclude from this that any myths or stereotypes we have about the elderly being less able to cope or adapt are not supported. The elderly may, indeed, be more capable of handling the loss of a loved one than are the younger bereaved.

FACTORS AFFECTING BEREAVEMENT ADJUSTMENT

In the vast literature on the effect of social support on the bereaved, two terms stand out as primary in regards to adjustment. The first term is social network and the second is social support. These terms are generally defined as separate, but related. Below are some general definitions to facilitate understanding of these terms.

Social Networks

The bereaved woman's social network plays a large role in how effectively she copes with the loss of a loved one. A support network can be defined as all the people and groups who provide support, including family, friends, co-workers, neighbours, and organisations (Lopata, 1993). Generally, research focused on support networks looks at frequency of encounters and closeness to those in the network.

Social Support

Researchers and theorists have defined social support as having two functional types. The first type is affective or emotional support, such as people who are confided in, talked to when upset, and who call often; while the second is instrumental or task-oriented support, for example help with tasks such as finances, chores, and errands (Schuster & Butler, 1989).

Schuster & Butler (1989), in their study on the effects of social network and social support on overall mental health adjustment of the bereaved, found that they contributed to all five areas of mental health studied, but in varying degrees. These areas included anomie (i.e. self-to-others alienation and desire to withdraw), anxiety, life satisfaction, future orientation, and perceived mental health. They concluded that both social networks, which generally refers to closeness of network and frequency of contact, and social support are important to adjustment in their own ways. Therefore, we cannot assume that a person will adjust adequately solely based on the number of supportive contacts they have, or the closeness to the people in their network, as previously thought.

In another study, Duran et al. (1989) also looked at social support in general and how it can serve as a buffer to stressful life experience such as bereavement. They hypothesised that if social support remains intact, a stressful event may have a less severe impact. Interestingly, the findings of this study identified no relationship between social support and stress measured right after the loss (at 6 months or 1 year), but the enduring social support system did show positive effects on stress after 2 years. Because we understand from other research that bereavement is a long-term process (Parkes & Weiss, 1983), this study provides more evidence for effects of social support in the process of bereavement. The study by Schuster & Butler (1989) found that the timing of when support was received had some different effects. For instance, support received at the time of death appears to have greater impact on the bereaved person's current mental health than current support or network closeness and frequency of contact.

Cognitive Appraisal and Coping

How one thinks about bereavement has been examined in the literature as a marker associated with the health outcomes of widows and widowers following bereavement. Some of the thinking processes involved include the meaning assigned to bereavement by the individual and the degree of perceived threat experienced. In a study looking at this appraisal (Gass, 1989), women who described their bereavement experience as "a harmful loss with other anticipated threats" were at a greater risk for health problems than women who described their experience as "a harmful loss without other losses" or "a challenge". These women had more psychosocial difficulties as well as health problems, but the more significant problems were in the psychosocial arena.

Gass (1989) explains that this style of thinking about bereavement can lead to poor coping strategies. She states that the women who endorsed the "other anticipated threats" category had a tendency to engage in more self-blame, wishful thinking, and mixed coping than other widows. These women defined their bereavement as a loss with many additional losses and fears, as well as anticipated problems that they believed they would be unable to manage. The widows who made a higher threat appraisal did use more coping strategies than women in the other categories and were associated with higher levels of psychosocial dysfunction.

DIVERSITY ISSUES

Grief is a human response to bereavement that occurs universally across all age groups and throughout all cultures. This inevitable experience has received much interest from professionals across a variety of disciplines. However, there are some aspects of the bereavement process about which relatively little is known. One of the most important aspects is the role that culture and heritage plays in an individual's grief experience and bereavement rituals and practices (Cowels, 1996). In the past, bereavement experiences and processes have largely been studied and discussed with reference to the Anglo-American culture. On the other hand, the interrelationship of culture and bereavement process, rituals, and practice has only recently received substantial research interest. Consequently, much of the available psychological literature regarding bereavement reflects that which is understood about Anglo-Americans.

Some anthropologists, physicians, sociologists, and psychologists, on the other hand have focused on a broad range of what are considered "appropriate" bereavement rituals and practices that highlight important cultural beliefs (Buchwald et al., 1994; Irish et al., 1993; Kleinman et al., 1978). Literature from this field underscores the need to pay close attention to the many factors that vary across cultures and impact upon the bereavement process. First and foremost are differences in meanings about the loss. As Lofland (1978) pointed out over a decade ago and others have more recently affirmed (Landrine & Klonoff, 1992), losses have different meanings from person to person and from culture to culture. For example, a spouse may or may not be a person on whom one depends economically or with whom one shares intimate thoughts and feelings. Depending upon the type(s) of connectedness experienced, a spouse's death may signify a wide range of losses or a narrower range of less crucial losses, some of which may easily be replaced. Furthermore, differences in cognitive interpretations of the meaning of one's loss lead to different behavioral manifestations of grief. Rosenblatt (1988) described what he terms a striking difference between grief in acculturated Americans and that expressed in many other cultures: among Americans, grief is often psychologised whereas in China and many other Asian societies, for example, grief is more likely to be expressed in somatic form. "People experience serious personal and social problems but interpret and articulate them and come to experience and respond to them through the medium of the body" (Kleinman, 1986, p.51).

Since so little research has been done on the positive and negative impacts of bereavement in groups such as Chinese Americans (and other ethnic minority groups in the United States), we have to be extremely cautious in generalising what we know from Anglo-Americans to the other groups. In fact, as Rosenblatt (1993) concluded, it may be "patently absurd" to use notions of pathology derived from one culture to evaluate people from another. His work includes numerous examples of how ethnocentric perspectives can be misleading, such as the Balinese mother who, after sudden death of her child remains calm and cheerful based on the belief that the gods will not heed one's prayers if one is not calm, at least on the surface. That behavior would probably be judged pathological by Northern American standards, yet for many recent immigrants (and for those who maintain strong ties with their culture of origin even though they have resided in the United States for a number of years), it would be expected by their social network of family and friends.

Factors for particular consideration when working with bereaved women include the role of the family, family structure (extended versus nuclear), the bereaved individual's and family's level of acculturation, as well as funeral and death anniversary rituals. For example, to a greater degree than for Anglo-Americans, the family is the central institution for many Mexican-Americans even though the impact of family has been eroded somewhat by assimilation, acculturation, and societal changes that have presented conflicting values (Portillo, 1989). Mexican-American families are often large systems consisting of parents, children, spouses, grandchildren, siblings, nieces and nephews, and, unlike Anglo-Americans, friends who are symbolically incorporated into the family via the *compadrazgo* (co-parenthood) system (Velez, 1980). Because these families are often warm, nurturing, and cohesive (Murillo, 1971), they are likely to be a powerful source of social support and play a critical role in the adjustment process of bereaved elderly women of Mexican-American identity.

Acculturation, similarly, is an important factor determining how women respond to major losses in their lives. Acculturation is generally viewed as a continuum reflecting the extent to which immigrants modify cultural beliefs, attitudes, and practices as a result of contact with the dominant culture until they assimilate and incorporate more and more characteristics of the prevailing culture (e.g. language, food preferences, celebration of holidays, and health care beliefs and practices) (Purnell & Paulanka, 1998). Generally, acculturation increases with length of residence, so that second and third generation Japanese or Chinese Americans, for example tend to be much more "Americanised" than first generation families from Vietnam or other Southeast Asia countries (Kitano & Daniels, 1988; Matocha, 1998). It is similar for other groups: for example, Mexican-Americans who have lived in the United States for many years have different views of death, dying, and bereavement, and different death rituals and practices from those who have more recently arrived from Mexico (Moore, 1970; Younoszai, 1993). It is said that death is present everywhere in Mexico: in the literature, on murals and in the streets. According to Younoszai (1993) death is seen as a part of life and an everyday occurrence, particularly in poor and rural areas. When death occurs in Mexico, the extended family is united, the body is on view at home (open casket) and food and drink are served while family and friends socialise. In contrast, in the United States, Mexican-Americans who are practicing Catholics may follow some similar rituals, but death is more often due to violence (homicide or drug-related) and so less peaceful acceptance and religious comfort can occur. Belief in an afterlife, where families will be reunited, appears to be more typical of less acculturated Mexican-Americans (who are often orthodox Catholics) while those who are more acculturated and/or better educated may have different beliefs, thus strongly influencing how death is perceived and how it is responded to. Cuban-Americans, in contrast, are often regarded as being more bi-cultural than many other Hispanic groups: they adjust well to mainstream American culture while remaining close to their Cuban roots (Grossman, 1998). They tend to be highly educated, religiously diverse (e.g. a fair proportion are of the Jewish faith), and economically advantaged. Yet as far as death rituals are concerned Cubans tend to be highly emotionally demonstrative and, thus, tend to be similar to other Hispanic groups. Some, however, practice a unique religious system called *santeria*, which is a blend of African and Roman Catholic elements that has its own set of practices around bereavement including, for example, use of animal sacrifice and related rites (called "ebo") to appease the gods and solicit their support.

Of course, generalisations about beliefs and practices should be avoided when actually conducting research or working directly with bereaved women of varying ethnic backgrounds. There is no substitute for directly asking the person what their cultural beliefs and practices are, and how these may positively (or negatively) impact on the bereavement process (see Buchwald et al., 1994, for specific suggestions). Based on literature presented thus far, it is clear that the interaction of culture and loss can create differences in the process of grief and bereavement that are very real. In order to better understand these interrelationships and to better serve older bereaved women of varying ethnic identities, further study is required.

HEALTH CARE COSTS RELATED TO BEREAVEMENT

Health care utilisation can be perceived as a consequence of bereavement that has important implications for the health care delivery system. Given the aging of the population and the associated increase in the prevalence of bereavement, the role that bereavement plays in physician visits and hospitalisations is highly salient for understanding and anticipating demands on the health care system. The percentage of bereaved who visit a physician during the first year of bereavement ranges from 40 to 85%, while the proportion of bereaved who make more than three physician visits during the year is approximately 20%. Similarly, approximately one-fifth of bereaved individuals are hospitalised (Mor et al., 1986; Steen, 1998).

While most studies find that the bereaved report declines in physical and mental health compared to married controls, other studies yield inconsistent findings regarding differential utilisation of mental health services, physician services, and hospitalisations (Carey, 1977; Clayton, 1974, 1975; Gallagher et al., 1983; Osterweis et al., 1984; Parkes & Brown, 1972; Steen, 1998; Thompson et al., 1984; Williams & Polak, 1979; Yeaworth & Valanis, 1985). In comparison with women whose husbands had experienced a myocardial infarction, the prevalence rate of primary care visits for physiological causes among a group of bereaved wives was almost three times higher (54.2 versus 19%; Surtees, 1995). When compared with age- and sex-adjusted national norms, Mor et al. (1986) found that the bereaved show higher rates of physician visits but lower hospitalisation rates. The elevated number of physician visits may reflect pent-up demand following deferred use of physician services during the period of intensive care giving. Alternatively, higher-than-expected utilisation of physician visits may reflect attempts to seek social support and/or a somatisation of the emotional distress associated with grief (Mor et al., 1986).

Research on bereavement outcomes has yielded a number of risk factors that may also be associated with health care utilisation among the bereaved, such as type of loss (conjugal versus other), age, gender, education, primary care giver health status, and depressive symptoms. Mor et al. (1986) found that physical limitations and depressed mood among bereaved care givers are associated with increased physician visits, while physical limitations and being the spouse of the deceased were important predictors of depressive symptoms and of hospitalisation. The increased risk associated with being a spouse of the deceased may be due to the greater disruption in fundamental life domains, such as family roles and finances (McHorney & Mor, 1988).

Social support may also play an important stress-buffering role in the association between bereavement and health care utilisation. Krause (1988) found that elderly people who experienced strong social support systems during bereavement make fewer visits to a physician for symptoms, while those with low social support reported more physician visits for symptoms. These findings point to the potential value of social resources in reducing physician visits among elderly adults during bereavement.

In summary, bereaved individuals are at risk for increased physician visits. Other than physical limitations, risk factors among the bereaved that are associated with increased utilisation include being the spouse of the deceased, depression-related somatisation, and low social support. Given the expected growth of the bereaved population, more research is needed on identifying risk factors for increased health care utilisation. Timely and appropriate treatment aimed at alleviating and preventing the morbidity brought on by bereavement may also be cost-effective in averting significant costs to the health care system.

INTERVENTION PROGRAMS

Roles of Health Professionals

Generally speaking, health professionals assume a variety of roles and responsibilities when caring for a dying patient and their family members. These responsibilities do not end when the patient is gone, but change to a focus on the grieving family. According to Osterweis et al. (1984), in their report on research findings on bereavement, it is vital that all health professionals develop an approach to addressing the bereavement process in the family members of their patients. The health professional's reaction will undoubtedly leave some impact on the family member, so it is best to have some guidelines on how to handle the grieving person. At a minimum, it is important to inform and educate the recently bereaved, keeping in mind that people differ regarding the type of information they want and how much they are able to take in at a given time. An additional minimum requirement is to provide emotional support, recognise when an individual's bereavement reaction is abnormal, and provide appropriate referrals to mental health professionals.

Given that increasing numbers of deaths are occurring in hospitals, for patients in medical facilities special considerations should be made around the time of death, such as allowing family members to be in the room with their loved one while her or she is dying and after the death as well. If family are not present, informing them immediately is recommended, and postponing the movement of the body until family have arrived and made their wishes known is beneficial to the grieving process. It is helpful to discuss with the family in advance their differing cultural and/or religious beliefs and practices regarding the dead, to avoid causing additional difficulties for the family by doing something inappropriate. Following the death of a patient, health professionals need to continue their contact with the family members of the deceased. The bereaved often need to go over aspects of the illness and the death of their loved ones.

Mutual Support Interventions

From 1964 to 1974, Phyllis Silverman, under the direction of Gerald Caplan at the Laboratory of Community Psychiatry at Harvard University, created the widow-to-widow program. During their research on widows, Silverman discovered that the best time to offer help to widows was 3–6 weeks after the death (a time when they are more open to help), and that the help should be offered one-on-one with another widow who could serve as a role model. This can eventually lead to participating in groups with other widows to gain knowledge and support. Groups all over the country now use Silverman's model, although each has adapted the model to fit their needs.

A number of researchers since Silverman have looked at the widow-to-widow approach to determine its effectiveness. Vachon et al. (1980) and others looked at self-help interventions for widows and found that Silverman's approach helped widows reduce symptoms of sadness and grief by 6 months after the death of their spouse. In addition, by 12 months they were actively involved at an interpersonal level and participating in new activities. Those who participated in the intervention progressed in their pattern of adaptation faster than those in the control group did.

Psychotherapeutic Interventions

It is always difficult to draw the line between where support ends and therapy begins for a bereaved person. It seems to depend most on whether the bereavement becomes complicated or not, or is present simultaneously with a previously existing psychological disorder. A more in-depth discussion of complicated bereavement can be found earlier in this chapter.

Regardless of when it occurs, psychotherapeutic management of bereavement pathology is a vital undertaking. It is also important to utilise psychotherapy techniques that have been shown to be effective in the literature. Dynamic psychotherapy approaches have been shown to increase symptomatic relief in bereaved individuals, but they did not significantly improve work and relationship functioning, although those who prior to treatment had a more stable and mature self-concept performed better after treatment in work and interpersonal functioning (Horowitz et al., 1984).

There are a variety of behavioral treatments that have been tested to determine their effectiveness on the management of bereavement pathologies. Mawson et al. (1981) designed an intervention called "guided mourning" which involved confronting aspects of loss repeatedly until their affects diminished and using homework that involved daily writing about the deceased. The participants in the treatment group improved in their approach to bereavement, but their depressed mood did not improve. Other behavioral approaches have focused on cognitive restructuring, behavioral skills, and self-help. In their study looking at these three approaches, Walls & Meyers (1985) found that the cognitive restructuring group had some effect on symptoms of depression, but otherwise the groups faired no better in their adjustment to bereavement than did the control group.

Others such as Kavanagh (1990) have suggested that we need to look at a combination of cognitive and behavioral therapies to treat complicated bereavement. His model proposes the use of controlled exposure, and graded involvement in roles and activities, focusing on encouragement of achievement and attention to positive aspects. Kavanagh suggests that it is important in the bereaved to focus on cognitions related to hopelessness, guilt, or personal worthlessness. In addition, he suggests reinforcement of social support and control of drug and alcohol use.

Currently, techniques are being developed that integrate cognitive–behavioral techniques with attachment concepts. In this type of approach, the focus would be to correct the cognitive distortions associated with an insecure attachment style that tends to lead to complicated grief (Rosenzweig et al., 1997).

Psychopharmacological Interventions

Medications can be used to address the episodes of anxiety, insomnia, and depression that often occur simultaneously with bereavement. Medications intended to reduce anxiety are referred to as tranquillisers, anxiolitics, or sedatives. Generally, physicians will prescribe the most common of the anti-anxiety medications – benzodiazepines to reduce symptoms of anxiety, fear and tension, which are often present in bereavement, especially in the early weeks of the grieving process.

Hypnotics are generally prescribed when an individual is having trouble getting to sleep at night. This is quite common among the recently bereaved. Grieving individuals regularly exhibit grief symptoms that mimic depression, such as sadness, hopelessness, somatic complaints, and sleep disturbances. Therefore, antidepressants such as selective serotonin re-uptake inhibitors, tricyclics, and monoamine oxidase inhibitors are sometimes prescribed to relieve symptoms of the bereaved individual. There is some evidence to support that antidepressants could reduce symptoms of grief, which include intrusive thoughts, avoidance behaviours, and hyperarousal, given that they have been effective in doing so in post-traumatic stress disorder patients (Rosenzweig et. al., 1997).

There is controversy regarding whether the symptoms of bereavement are "normal" or whether they need to be treated with medication. Many health professionals believe that grief has a normal adaptive process that can be inhibited by the use of prescription drugs. Some go as far as to say that suppressing the grief process could lead to later mental or physical problems.

Although it is important to understand which interventions are most helpful for bereaved women, it is also important to realise that although women tend to report more anxiety, tension, and apprehension than males within the first 6 months of the death of a spouse, by the end of a year, both males and females report adequate functioning in their daily lives. This finding reported by Farberow et al. (1992) was accompanied by the conclusion that bereavement was more difficult for those who lost their spouses to suicide, and generally speaking these women and men may need more professional assistance.

SUMMARY AND CONCLUSIONS

Over the past few decades, bereavement theory, research, and anecdotes have provided invaluable information in the areas of loss, importance of social support, effective and ineffective methods of coping, role of culture and heritage, and interventions to ameliorate the negative effects of loss on psychological well-being. However, given the expected explosion of bereaved elderly in the next century and recent social changes affecting women and their life-styles, it is clear that more research is needed.

In particular, it is critical that we gain a clearer understanding of the role of culture in the bereavement process so that culturally competent and sensitive interventions may be developed and implemented. Secondly, given that future waves of elderly are expected to exhaust social resources (Hobbs & Damon, 1996), more researchers need to address the impact of bereavement on patterns of health care utilisation. In addition, the effectiveness of intervention programs to prevent or ameliorate a complicated bereavement process that is likely to cause increased health care utilisation (e.g. physician visits and hospital stays) needs further investigation. Finally, bereavement research must continue to take into account the dynamic social and economic environments that affect women of all cultures, because these factors will continue to impact our conceptualisation of normal and complicated grief, health service utilisation by women, and the development of bereavement programs sensitive to the needs of future generations of women

REFERENCES

Anderson, K.L., & Dimond, M.F. (1995). The experience of bereavement in older adults. *Journal of Advanced Nursing, 22*, 308–315.

Bowlby, J. (1971). *Attachment and Loss. Volume I: Attachment.* New York: Basic Books.

Bowlby, J. (1980). *Attachment and Loss. Volume III: Loss: Sadness and Depression.* New York: Basic Books.

Buchwald, D., Caralis, P., Gany, F., Hardt, E., Johnson, T., Muecke, M., & Putsch, R. (1994). Caring for patients in a multicultural society. *Patient Care,* 105–123.

Cacace M.F., & Williamson, E. (1996). Grieving the death of an adult child. *Journal of Gerontologic Nursing, 22*, 16–22.

Carey, R.G. (1977). The widowed: a year later. *Journal of Counseling Psychology, 24*, 125–131.

Clayton, P.J. (1974). Mortality and morbidity in the first year of widowhood. *Archives of General Psychiatry, 30*, 747–750.

Cline, S. (1995). *Lifting the Taboo: Women, Death and Dying.* London: Little, Brown.

Cowels, K. (1996). Cultural perspectives of grief: an expanded concept analysis. *Journal of Advanced Nursing, 23*, 287–294.

Duran, A., Turner, C.W., & Lund, D.A. (1989). Social support, perceived stress, and depression following the death of a spouse in later life. In Lund, D.A. (Ed.), *Older Bereaved Spouses: Research with Practical Applications.* New York: Hemisphere Publishing Corporation.

Farberow, N.L., Gallagher-Thompson, D., Gilewski, M., & Thompson, L. (1992). Changes in grief and mental health of bereaved spouses of older suicides. *Journal of Gerontology, 47*, 357–366.

Freud, S. (1917). Mourning and melancholia. In Strachey, J. (Ed.), *The Standard Edition of the Complete Psychological Works of Sigmund Freud,* Volume 14. London: Hogarth Press and Institute for Psychoanalysis.

Gallagher, D.E., Breckenridge, J.N., Thompson, L.W., & Peterson, J.A. (1983). Effects of bereavement on indicators of mental health in elderly widows and widowers. *Journal of Gerontology, 38*, 565–571.

Gass, K.A. (1989). Appraisal, coping, and resources: markers associated with the health of aged widows and widowers. In Lund, D.A. (Ed.), *Older Bereaved Spouses: Research with Practical Applications.* New York: Hemisphere Publishing Corporation.

Glick, I., Weiss, R., & Parkes, C. (1974). *The First Year of Bereavement.* New York: John Wiley & Sons Ltd.

Goodman, M., Rubinstein, R.L., Alexander, B.B., & Luborsky, M. (1991). Cultural differences among elderly women in coping with the death of an adult child. *Journal of Gerontology, 46*(6) S321–329.

Grossman, J. (1998). Cuban-Americans. In Purnell, L., & Paulanka, B. (Eds.), *Transcultural Health Care: A Culturally Competent Approach.* Philadelphia: F.A. Davis Company.

Hobbs, F., & Damon, B. (1996). *65+ in the United States. U.S. Bureau of the Census. Current Population Reports, Special Studies.* Washington: US Government Printing Office.

Hocker, W. (1988). Parental loss of an adult child. In Margolis, O., Kutscher, A., Marcus, E., Raether, H., Pine, V., Seeland, I., & Cherics, D. (Eds.), *Grief and the Loss of an Adult Child.* New York: Praeger.

Holmes, T., & Rahe, R. (1967). The social readjustment rating scale. *Journal of Psychosomatic Research, 11,* 213–218.

Horowitz, M., Marmar, C., Weiss, D., DeWitt, K., & Rosenbaum, R. (1984). Brief psychotherapy of bereavement reactions. *Archives of General Psychiatry, 41,* 438–448.

Irish, D., Lundquist, K., & Nelson, V. (1993). *Ethnic Variations in Dying, Death and Grief: Diversity in Universality.* Washington DC: Taylor & Francis.

Karlan, F. (1988). One parent's experience with the death of an adult child. In Margolis, O., Kutscher, A., Marcus, E., Raether, H., Pine, V., Seeland, I., & Cherics, D. (Eds.), *Grief and the Loss of an Adult Child.* New York: Praeger.

Kavanagh, D. (1990). Towards a cognitive–behavioral intervention for adult grief reactions. *British Journal of Psychiatry, 157,* 373–383.

Kitano, H., & Daniels, R. (1988). *Asian Americans.* Englewood Cliffs, NJ: Prentice Hall.

Klass, D. (1996). *Parental Grief: Solace and Resolution.* New York: Springer Verlag.

Kleinman, A. (1986). *Social Origins of Distress and Disease: Depression, Neurasthenia, and Pain in Modern China.* New Haven: Yale University Press.

Kleinman, A., Eisenberg, L., & Good, B. (1978). Culture, illness, and care: clinical lessons from anthropologic and cross-cultural research. *Annals of Internal Medicine, 88,* 251–258.

Krause, N. (1988). Stressful life events and physician utilization. *Journal of Gerontology, 43,* 553–561.

Kubler-Ross, E. (1968). *On Death and Dying.* New York: Macmillan.

Landrine, H., & Klonoff, E. (1992). Culture and health-related schemas: a review and proposal for interdisciplinary integration. *Health Psychology, 11,* 267–276.

Leshner, E., & Bergey, K. (1988). Bereaved elderly mothers: changes in health, functional activities, family cohesion, and psychological well-being. *International Journal of Aging and Human Development, 26,* 81–91.

Lofland, L.H. (1978). *The Craft of Dying: The Modern Face of Death.* Beverley Hills: Sage.

Lopata, H.Z. (1993). The support systems of American urban widows. In Strobe, M.S., Stroebe, W., & Hansson, R.O. (Eds.), *Handbook of Bereavement* (pp.181–396). New York: Cambridge University Press.

Matocha, M. (1998). Chinese-Americans. In Purnell, L., & Paulanka, B. (Eds.), *Transcultural Health Care: A Culturally Competent Approach*. Philadelphia: F.A. Davis Company.

Mawson, D., Marks, I., Ramm, L., & Stern, R. (1981). Guided mourning for morbid grief: a controlled study. *British Journal of Psychiatry, 138,* 185–193.

McHorney, C.A., & Mor, V. (1988). Predictors of bereavement depression and its health services consequences. *Medical Care, 26,* 882–893.

Miles, M., & Demi, A. (1986). Guilt in bereaved parents. In Rando, T. (Ed.), *Parental Loss of a Child*. Champaign, IL: Research Press.

Moore, J. (1970). The death culture of Mexicans and Mexican Americans. *Omega, 1,* 271–291.

Mor, V., McHorney, C., & Sherwood, S. (1986). Secondary morbidity among the recently bereaved. *American Journal of Psychiatry, 143,* 158–163.

Moss, M., Leschner, E., & Moss, S. (1984). Impact of the death of an adult child on elderly parents: some observations. *Omega, 17,* 209–218.

Murillo, N. (1971). The Mexican American family. In Wagner, N., & Haug, M. (Eds.), *Chicanos: Social and Psychological Perspectives* (pp.97–108). Saint Louis: Mosby.

Osterweis, M., Solomon, F., & Green, M. (Eds.) (1984). *Bereavement: Reactions, Consequences, and Care*. Washington DC: National Academy Press.

Parkes, C.M. (1965). Bereavement and mental illness. *British Journal of Medical Psychology, 38,* 388–397.

Parkes, C.M., & Brown, R. (1972). Health after bereavement: a controlled study of young Boston widows and widowers. *Psychosomatic Medicine, 34,* 449–461.

Parkes, C.M., & Weiss, R.S. (1983). *Recovery from Bereavement*. New York: Basic Books.

Pollock, G. (1987). The mourning–liberation process in health and disease. *Psychiatric Clinics of North America, 10,* 345–354.

Portillo, C. (1989). Treatment of Mexican American widows. In Kay, M. (Chair), Efficacy of support groups for Mexican American widows. Symposium conducted at the 22nd Annual Communicating Nursing Research Conference, San Diego, CA.

Prigerson, H.G., Maciejewski, P.K., Reynolds, C.F., III, Bierhals, A.J., Newsom, J.T., Fasiczka, A., Frank, E., Doman, J., & Miller, M. (1995). Inventory of complicated grief: a scale to measure maladaptive symptoms of loss. *Psychiatry Research, 59,* 65–79.

Prigerson, H., Bierhals, A., Kasl, S., Reynolds, C.F., III, Shear, M., Newsom, J., & Jacobs, S. (1996). Complicated grief as a disorder distinct from bereavement-related depression and anxiety: a replication study. *American Journal of Psychiatry, 153,* 1484–1486.

Purnell, L., & Paulanka, B. (1998). *Transcultural Health Care: A Culturally Competent Approach*. Philadelphia: F.A. Davis Company.

Rando, T. (1986). Parental bereavement: an exception to the general conceptualization of mourning. In Rando, T. (Ed.), *Parental Loss of a Child*. Champaign, IL: Research Press.

Rosenblatt, P. (1988). Grief: the social context of private feelings. *Journal of Social Issues, 44*, 67–78.

Rosenblatt, P. (1993). Cross-cultural variation in the experience, expression, and understanding of grief. In Irish, D., Lundquist, K., & Nelson, V. (Eds.), *Ethnic Variations in Dying, Death, and Grief: Diversity in Universality* (pp.13–19). Washington DC: Taylor & Francis.

Rozenzweig, A., Prigerson, H., Miller, M.D., & Reynolds, C.F., III (1997). Bereavement and the late-life depression: grief and its complications in the elderly. *Annual Review of Medicine, 48*, 421–428.

Rubin, S. (1993). The death of a child is forever: The life course impact of child loss. In Stroebe, M., Stroebe, W., & Hansson, R. (Eds.), *Handbook of Bereavement*. New York: Cambridge University Press.

Scrutton, S. (1995). *Bereavement and Grief: Supporting Older People Through Loss*. London: Edward Arnold.

Schatz, B. (1986). Grief of mothers. In Rando, T. (Ed.), *Parental Loss of a Child*. Champaign, IL: Research Press.

Schuster, T.A., & Butler, E.W. (1989). In Lund, D.A. (Ed.), *Older Bereaved Spouses: Research with Practical Applications*. New York: Hemisphere Publishing Corporation.

Steen, K.R. (1998). A comprehensive approach to bereavement. *The Nurse Practitioner, 23*, 54–68.

Stevenson, R. (1988). Parental and grandparental grief for the loss of an adult child. In Margolis, O., Kutscher, A., Marcus, E., Raether, H., Pine, V., Seeland, I., & Cherics, D. (Eds.), *Grief and the Loss of an Adult Child*. New York: Praeger.

Stroebe, M., Stroebe, W., & Hansson, R. (1988). Bereavement research: an historical introduction. *Journal of Social Issues, 44*, 1–18.

Stroebe, M., Stroebe, W., & Hansson, R. (1993). *Handbook of Bereavement Theory Research and Intervention*. Cambridge: Cambridge University Press.

Surtees, P.G. (1995). In the shadow of adversity: the evolution and resolution of anxiety and depressive disorder. *British Journal of Psychiatry, 166*, 583–594.

Thompson, L.W., Breckenridge, J. N., Gallagher, D., & Peterson, J. (1984). Effects of bereavement on self-perceptions of physical health in elderly widows and widowers. *Journal of Gerontology, 39*, 309–314.

United States Bureau of the Census (1993). *Current Population Reports. Special Studies. Sixty-five Plus in America*. Washington DC: Superintendent of Documents, US Government Printing Office.

Vachon, M.L., Lyall, W.A., Rogers, J., Freedman-Letofsky, K., & Freeman, S.J. (1980). A controlled study of self-help intervention for widows. *American Journal of Psychiatry, 137*, 1380–1384.

Velez, C. (1980). Mexicano/Hispano support systems and confianza: theoretical issues of cultural adaptation. In Valle, R., & Vega, W.

(Eds.), *Hispanic Natural Support Systems* (pp.45–54). Sacramento, CA: Office of Prevention, State of California, Department of Mental Health.

Walls, N., & Meyers, A. (1985). Outcome in group treatments for bereavement: experimental results and recommendations for clinical practice. *International Journal of Mental Health, 13,* 126–147.

Williams, W.V., & Polak, P.R. (1979). Follow-up research in primary prevention: a model of adjustment in acute grief. *Journal of Clinical Psychology, 35,* 35–45.

Yeaworth, R., & Valanis, B. (1985). Health status and resources of recently bereaved older persons. *Public Health Nursing, 2,* 232–244.

Younoszai, B. (1993). Mexican American perspectives related to death. In Irish, D., Lundquist, K., & Nelsen, V. (Eds.), *Ethnic Variations in Dying, Death, and Grief: Diversity in Universality* (pp.67–78). Washington DC: Taylor & Francis.

Zisook, S., Shuchter, S.R., & Lyons, L.E. (1987). Predictors of psychological reactions during the early stages of widowhood. *Pyschiatric Clinics North America, 10,* 355–368.

Zisook, S., Shuchter, S.R., Sledge, P., & Mulvihill, M. (1993). Aging and bereavement. *Journal of Geriatric Psychiatry and Neurology, 6,* 137–143.

Chapter 11

Working Conditions and Mental Health Among Women

Carina Bildt Thorbjörnsson

National Institute for Working Life, Sweden

This chapter reviews the relationship between working conditions and women's mental health. Mental health has been measured in a number of different ways, resulting in large differences between the reported prevalences of emotional and behavioural disorders in different study populations. Many of the studies published in the 1960s and 1970s were based solely on case studies using anecdotal records of treatment (Chester, 1972). Subsequently, objections were voiced about the way in which information on mental health was collected and reported. For example, critics noted that most of the psychological problems in a society are never diagnosed or treated, thus were being overlooked in much of the extant literature. These objections were supported in a study which clearly showed that women sought treatment for psychological disorders to a greater degree than men (Bygren, 1974). Other disparities in access to care and in health care utilisation were also identified, showing reduced care for middle-aged people and working class men and women. Subsequently more reliable data has emerged on the prevalence of common emotional and behavioural disorders (Hällström 1996). Yet current indices of prevalence may still retain some

Women, Health and the Mind
Edited by L. Sherr and J.S. St Lawrence. © 2000 John Wiley & Sons, Ltd

implicit gender bias. A carefully controlled 1991 study found that psychiatric diagnoses were assigned to 34% of the women, but only 20% of the men, who obtained comparable scores on the General Health Questionnaire (Redman et al., 1991).

Sources of bias when investigating mental health at the population level are (a) biases inherent in the questionnaire that collects the information and (b) gender differences in responding to questions about mental health. Women and men are assigned different roles in society, with certain personality characteristics more valued in women and others in men (Lindelöw & Bildt Thorbjörnsson, 1998). Questionnaires can be inadvertently skewed by socially embedded prejudices to yield results that suggest that women are more disturbed than men. [For a more extensive discussion of this issue, see Alexandersson (1998).] Assertiveness, for example, has been considered a masculine attribute for many decades, a fact that may result in lower evaluations for women who endorse items reflecting assertive behaviour. Ultimately, such inherent instrumentation biases can lead to female subjects becoming falsely classified as evincing emotional or behavioural disorders. This finding was common in studies reviewed for this chapter.

GENERAL EFFECTS OF GAINFUL EMPLOYMENT ON WOMEN'S HEALTH

During the last few decades, the effects of gainful employment on women's mental health have been studied extensively as a consequence of interest in clarifying the relationship between women's increasing participation in the labour force and their mental and physical health. No parallel focus on the relationship between men's health and employment has been seen.

As the proportion of women in the labour force increased, researchers compared the health of gainfully employed women to that of housewives. The results generally showed that gainfully employed women reported better mental health than housewives (Dennerstein, 1995; Parry, 1986). These findings may well have been affected by a selection bias, given that the healthiest women were more likely to become gainfully employed. Longitudinal studies, however, found that working women and housewives who had similar mental health status at baseline still differed from one another at follow-up, suggesting that the effect of employment on women's mental and physical health was a robust positive effect that could not be attributed solely to pre-existing differences. The positive effects of access to multiple social roles and multiple support systems were two explanations for these findings (Barnett et al., 1992; Pietromonaco & Frohardt-Lane, 1986; Pugliese, 1992). Multiple social roles and support systems can supply increased sources for gratification and decrease a person's vulnerability to disturbances and distress. However, the larger number of interpersonal relations resulting from the strain of sustaining multiple roles may also generate higher total demands for caring, emotional and instrumental support, thereby potentially affecting women's health in a negative way. Gainful employment produces increased financial resources and hence a higher standard of living. The increased resources could affect mental health and psychological well-being positively, as would the resulting economic autonomy.

Commonly studied aspects of women's mental health include depression and decreased psychological well-being. Differences have been noted in the prevalence of mental health problems between women in different ethnic and social groups (Dennerstein, 1995; Waldron & Jacobs, 1998), as well as between women in different occupational sectors (Ågren, et al. 1995; Jenkins et al., 1996). For example, the prevalence of reduced psychological well-being differed between women who were in different occupational groups in the county of Stockholm (Ågren, et al. 1995). Occupational groups with high prevalence (29–43%) included cleaners, science teachers, waitresses and journalists. Low-prevalence groups (8–18%) were business administrators, shop attendants, pre-school teachers, home care workers and programmers.

EFFECTS OF WORKING CONDITIONS ON WOMEN'S MENTAL HEALTH

The general positive effects of gainful employment on women's mental health do not preclude negative reactions to the stresses within individual work places (Bildt Thorbjörnsson, 1998). In many of the studies that evaluated the effects of working conditions on mental health, women were not included in the sample. Where they were included the analyses invariably failed to address gender differences and could not, therefore, identify effects specific to women's mental health. A further limitation in this area of research is that the major psychological disorders such as schizophrenia, bipolar disorder and major depression have not been included in studies evaluating the mental health effects that result from demanding working conditions. Many of the individuals who are diagnosed with these severe disorders are hospitalised or unemployed.

The following discussion will be confined to those studies that evaluated associations between working conditions and women's mental health. The outcomes in the reviewed studies are organised in this discussion according to their assumed severity. Psychological distress (severe category) includes subclinical depression and anxiety disorders, which in most studies were measured by paper-and-pencil questionnaires. Reduced psychological well-being (less severe) includes studies that assessed decreased psychological well-being, physical stress reactions and minor morbidity measured by questionnaires such as the General Health Questionnaire or similar paper-and-pencil measures.

Factors associated with family life and personality traits (examined in studies focusing on occupational risk factors) and possible interactions between work and family life will be discussed in a separate section. Studies that looked directly at personality traits or stress within the home as a cause of psychological morbidity among women are not reviewed here.

Classifications of Working Conditions

Common categories used to classify working conditions are psychosocial, organisational and physical conditions inherent in the employment setting (Bildt Thorbjörnsson, 1998).

Psychosocial conditions include social support factors such as emotional, instrumental and informative support in the work place, as well as job satisfaction, job stress and time pressure. The individual's subjective experience of the work environment is another way that psychosocial working conditions have been defined (Bongers, 1995). The category of organisational conditions is usually defined by the individual's working conditions, such as shift work, supervisory position and ability to influence the pace of work. Physical working conditions are easier to define. Tasks that are physically demanding, for example heavy lifting, pushing, and work with arms above shoulder level or below knee level, are categorised as physical working conditions. Also factors such as exposure to vibrations, noise, solvents and dust are categorised as physical working conditions.

Psychosocial Working Conditions and Mental Health

Psychosocial working conditions are the aspects of working that have been most frequently examined in relation to women's mental health, and many psychosocial risk factors have been identified. Occupational stress was examined in nearly half of the reviewed studies. Occupational stress is related to the individual's position or status in the organisation and is higher among women in lower positions (Noborisaka & Yamada, 1995). Many typical "women's" occupations are characterised by low status and are therefore assumed to have a high level of occupational stress. Across studies, occupational stress is measured in a variety of different ways and is often poorly defined. However, unbalanced role demands were risk factors for both emotional distress and reduced psychological well-being across many of the studies (Aro & Hasan, 1987; Barnett & Baruch, 1987; Bromet et al., 1992; Cooper & Melhuish, 1984; Cooper et al., 1987; Davidson et al., 1995; Estryn-Behar et al., 1990; Iwata et al., 1988, 1989; Kandel et al., 1985; Kandolin, 1993; Lam et al., 1985; Lundberg et al., 1994; O'Neill & Zeichner, 1985; Reifman et al., 1991; Schonfeld & Ruan, 1991; Schonfeld, 1992; Shigemi et al.,

1997; Stansfeld et al., 1995). High mental demands and time pressure also were risk factors for distress and reduced psychological well-being (Amick et al., 1998; Braun & Hollander, 1988; Eshelinen et al., 1991; Estryn-Behar et al., 1990; Kandolin, 1993; Makowska, 1995; Noor, 1995; Reifman et al., 1991). These relationships emerged from both cross-sectional and prospective studies, and there seems to be a clear causal link to mental health.

Some psychosocial factors have been examined only in cross-sectional studies and their long-term effects on mental health are less clear. Lack of social support, low job satisfaction, interpersonal conflict, fear of making mistakes, conflicts between personal beliefs and organisational values, sexual harassment and sex discrimination are all risk factors that have been associated with either distress or reduced psychological well-being, although the findings are somewhat equivocal (Bromet et al., 1992; Chevalier et al., 1996; Cooper et al., 1987; Davidson et al., 1995; Goldberg et al., 1996; Goldenhar et al., 1998; Kandolin, 1993; Makowska, 1995; Piotrowksi, 1998; Reifman et al., 1991; Shigemi et al., 1997; Stansfeld et al., 1995, 1997).

These psychosocial variables have been criticised because they are often derived from studies of men who were engaged in industrial work (Bildt Thorbjörnsson, 1998) and their appropriateness for women remains unclear. In addition, many of the questionnaires used to assess these constructs are gender neutral. If the aim of a study were to detect occupational impact on women's mental health, then selecting instruments that have gender sensitivity would improve the quality of measurement. Women and men in different occupations may perceive and express their working conditions in different ways, and there is some research support for such an assumption – in studies of how the genders defined job satisfaction (Barnett & Baruch, 1987; Miller & Kirsch, 1987). In order to experience job satisfaction, women wanted to use their resources and competence and to have an opportunity to help colleagues. Men underlined the importance of exerting personal influence over their job situations. The commonly used definition of social support as frequency of social interaction, rather than quality of the contacts, can also be criticised. Women take greater responsibility for their social relations (Lindelöw & Bildt Thorbjörnsson, 1998); frequent social contacts may therefore be a burden rather than a support for women. This "responsibility tendency" among women has been suggested as an explanation for the findings in studies of heart disease, in which, among women, a high frequency of social contacts was related to an increased risk for myocardial infarction, rather than a decreased risk (Jung, 1984; Rook, 1984). There is good reason to measure both the quantitative and qualitative aspects of social support in relation to mental health among women, although it is rarely done.

Sexual harassment and sex discrimination, both risk factors for mental illness, are often present simultaneously and sexual harassment often reflects the organisational climate rather than a co-worker's behaviour

(Bursten, 1985). A recent study of the health consequences of sexual harassment (Decker & Barling, 1998) found that there was a higher occurrence of sexual harassment in organisations where there were few sanctions against sexual harassment and where women had lower status and lower pay than men. Definitions of sexual harassment differ between different studies, as does the reported occurrence, and it is possible that qualitative studies will be needed to refine the definitional issues before further research can be worthwhile. Currently, information from both an individual and an organisational level should be collected to understand interaction effects and to develop appropriate and effective interventions.

The psychosocial aspect of working conditions may be influenced by individual characteristics and personality, just as personality traits influence an individual's experience and reports of psychosocial working conditions. An individual with weak coping strategies may experience more mental demands at work because of the lack of personal resources to solve problems as they arise. An individual with a negative attitude to life may see more problems in the daily working situation, whereas a more positive person would perceive challenges or opportunities. Individuals with poor ability to initiate and maintain social relationships may report a lack of social support at work because of their lack of social competence, rather than because of colleagues and superiors. Similarly, individuals who display type-A behaviour may rush through each work day without taking advantage of the available possibilities for support.

Type-A behaviour has been related to reduced psychological well-being, but not to psychiatric distress (Cooper et al., 1984; Davidson et al., 1995). However, because the study that showed this was cross-sectional, the long-term implications for psychological well-being remain unclear. Negative affect (negative attitude to life) has been examined in both cross-sectional and prospective designs and was only a risk factor for reduced psychological well-being in the cross-sectional analyses. This raises the possibility that reduced psychological well-being may generate negative reports, rather than the opposite.

Organisational Conditions and Mental Health

Relative to psychosocial factors, fewer organisational factors have been examined. Lack of influence over working conditions or the pace of work are risk factors for both psychiatric distress and reduced psychological well-being (Amick et al., 1998; Barnett et al., 1992; Eshelinen et al., 1991; Goldenhar et al., 1998; Makowksa, 1995; Reifman et al., 1991; Stansfeld et al., 1995, 1997). The links for these risk factors appear to be causal. Limited authority to influence working conditions or working pace are common in many of the occupations dominated by women, as are high mental demands (a psychosocial risk factor for mental illness) and a combination of these two (Westberg, 1998).

Shift work has been described as being more stressful to women (Costa, 1997). The effects of shift work on mental illness have been examined in several studies that yielded positive correlations (Estryn-Behar et al., 1990; Goldberg et al., 1996; Kandolin, 1993). A poor match between the individual's ability and the demands of the work and stress due to a fixed time schedule have been shown to be risk factors for distress and/or reduced psychological well-being (Estryn-Behar et al., 1990; Shigemi et al., 1997).

Other organisational factors – such as having a supervisory position, heavy work-related responsibility and frequent transfers – have emerged as risk factors for psychiatric distress and/or reduced psychological well-being only in cross-sectional studies, thus no cause-and-effect conclusions are warranted at this time. The long-term consequences remain unclear.

Physical Factors and Mental Health

Physical demands of work have been associated with the subjects' mental health. High physical load is a risk factor for both psychological distress and reduced psychological well-being (Amick et al., 1998; Eshelinen et al., 1991; Estryn-Behar et al., 1990), and the combination of high physical load and few possibilities to influence working conditions increases the risk for psychological distress (Eshelinen et al., 1991). This suggests that it is in interaction with other factors in the workplace that physical factors affect mental health. This assumption is supported by the results from a study of mental health among nurses working on different wards; nurses on wards that were both physically and psychologically demanding had a higher levels of distress (Petterson et al., 1995). Piece work has also been identified as a risk factor for psychiatric distress (Eshelinen et al., 1991).

One aspect of physical working conditions that is rarely investigated in relation to women's health is work place exposure to toxic substances (Hansson, 1998). In one cross-sectional study, exposure to solvents was a risk factor for psychological distress (Bromet et al., 1992).

The Interaction Between Working Conditions and Family

Studies assessing the relationships among working conditions, mental health and non-occupational areas of women's life have also been of interest. Both family life and factors intermediary between work and family have been examined. Being unmarried was found to be a risk factor for distress in cross-sectional, but not in prospective, studies (Iwata et al., 1988; Kandel et al., 1985; Snapp, 1992). This suggests that women with poorer mental health tend to live alone, rather than implying that poor mental health is caused by the single life. The presence of young children in the home has not been convincingly related to either distress or reduced psychological well-being, despite being identified as a risk factor in the epidemiological literature (Beatty, 1996; Goldberg et al., 1996; Iwata et al., 1988, 1989; Kandel et al., 1985: Kandolin, 1993; Lennon & Rosenfield, 1992; Noor, 1995: Snapp, 1992). This may be because of the narrow research perspective in many studies, where there was little consideration of the individual's entire situation. A number of studies found that limited social support from family and friends was not related to distress or reduced psychological well-being (Bromet et al., 1992; Davidson et al., 1995; Makowska, 1995; Schonfeld & Ruan, 1991; Snapp, 1992), perhaps because most of the studies defined poor social support as low frequency of social contacts rather than poor quality of social interactions. Demanding life events were related to both distress and reduced psychological well-being in cross-sectional studies, but not in prospective studies (Bromet et al., 1992; Cooper & Melhuish, 1984; Makowska, 1995; Noor, 1995; Schonfeld & Ruan, 1991; Schonfeld, 1992). Other factors, such as being responsible for children and home, having marital problems and having very little time for personal interests have only been studied in cross-sectional studies and were found to be related to distress (Iwata et al., 1988, 1989; Kandel et al., 1985; Lennon & Rosenfield, 1992; Reifman et al., 1991).

Role conflicts between the demands of work and family life in relation to mental health have also been examined. Assumptions that children were negatively affected by the mother's work outside the home and that work intruded on family life were related to distress in cross-sectional analyses, but not in prospective analyses (Beatty, 1996; Reifman et al., 1991). That family life did intrude on work was a risk factor in both types of analyses (Reifman et al., 1991).

Several factors from family life and leisure time may interact with occupational factors but the interactive pathways are not clear.

NEEDS FOR FURTHER RESEARCH

In further research addressing mental health among women it would be valuable to include information from broader spheres of women's lives. Indicators from sub-systems such as work, family life and leisure time, and from the local labour market, can increase our understanding of the interactive relationships among factors that are most important in relation to women's mental health. This would also allow preventive interventions to be more carefully tailored to meet women's needs. Prospective studies are needed as well, to investigate the long-term effects of many of the factors from work and family life that emerged in cross-sectional studies but have not been verified by longitudinal research.

REFERENCES

Ågren, G., Lundberg, I., Ekenvall, L., & Hogstedt, C. (1995). *Arbetshälsorapport om Samband Mellan Arbetsvillkor Och Ohälsa i Stockholms Län!* Stockholms läns landsting.

Alexandersson, K. (1998). Measuring health: indicators for working women. In Kilbom, K., Messing, K., & Bildt Thorbjörnsson, C. (Eds.), *Women's Health at Work.* Stockholm: National Institute for Working Life.

Amick, B., Kawachi, I., Coakley, E., Lerner, D., & Colditz, G. (1998). Relationship of job strain and iso-strain to health status in a cohort of women in the United States. *Scandinavian Journal of Work and Environment, 24,* 54–61.

Aro, S., & Hasan, J. (1987). Occupational class, psychosocial stress and morbidity. *Annals of Clinical Research, 19,* 62–68.

Barnett, R., & Baruch, G. (1987). Social roles, gender and psychological distress. In Barnett, C., Biener, L., & Baruch, G. (Eds.), *Gender and Stress.* New York: Free Press.

Barnett, R., Marchall, N., & Singer, J. (1992). Job experiences over time, multiple roles, and women's mental health: a longitudinal study. *Journal of Personality and Social Psychology, 62,* 634–644.

Beatty, C. (1996). The stress of managerial and professional women: Is the price too high? *Journal of Organisational Behaviour, 17,* 233–251.

Bildt Thorbjörnsson, C. (1998). Job stress differs between sub groups of women: psychiatric ill health and conditions at work. In Kilbom, K., Messing, K., & Bildt Thorbjörnsson, C. (Eds.), *Women's Health at Work.* Stockholm: National Institute for Working Life.

Bongers, P. (1995). Psychosocial factors and musculoskeletal disease. Presentation at the PREMUS conference in Montreal.

Braun, S., & Hollander, R. (1988). Work and depression among women in the Federal Republic of Germany. *Women and Health, 14,* 3–26.

Bromet, E., Dew, M., Parkinson, D., Cohen, S., & Schwartz, J. (1992). Effects of occupational stress on the physical and psychological health of women in a microelectronics plant. *Social Science and Medicine, 34,* 1377–1383.

Bursten, B. (1985). Psychiatric injury in the women's workplace. *Bulletin of the American Academy of Psychiatry and the Law, 13,* 399–406.

Bygren, L.O. (1974). Met and unmet needs for medical and social services. *Scandinavian Journal of Social Medicine, Suppl. 8,* 1–134.

Chester, P. (1972). *Women and Madness.* New York: Doubleday.

Chevalier, A., Bonenfant, S., Picot, M., Chastang, J., & Luce, D. (1996). Occupational factors of anxiety and depressive disorders in the French national electricity and gas company. The anxiety-depression group. *Journal of Occupational and Environmental Medicine, 38,* 1098–1107.

Cooper, C., & Melhuish, A. (1984). Executive stress and health. Differences between men and women. *Journal of Occupational Medicine, 26,* 99–104.

Cooper, C., Watts, J., & Kelly, M. (1987). Job satisfaction, mental health, and job stressors among general dental practitioners in the UK. *British Dental Journal, 162,* 77–81.

Costa, G. (1997). The problem; shift work. *Chronobiology International, 14,* 89–98.

Davidson, M., Cooper, G., & Baldini, V. (1995). Occupational stress in female and male graduate managers – a comparative study. *Stress Medicine, 11,* 157–175.

Decker, I., & Barling, J. (1998). Personal and organizational predictors of workplace sex harassment of women by men. *Journal of Occupational Health Psychology, 3,* 7–18.

Dennerstein, L. (1995). Mental health, work and gender. *International Journal of Health Services, 25,* 503–509.

Eshelinen, L., Toikkanen, J., Tuomi, K., Mauno, I., Nygård, C.-L., Klockars, M., & Illmarinen, J. (1991). Work-related stress symptoms of aging employees in municipal occupation. *Scandinavian Journal of Work, Environment and Health, 17,* 87–93.

Estryn-Behar, M., Kaminski, M., Peigne, E., Bonnet, N., Vaichere, E., Gozlan, C., Azoulay, S., & Giorgi, M. (1990). Stress at work and mental health status among female hospital workers. *British Journal of Industrial Medicine, 4,* 20–28.

Goldberg, P., David, S., Landre, M., Goldberg, M., Dassa, S., & Fuhrer, R. (1996). Work conditions and mental health among prison staff in France. *Scandinavian Journal of Work, Environment and Health, 22,* 45–54.

Goldenhar, L., Swanson, N., Hurrell, J., Ruder, A., & Deddens, J. (1998). Stressors and adverse outcomes for female construction workers. *Journal of Occupational Health Psychology, 3,* 19–32.

Gutek, B., & Koss, M. (1993). Effects of sexual harassment on women and organizations. *Occupational Medicine, 8,* 807–819.

Hansson, S.-O. (1998). Neglect of women? Occupational toxicology. In Kilbom, K., Messing, K., & Bildt Thorbjörnsson, C. (Eds.), *Women's Health at Work.* Stockholm: National Institute for Working Life.

Hällström, T. (1996). Psykisk ohälsa – könsskillnader [Mental disorders – gender differences]. In Östlin, P., Danielsson, M., Diderichsen, F., Härenstam, A., & Lindberg, G. (Eds.), *Kön och Ohälsa – en Antologi om Könskillnader ur ett Folkhälsoperspektiv [Gender and Health – An Anthology about Gender Differences from a Public Health Perspective],* Vol. 1 (pp.127–148). Lund: Studentlitteratur.

Iwata, N., Okuyama, Y., Kawakami, Y., & Saito, K. (1988). Psychiatric symptoms and related factors in a sample of Japanese workers. *Psychological Medicine, 88,* 659–663.

Iwata, N., Okumyama, Y., Kawakami, Y., & Saito, K. (1989). Prevalence of depressive symptoms in a Japanese occupational setting: a preliminary study. *American Journal of Public Health, 79,* 1486–1489.

Jenkins, R., Harvey, S., Butler, T., & Thomas, R. (1996). Minor psychiatric morbidity, its prevalence and outcome in a cohort of civil servants in a seven-year follow-up study. *Occupational Medicine, 46,* 209–215.

Jung, J. (1984). Social support and relation to health: a critical evaluation. *Basic and Applied Social Psychology*, 5, 143–169.

Kandel, D., Davies, M., & Raveis, V. (1985). The stressfulness of daily social roles for women: marital, occupational and household roles. *Journal of Health and Social Behavior*, 26, 64–78.

Kandolin, I. (1993). Burnout of female and male nurses in shiftwork. *Ergonomics*, 36, 141–147.

Lam, T., Ong, M., Wong, C., Lee, P., & Kleevens, J. (1985). Mental health and work stress in office workers in Hong Kong. *Journal of Occupational Medicine*, 27, 199–205.

Lennon, M., & Rosenfield, S. (1992). Women and mental health: the interaction of job and family conditions. *Journal of Health and Social Behavior*, 33, 316–327.

Lindelöw, M., & Bildt Thorbjörnsson, C. (1998). Facts and prejudice, psychological differences between women and men. In Kilbom, K., Messing, K., & Bildt Thorbjörnsson, C. (Eds.), *Women's Health at Work*. Stockholm: National Institute for Working Life.

Lundberg, U., Mårdberg, B., & Frankenhauser, M. (1994). The total workload of male and female white collar workers as related to age, occupational level, and number of children. *Scandinavian Journal of Psychology*, 35, 315–327.

Makowska, Z. (1995). Psychosocial characteristics of work and family as determinants of stress and well-being of women – a preliminary study. *International Journal of Occupational Medicine and Environmental Health*, 8, 215–222.

Miller, S., & Kirsch, N. (1987). Sex differences in cognitive coping with stress. In Barnett, C., Biener, L., & Baruch, G. (Eds.), *Gender and Stress*. New York: Free Press.

Noborisaka, Y., & Yamada, Y. (1995). The relationship between job status, gender and work related stress among middle-aged employees in a computer manufacturing company. *Journal of Occupational Health*, 37, 167–168.

Noor, N. (1995). Work and family roles in relation to women's well-being: a longitudinal study. *British Journal of Social Psychology*, 34, 87–106.

O'Neill, C., & Zeichner, A. (1985). Working women in a study of relationship between stress, coping and health. *Journal of Psychosomatic Obstetrics and Gynaecology*, 4, 105–116.

Parry, G. (1986). Paid employment, life events, social support, and mental health in working-class women. *Journal of Health and Social Behavior*, 27, 193–208.

Petterson, I., Arnetz, B., Arnetz, J., & Hörte, L. (1995). Work environment, skills utilization and health of Swedish nurses – results from a national questionnaire study. *Psychotherapy and Psychosomatics*, 64, 20–31.

Pietromonaco, P., & Frohardt-Lane, K. (1986). Psychological consequences of multiple social roles. *Psychological Woman's Quarterly*, 10, 373–381.

Piotrkowski, C. (1998). Gender harassment, job satisfaction, and distress among employed white and minority women. *Journal of Occupational Health Psychology, 3*, 33–43.

Pugliese, K. (1992). Women and mental health; two traditions of feminist research. *Women and Health, 19*, 43–68.

Redman, S., Webb, G., Hennrikus, D., Gordon, J., & Sanson-Fisher, R. (1991). The effect of gender on diagnosis of psychological disturbances. *Journal of Behavioral Medicine, 14*, 527–540.

Reifman, A., Biernat, M., & Lang, E. (1991). Stress, social support, and health in married professional women with small children. *Psychological Women's Quarterly, 15*, 431–445.

Rook, K.S. (1984). The negative side of social interaction: impact on psychological well-being. *Journal of Personality and Social Psychology, 46*, 1097–1108.

Schonfeld, I.S. (1992). A longitudinal study of occupational stressors and depressive symptoms in first-year female teachers. *Teaching and Education, 8*, 151–158.

Schonfeld, I., & Ruan, D. (1991). Occupational stress and preemployment measures of depressive symptoms: the case of teachers. *Journal of the Society of Behavior and Personality, 6*, 95–114.

Shigemi, J., Minno, Y., Tsuda, T., Babazono, A., & Aoyama, H. (1997). The relationship between job stress and mental health at work. *Industrial Health, 35*, 29–35.

Snapp, M. (1992). Occupational stress, social support, and depression among black and white professional-managerial women. *Women and Health, 18*, 41–79.

Stansfeld, S., North, F., White, I., & Marmot, M. (1995). Work characteristics and psychiatric disorder in civil servants in London. *Journal of Epidemiology and Community Health, 49*, 48–53.

Stansfeld, S., Rael, E., Head, J., Shipley, M., & Marmot, M. (1997). Social support and psychiatric sickness absence: a prospective study of British civil servants. *Psychological Medicine, 27*, 35–48.

Waldron, I., & Jacobs, J. (1988). Effects of labor force participation on women's health: new evidence from a longitudinal study. *Journal of Occupational Medicine, 30*, 977–983.

Westberg, H. (1998). Different worlds: Where are women in today's workplace? In Kilbom, K., Messing, K., & Bildt Thorbjörnsson, C. (Eds.) Women's Health at Work. Stockholm: National Institute for Working Life.

Chapter 12

Women and Depression

Margarita Alegría and Glorisa Canino

University of Puerto Rico Medical Sciences Campus

Depression, the fourth leading cause of disability in the world (Murray & López, 1996), has been the focus of numerous studies. This chapter examines the findings in three interrelated areas. The first deals with the higher prevalence of depression in women and the findings from epidemiological studies about the possible explanations for these higher rates. The second area examines whether there are gender differences in the clinical expression of depression, in the course of illness, and in the associated co-morbidities. The third and last area centres on the need to attend to gender differences in the management and treatment of depression.

WHAT IS DEPRESSION?

Typically, depressed patients report feeling persistently sad, blue or hopeless, and experience difficulties in perception, cognition, behaviour and functioning (Rehm & Tyndall, 1993). Also common in depression are changes in sleep patterns and appetite, and fluctuations in energy level and libido (Montano, 1994; Pies, 1994). Several nomenclatures are used to define depression. Evolving changes in diagnostic categories, divergent approaches to defining depression (disorder versus symptom level approaches) and multiple classification systems (ICD versus DSM) obviate a consensus about a single definition of

Women, Health and the Mind
Edited by L. Sherr and J.S. St Lawrence. © 2000 John Wiley & Sons, Ltd

depression. It is safe to say that depression represents a heterogeneous disorder composed of several subtypes with overlapping diagnostic criteria. As a consequence, depressed patients have shared but also divergent features.

Several types of depression within mood disorders are depicted in Table 12.1, which illustrates the most common subgroups included under the clinical term "depression". A diagnosis of depression may define a diverse group of patients, with great variation in their ability to function, in the expected course of illness and in the responses to treatment. In this review, we include studies from the fields of epidemiology, psychology, mental health services research and clinical treatment research that use different definitions of depression. For the purposes of this chapter, we will not confine ourselves to a single definition but will attempt to identify the one employed in the context of the original research.

PREVALENCE OF DEPRESSION IN WOMEN

One of the most consistent findings of epidemiological studies of mental disorders (Weissman et al., 1993, 1994) is that women report significantly higher rates of major depression and dysthymia as compared to men (see Figure 12.1). This finding has been consistently replicated since the early 1970s in clinical settings in the United States and other parts of the world (Weissman & Klerman, 1977), community studies in the United States, Europe, Asia and the Caribbean (Bebbington et al., 1981; Bland et al., 1988; Blazer et al., 1994; Canino et al., 1987; Kessler et al., 1993; Weissman & Myers, 1978; Weissman et al., 1984, 1991, 1993;

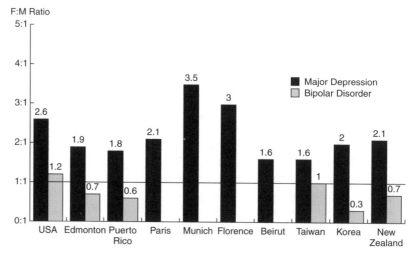

Figure 12.1 Female to male ratio of major depression and bipolar disorder
Source: Weissman et. al. (1994)

Table 12.1 Most common types of depressive disorders

	Major depression	Dysthymic disorder	Bipolar disorder, mixed type
General characteristics	Manifestation of a combination of symptoms that have been present during the same 2-week period provoking a change in the level of previous functioning	Symptoms similar to major depression, but milder in intensity and persisting for a longer period of time	Alternating cycles of depression and elation or mania
	At least 1 of the symptoms is either depressed mood or loss of interest or pleasure	Person presents a depressed mood for more days than not, during a period of at least 2 years	The mood switches usually occurs gradually, but can happen in a dramatic and rapid way
		The person has never been without these symptoms and a depressed mood for more than 2 months at a time.	When an episode occurs, the person meets the criteria for a manic episode and for a major depressive episode
Symptoms	At least 5 of the following symptoms: a. Depressed mood b. Marked diminished interest or pleasure in activities c. Significant weight lost/gain or decreased/increased appetite d. Insomnia or hypersomnia e. Psychomotor retardation or agitation f. Fatigue or loss of energy g. Feelings of worthlessness or excessive guilt h. Diminished ability to think or concentrate, or indecisiveness	At least 2 of the following symptoms: a. Poor appetite or overeating b. Insomnia or hypersomnia c. Low energy or fatigue d. Low self-esteem e. Poor concentration or difficulty making decisions f. Feelings of hopelessness	Symptoms manifested frequently: a. Agitation b. Insomnia c. Psychotic features d. Suicidal thinking e. Disturbance with appetite

(continued overleaf)

Table 12.1 *(continued)*

	Major depression	Dysthymic disorder	Bipolar disorder, mixed type
Symptoms *(Continued)*	i. Recurrent thoughts of death, recurrent suicidal ideation or a suicidal attempt or a specific plan for committing suicide		
Level of impairment	Symptoms cause clinically significant distress or impairment in occupational, social or other important areas of functioning	Symptoms cause clinically significant distress or impairment in social, occupational or other important areas of functioning	Symptoms are sufficiently severe to cause marked impairment in occupational or social functioning or to require hospitalisation to prevent harm to self or others, or there are psychotic features

Source: American Psychiatric Association (1995). *Diagnostic and Statistical Manual of Mental Disorders*

Wells et al., 1989a,b,c; Wittchen et al., 1992;) and high-risk samples such as first-degree relatives of probands with affective disorder (Leon et al., 1993; Merikangas et al., 1985). The prevalence of major depression in women has been found to vary from one and a half to three and a half times that of men, depending on the country (see Figure 12.1). These findings have been replicated using a variety of methods and instruments and in both clinical and community samples, and thus cannot be explained simply by the fact that women engage in more help seeking behaviour than men (Paykel, 1991). Consistent with previous research (Culbertson, 1997; Paykel, 1991; Weissman et al., 1992, 1993) Kessler et al. (1994) reported that women are approximately 1.7 times more likely than men to have a lifetime history of major depression as well as a 12-month episode of major depression. Several reasons are proposed for this higher prevalence of depression in women.

POSSIBLE EXPLANATIONS FOR THE HIGHER RATES OF DEPRESSION IN WOMEN

Methodological Artefacts

Most investigators agree that the overwhelming evidence showing higher prevalence of depression in women is probably accurate. However, this finding has been disputed by several investigators (see Ernst & Angst, 1992; Frank et al., 1988; Wilhelm & Parker, 1994), who argue that the apparent differences in depression are due to methodological artefacts. These investigators claim that men are subjected to more stigma associated with depression, and, because of this, are less likely than women to admit to a depressive episode. Under this hypothesis, the predominance of women with depression is explained by response bias. However, several investigators have presented evidence against this hypothesis (Clancy & Gove, 1974; Weissman & Klerman, 1977, 1985). The most recent data against this hypothesis are the results of the National Comorbidity Survey (NCS), which show that men report current depressive episodes as much as women (Kessler et al., 1993). Other methodological explanations are that men are more likely than women to forget past episodes of depression, or that men tend to under-report symptoms (Ernst & Angst, 1992; Wilhelm & Parker, 1994; Wittchen et al., 1989). Although Kessler et al. (1993) acknowledged that some of the reported differences may be due to recall bias and under reporting, the sex differences in the rates of major depression cannot be completely explained by these. Data from the NCS showed that women were not much more likely than men to recall the lifetime occurrence of a 2-week episode of dysphoria (Kessler et al., 1993). Instead, the higher annual prevalence of major depression observed in women in the United States who met diagnostic criteria for major depression was due to the fact that women were more likely than men to report symptoms that occurred during their worst 2-week episode. Other studies have shown that males and females equally under-report symptoms for remote episodes and that a more restrictive cut off point for number of symptoms for women does not eliminate the differential rates (Fennig et al., 1994; Young et al., 1990). Research that followed 156 depressed community subjects over 15 years found no sex differences in the number or duration of episodes between men and women (Wilhelm et al., 1998). Women nevertheless reported more symptoms per episode. Due to these findings, we are inclined to agree with Weissman & Klerman (1985) and Kessler et al. (1993), who concluded that the observed sex differences in depression in women are genuine rather than artifactual.

Higher Chronicity, Recurrence or Incidence?

There is evidence to suggest that women remain depressed longer than men and, therefore, may suffer more from chronic depression than men (Aneshensel, 1985; Ernst & Angst, 1992), thus accounting for the excess of depression in women. As stated by Kessler et al. (1993), chronicity could be due to a number of reasons:

- the individual may not recover from a first episode
- the individual without chronic depression may develop frequent episodes
- a combination of the two, slow recovery with multiple episodes

Results from the NCS show that women and men do not differ in their rates of acute recurrent episodes or the chronicity of episodes; however, significant differences were found in the risk of first onset of depression, with women exhibiting greater risk (Kessler et al., 1993). Their argument is, thus, that the main explanation for the higher prevalence rates of women is their greater risk of first onset.

Cohort Effects

In an attempt to explain the nature of these sex differences, a number of researchers have investigated the possibility that these may be due to cohort effects. People born in a certain time period are at greater or lower risk of a condition. Among the first to report cohort differences in depression were Wickramaratne et al. (1989) who observed that people living in five United States communities and who were more recently born had higher rates of depression than those born earlier in time. These results were later found in several other countries as well (Weissman et al., 1992). More recently, Kessler et al. (1993) found that the higher sex ratio of depression in women remained in the four age group cohorts examined (from 15 to 54 years). These authors interpreted this finding as meaning that the factors leading to increased depression in the younger cohorts (a finding replicated from the Epidemiologic Catchment Area study of five communities in the United States) have proportionally similar effects on men and women. Nevertheless, the sex ratio has diminished in the last decade from approximately 2.4 female to male ratio to 1.7 (Kessler et al., 1993; Weissman et al., 1991). This may be due in part to the finding reported by Weissman et al. (1993) that rates of major depression for males seem to be rising and for females the rates stabilised for birth cohorts born after 1945.

Gender-specific Socialisation

A frequent explanation for higher rates of depression in women is that women's social disadvantage in chronic social and labour status discrimination, role and life stress, and victimisation has led to learned helplessness and psychological consequences that express themselves in depressive symptomatology (Brown & Prudo, 1981; Brown et al., 1986; Parry, 1989; Paykel, 1991). Although there is a vast quantity of empirical data supporting the association between depression and past serious life events (Paykel & Cooper, 1991), women do not seem to experience more life events than men. However, Kessler et al. (1994) argued against the gender socialisation explanation because the higher risk of onset for women, compared with men, in the United States manifests mainly in pre-adolescence and early adolescence (10–14 years), before role stress, labour discrimination or victimisation is fully felt in women. However, NCS data provide just an indication that the gender specific socialisation theory might not be the only factor explaining the excess of depression in women. Several findings (Bebbington et al, 1991; Gater et al., 1989) point to increased rates of depression in women who are 20–40 years, married and with children, those for whom role-related stress is most acute. There is also epidemiological evidence that women in the child-bearing years who have children at home have higher and more severe rates of depression than women without children (Canino et al., 1987).

It might, therefore, be that higher female rates of depression in this age range are partly explained by a hypothesis of social causation. The excess of depression in women of 20–40 years may be linked to the problems of child rearing in "nuclear" families, particularly if women lack social, familial or partner support. Limited nurturance in intimate relations appears associated with increased risk for depression (Birtchnell, 1988), as does conflict-ridden or unhappy marriage (Weissman, 1987). Socio-environmental conditions such as lack of employment (Andrews & Brown, 1988; Brown & Bifulco, 1990; Monroe & Steiner, 1986), role conflict and overload (Bebbington, 1998), poor family support (Garmezy, 1985), low socio-economic status (Brown et al., 1986) and caring for children (Canino et al., 1987) are likely to increase vulnerability to depression. However, it may be the coexistence of personality factors (Aro, 1994; Boyce & Mason, 1996; Boyce et al., 1991, 1998) with socio-environmental conditions that differentially place women at risk for depression.

Findings by Teasdale (1988) suggest that maladaptive attitudes can be reactivated by certain experiences or by the residuals of prior depressive episodes. As such, an interacting cognitive system, particularly the ruminating styles more typically seen in women than in men (Nolen-Hoksemae et al., 1986), may result in more depression for women. More recent work suggests that negative childhood experiences may be more predisposing to depression in women than in men (Veijola et al., 1998). The nature, occurrence and quality of the childhood experiences do not differ much between the sexes (Veijola et al., 1998), which suggests than it is the reaction and coping with these experiences that varies between the sexes.

Biological Vulnerability

Few investigators would claim that biological vulnerability is the only explanation for the observed sex differences in depression, since it is obvious that men and women differ not only in their biological but on their social conditions as well. The argument between those who claim biological vulnerability and those who claim social causality is usually on the emphasis given to either of these two explanations. Several epidemiological studies have shown that depressive disorders are rare in childhood and no sex differences are observed (Angold & Rutter, 1992; Petersen et al., 1991). Yet, prevalence rises significantly in adolescence and early adulthood, particularly in females (Costello et al., 1996; Lewinshon et al., 1994). Some investigators have claimed that this rise in depression in women during adolescence is due to hormonal changes related to puberty (Cohen et al., 1993; Patton et al., 1996). On the other hand, it is claimed that this sex difference emerges in adolescence, a particularly difficult transition period for females when sex role differentiation begins to emerge more fully (Fombonne, 1995).

Other findings seem to support a biological explanation for sex differences in depression. For example, women seem to be at an increased risk for developing a seasonal pattern for depression (Leibenluft et al., 1995) and for experiencing hormonal triggers for depression (Endicott, 1993; Frank et al., 1987; Gotlib et al., 1989; Parry, 1989). Endicott (1993) finds increased vulnerability for the onset of a depressive episode during women's premenstrual phase. The biological susceptibility hypothesis has also been partly sustained by the evidence that a significant number of women developed post-partum depression, possibly associated with the hormonal changes associated with this period (O'Hara et al., 1991). Frank et al. (1987) reported that a third of women with children with recurrent depression experience at least one post-partum episode. Notwithstanding these studies, a controlled prospective study found that the prevalence of depression in pregnant and post-partum women is similar to non-pregnant and non-postpartum controls (O'Hara et al., 1991).

In 1977, Weissman & Klerman reviewed the available data and concluded there was substantial evidence that menopause had little effect on increasing the incidence of depression. However, there are more recent findings which suggest that many women experience mood changes during the perimenopausal or menopausal period, particularly those previously vulnerable to mood disturbances (Schmidt & Rubinow, 1991; Stewart & Boydell, 1993). Stowe et al. (1995) indicated that for many women, the post-partum period is the onset of their first depressive episode. In addition, hormonal contraceptives, hormonal treatments for infertility and hormone replacement therapy may also increase the risk for depressive episodes (Magos et al., 1986; Slap, 1981; Wagner & Berenson, 1994).

Bebbington et al. (1998b) provided evidence, from a national epidemiological study of the adult population of London, in favour of the influence of biological factors in explaining this sex difference. They found, that although sex differences in depression were apparent in all the adult cohorts studied, this difference was not apparent after the age of 55. After this age, which coincides with the completion of menopause in women, there was no difference in rates of depression among men and women. These investigators controlled statistically for possible confounding variables such as marital status, child care or employment status. In addition, they quoted other investigators who reported similar findings of no sex differences in depression after menopause (e.g. Kaufert et al., 1988). However, Bebbington et al. were cautious in their interpretation of the data and state that these findings do not necessarily imply biological causation. Although certain social variables were controlled in the analyses, this does not rule out the possibility of other social and psychological explanations not contemplated in their study, correlated with age of menopause. They suggested there is a need for a longitudinal study of women as they approach and pass through the menopause using detailed social, psychological and biological measures.

Furthermore, certain gender differences in neuropsychological function may predispose women to depression (Levy & Heller, 1992). Heller (1993) cogently argued that regional differences in brain activity could play a role in the observed female predominance in the rates of depression. Sex differences regarding aspects of brain organisation for cognitive function and brain–behaviour relationships could help address differential vulnerability of women to depression. Heller (1993) recommended longitudinal and cross-sectional studies comparing males and females in neuroendrocrine responses, neuropsychological performance and emotional status to further clarify the potential role of neuropsychology in depression.

However, as stated earlier, it is highly improbable that biological, endocrinological or neuropsychological susceptibility is the only explanation to the observed sex differences in depression. As eloquently stated by Weissman et al. (1993), it is unlikely that any of the explanations or hypotheses given would be the sole factor in accounting for the phenomenon. Similar to Bebbington et al. (1988b), they suggested the need for a study that would be prospective in nature and take into account social, psychological, endocrinological and biological variables to understand the differential risk of depression in women.

A recent editorial in *Psychological Medicine* (Bebbington, 1998) stated that the sex differential in depressive disorders has not been adequately explained, emphasising limitations in current research in terms of offering a comprehensive aetiological account of depression. A particularly important aspect for consideration in future research is that the factors accounting for the sex differences may diverge from the causes of depression itself, and may vary along the spectrum of the life span. We agree with this editorial regarding future areas of investigation that are needed to fully understand higher rates of depression in women: "... the epidemiological study of macro social variables and of age effects; temperament, personality, and attributional and coping styles; the experience of psychosocial adversity; and the possibility of increased susceptibility to some forms of stress in women" (p.1). Additional areas include women's differential response to the quality of intimate relations and social supports; the strains and role conflicts they experience; and socio-environmental circumstances; and women's biological and genetic vulnerability; as well as social and psychological experiences of puberty and menopause. Finally, a promising research focus is the examination of gender differences in neuropsychological functions in depression (see Heller, 1993).

SEX DIFFERENCES IN THE EXPRESSION, COURSE, AND ASSOCIATED CO-MORBIDITIES OF DEPRESSION

The second area to be examined centres on the debate of whether there are differences in how men and women conceptualise and experience their depression (Gater et al., 1998; Kornstein et al., 1995). Frank et al. (1988) argued that although male and female depressed patients are similar in clinical characteristics, including severity, there are differences in the type of depressive symptoms manifested. Compared with depressed men, women with depression report more appetite and weight increase, augmented levels of expressed anger and hostility, and more somatisation. Other investigators (Kornstein et al., 1995) confirmed the presence of gender differences in the manifestation of chronic major depression. In examining 96 males and 198 females with a DSM-III-R diagnosis of major depression of at least 2 years' duration, women were found to have increased severity of illness compared with their male counterparts. Women with major depression, in contrast to men, reported more psychomotor retardation (Kornstein et al., 1995).

Young et al. (1990) studied gender differences in the clinical features of unipolar major depressive disorder of 498 moderately to severely depressed patients. These authors found no significant gender difference in severity of depression, in impairment in functioning or in endogenous symptoms. Only increased appetite and weight gain differed between severely depressed men and women. Wilhelm et al. (1998) have replicated this finding. These researchers reported that women describe more symptoms of depression per episode and some specific symptoms (such as tearfulness, appetite and weight gain) more frequently than men. The findings of Gater et al. (1998) suggest differences in the way men and women may conceptualise the experience of depression.

Analysis of gender differences in the clinical manifestations of depression also depict women as being more likely than men to experience reverse vegetative or atypical symptoms as well as anxiety and somatic symptoms (Angst & Dobler-Mikola, 1984). Symptom presentation is reported to vary by gender, with women endorsing feelings of increased hostility and loss of libido more frequently than men (Schatzberg et al., 1999). Both the Collaborative Depression Study (Casper et al., 1985) and Hawkins et al. (1985) found hypersomnia to be more common in depressed men than women These published studies raise the question of whether depression looks different in men and women. Future research is needed to lay the foundation for gender differences in the clinical manifestations of depression. Such findings would be a crucial consideration in assessment, case-identification and treatment.

Course of Illness

The majority of research studies have reported no gender difference in age of onset of depression (Frank et al., 1988; Kessler et al., 1993; Weissman et al., 1993), while a few investigators have reported an earlier age of onset for women (Fava et al., 1996; Kornstein et al., 1996). In the NCS, women were found to be at an increased risk of first onset in comparison with men (Kessler et al., 1994). Regarding recurrence of depression, some cross-sectional studies have found no evidence of gender differential (Weissman et al., 1993), while the NCS found that among those with a history of depression, women had a higher 12-month recurrence risk than their male counterparts (Kessler et al., 1994). However, men with a history of depression had increased risk, compared with women with a history of depression, of becoming chronically depressed (Kessler et al., 1993). In contrast, several longitudinal studies have suggested longer episodes of depression in women that increase their likelihood for chronic and recurrent depression (Ernst & Angst, 1992; Keitner et al., 1991; Sargeant et al., 1990; Winokur et al., 1993). Prospective follow-up data from the Stirling Study (Murphy et al., 1986) also indicated that depression has a worse prognosis for men than for women, the risk of death being two times greater for depressed men than for depressed women (Murphy et al., 1987). These findings suggest possible gender differences regarding the course of illness.

Co-morbidities

Gender differences in the co-morbidities of depression have also been reported. Results from the NCS suggest that depressed women have augmented rates of co-morbidity (Blazer et al., 1994). According to the

Epidemiologic Catchment Area (ECA) Study, women were more likely to report a co-morbid anxiety disorder, typically phobia or panic disorder (Regier et al., 1990). A recent study by Fava et al. (1996) also described higher rates of co-morbid simple phobia and bulimia nervosa in women with major depression, compared with their male counterparts. Several published studies (Fava et al., 1996; Kornstein et al., 1996; Regier et al., 1990) found higher lifetime rates of alcohol and substance abuse and dependence in men with major depression than in women with the same disorder. Golomb et al. (1995) described an increased prevalence of antisocial, narcissistic and obsessive–compulsive personality disorders in depressed men compared with depressed women. In contrast, Shea et al. (1987) reported no significant gender differences in the prevalence of co-morbid personality disorders in depressed cases.

As can be seen from this review, significant gender differences in the co-morbidities linked to depression may be an important element in treatment. Given these potential gender differences, more research is needed that looks at differential patterns of co-morbidities on the effectiveness of treatments for depression.

Gender Differences in the Treatment of Depression

As many as one in every five women will become clinically depressed at some time during their lives (Weissman et al., 1993). However, the American Psychological Association's National Task Force on Women and Depression concluded that between 30 and 50% of women diagnosed as having a depressive disorder may be misdiagnosed (McGrath et al., 1990). Such data become disturbing in light of the fact that 70% of prescriptions of antidepressant medications are for women (Floyd, 1997). Some explanations of this high degree of diagnostic inaccuracy for women are:

- the presence of physical illnesses that closely resemble affective distress (Fava & Molnar, 1987)
- physician bias in diagnosing the nature of female patient's complaints (Friedlander & Phillips, 1984)
- medical treatments that induce symptoms which mimic depression (Pies, 1994)
- the low threshold that practitioners might adopt for case identification in women but not in men, because patients mention a depressed mood during consultation (Floyd, 1997).

Use of Services for Depression

Findings of recent studies (Lehtinen et al., 1991; Regier et al., 1993) suggest that between one-third and less than one-half (45%) of people suffering from a clinically defined depression were found to be receiving treatment. In the 16-year follow up to the Stirling Study, Murphy (1990) found that only 37% of depressed men had sought professional help while 83% of depressed women had done so. Others have found no difference in the rates of receiving treatment for depression between men and women (Jiménez et al., 1997). Another longitudinal study of factors affecting help-seeking during depression in a community sample found that only 40.6% of women experiencing a depressive episode sought professional help (Dew et al., 1988). This may be partly explained by the findings of Ginsberg & Brown (1982) in a sample of 45 depressed mothers who never received treatment. Their data suggests that the family and social network and general practitioners contacted by the women interpreted the depression as an expected response to recent stress. As such, they assumed the depression did not require formal treatment. Others (Monroe et al., 1991) have found that stresses before the onset of a depressive disorder are the strongest predictors of time to enter treatment. Those persons with severe life events in the year before the onset of the disorder sought treatment more rapidly than those without acute stress. Stressful events that started after onset of the disorder had no impact on treatment entry. The results of Monroe et al. (1991) suggested that individuals without any serious stress before onset may have difficulty recognising the presence of the disorder, or may believe it will abate shortly without the need for professional help.

However, little is known about whether there is differential recognition or referral for treatment by general practitioners, intermediary helping agencies, or family and friend networks, depending on the gender of the patient reporting the depression. Data from the World Health Organisation Collaborative Study on Psychological Problems in General Health Care (Gater et al., 1998) found no significant gender difference in the detection rates of ICD-10 depressive disorder. Gender did not seem to affect the odds of a depressive disorder being detected by a primary care physician. More empirical data are needed in this area.

There is also reason to believe that one of the main reasons why depression goes undetected in young women (15–44 years) is their decreased likelihood of receiving care by professional mental health systems or by general primary care physicians (Miranda & Muñoz, 1994). In their public sector sample, 87% of young women received care only from a gynaecologist. Frequently, young women select their gynaecologist or obstetrician as their primary care providers during their child-bearing years (Commonwealth Fund, 1993). A paper commissioned by the Commonwealth Fund in 1995 (Leiman, 1995) concluded that much of the care that women received for psychological or emotional problems occurred outside the professional mental health system, by physicians who have not been trained to provide this type of care.

Because insurers and employers have realised the height of costs and morbidity associated with depression, several managed care organisations have designed and implemented programmes to improve its diagnoses and treatment by primary care physicians (Gonen, 1997). To facilitate increased quality of care, several agencies and professional groups (such as the American Psychiatric Association) have developed treatment guidelines for depression. The Agency for Health Care Policy and Research (AHCPR) Guidelines (1993) for Depression include an extremely comprehensive and detailed summary of the treatments for depression, the current evidence on the efficacy of available treatments and recommendations for treatment of depression in primary care practice. Yet, available guidelines, promulgated to improve detection and management of depression by primary care providers (such as the AHCPR guidelines), offer minimal attention to gender differences (Hoffman, 1996).

MANAGEMENT OF DEPRESSION

Currently, primary care physicians and mental health specialists treat depression with psychotherapy, drugs, electroconvulsive therapy, light therapy and other techniques. For patients who are appropriately matched to the therapy that is effective for them, these treatments can alleviate symptoms, delay or prevent relapse and recurrence, diminish impairment and disability, and shorten the course of a depressive episode.

The new emphasis on gender differences in treatment response of depression (Schatzberg et al., 1999) provides impetus for paying attention to these differences in the evaluation and management of depressive disorders. Recently there has been a growing interest in examining gender differences in response to depression treatments (Kornstein, 1997), including psychotropic medications (Dawkins & Potter, 1991; Yonkers et al., 1992), psychotherapy (Jarrett et al., 1991; Thase et al., 1994), combined pharmacotherapy and psychotherapy (Frank et al., 1987), and electroconvulsive therapy (Lawson, 1996; Sackeim et al., 1987).

A review of the literature on pharmacotherapy for depression suggests potential gender differences in drug absorption, metabolism and elimination (Dawkins & Potter, 1991; Yonkers et al., 1992). Some examples of sex-related differences in pharmacokenetics of antidepressants included women's higher plasma levels of imipramine (Hamilton et al., 1996) and amitriptyline (Perkson & Mac, 1985). Oral contraceptives (Abernethy et al., 1984) and endogenous hormones (Jensvold et al., 1992) may also impact the dosage requirements of antidepressant medication. Tricyclic dose requirements have also been shown to vary across pregnancy (Wisner et al., 1993). Studies assessing differential treatment response to antidepressant medications have suggested that women have a poorer response than men to tricyclics (Glassman et al., 1977; Raskin, 1974) but better response to selective serotonin reuptake inhibitors (SSRIs) (Davidson & Pelton, 1986). It is believed that gender differences in absorption, metabolism, side-effects, toxicity and efficacy of antidepressant medication may have significant clinical implications for treatment.

Issues of safety, efficacy and compliance with pharmacotherapy of depressive disorders are raised due to women's reproductive cycle. For example, antidepressant discontinuation during pregnancy in women with recurrent major depression appears correlated to an augmented risk for relapse (Schatzberg et al., 1999). Vulnerability to mood disorders does not appear to diminish during pregnancy for women with a history of depression. Furthermore, women with bipolar disorders evidence an increased risk for psychiatric admission during the first 90 days post-partum (Kendell et al., 1987). Because depression during pregnancy may elevate the odds for relapse post-partum, investigators have recommended that pregnant women do not stop antidepressant medication during labour or delivery (Schatzberg et al., 1999).

Another area of concern has been the use of antidepressants during pregnancy. A recent study evaluated the exposure to Prozac (fluoxetine) during the first trimester of pregnancy in terms of risk of major congenital malformations (Pastuszack et al., 1993). These authors report no apparent increased risk of malformations due to prozac as compared to tricyclic antidepressants. Because of limitations regarding the aggregate nature of the analyses (the results from the three medications were collapsed for analysis), these results should be taken with caution. There is still much heated debate on the medical decisions involved treating depressed women during pregnancy. A study by Chambers et al. (1996) found that women who delivered while on fluoxetine or who had taken it during the third trimester of pregnancy had elevated rates of perinatal complications; however, this study has been severely criticized on methodological grounds. As such, there is conflicting clinical advice regarding whether women should take fluoxetine during the third trimester period.

Limited studies of psychotherapy in depression have examined the differential treatment response by gender (Kornstein, 1997). Of the few studies in this area, Thase et al. (1994) reported similar outcomes in depressed men and women treated with cognitive–behaviour therapy (CBT). The only differential impact of CBT by sex was observed in those patients with severe depression: women exhibited significantly poorer outcomes when compared with men who had a similar clinical profile. Jarrett et al. (1991) also found similar treatment effects in depressed men and women receiving cognitive therapy. However, less is known regarding differential treatment response by gender to other types of psychotherapy (such as interpersonal therapy). Studies addressing gender differences in outcomes in specific types of psychotherapy are necessary to adequately match patients to effective treatments.

There is also a void in the empirical research examining gender differences in the effects of combination pharmacotherapy and psychotherapy. Frank et al. (1987) compared the treatment response of men and women treated by imipramine and interpersonal psychotherapy. Interpersonal therapy is typically a time-limited approach that aims at clarification and resolution of interpersonal difficulties such as role disputes, role transition, prolonged grief, social isolation and others. The findings of Frank et al. (1987) suggested that men experienced a fast and sustained clinical response in comparison with women. The authors argued that males were possibly showing an improvement due to the action of imipramine, while women showing a delayed improvement needed both the imipramine and psychotherapy to positively respond to treatment.

Gender differences have also been studied with regards to electroconvulsive therapy (ECT). This is a treatment modality in which a low-voltage alternating current is briefly applied to induce a convulsion or seizure. This is a treatment option for patients suffering from severe or psychotic forms of major depressive disorder, whose symptoms are intense and prolonged. In looking at gender differences in the response to ECT, Lawson (1996) found that women could have lower seizure thresholds during ECT than men. Several studies (see for example McCall et al., 1993) have implied that males require a higher dose of electrical stimulus for seizure than women.

Further research on the differential gender response to treatments for depression is needed. Nevertheless, the review presented by this chapter emphasises the importance of attending to these differences to increase the efficacy and effectiveness of depression treatments. Recently, concerns have been raised about patients who, although in depression treatment, fail to respond and improve in psychological wellness and functioning (Fava et al., 1996). The lack of an appropriate match between treatment dose or intensity and patient has been identified as a source likely to cause "treatment-resistant depression" (Fava et al., 1996). It, therefore, seems imperative to consider gender differences with regards to depression treatment.

CONCLUSIONS

The literature reviewed in this chapter emphasises notable gender differences that appear to exist in the prevalence of depression, in the manifestation and experience of the illness, in the course of the condition and associated co-morbidities, and in the responses to various treatments. Enormous advances have been accomplished in rejecting potential explanations for the higher prevalence rates of depression in women and in identifying possible mechanisms that are likely to differentially increase the risk for women. Treatment efficacy and effectiveness studies in pharmacotherapy to treat depression have started to provide essential information on treatment issues for women. However, more knowledge in this area is urgently needed to guarantee that depression treatments for women restore and improve their functioning. Additional research is needed to better understand what causes and triggers depression, which are the most effective depression treatments depending on the woman's clinical, medical and social profile, and how we can ameliorate the negative consequences of depression.

ACKNOWLEDGEMENTS

We are grateful for financial support from the National Institute of Mental Health (MH R01–42655). We thank Mildred Vera and Thomas McGuire for comments on earlier versions of this chapter, and Leida Matías, Abigaíl González and María Lebrón for help with the preparation of the manuscript.

REFERENCES

Abernethy, D.R., Greenblatt, D.J., & Shader, R.I. (1984). Imipramine disposition in users of oral contraceptives. *Clinical Pharmacology and Therapeutics*, *35*, 792–797.

Agency for Health Care Policy and Research (1993). *Depression in Primary Care: Clinical Practice Guidelines (AHCPR Publication No. 93–0550)*. Rockville, MD: Agency for Health Care Policy and Research.

Ahnlud, K., & Frodi, A. (1996). Gender differences in the development of depression. *Scandinavian Journal of Psychology*, *37*, 229–237.

American Psychiatric Association (1995). *Diagnostic and Statistical Manual of Mental Disorders*, 4th Edition. Washington DC: American Psychiatric Association.

Andrews, B., & Brown, G.W. (1988). Marital violence in the community. *British Journal of Psychiatry*, *153*, 305–312.

Aneshensel, C. (1985). The natural history of depressive symptoms. *Research and Community Mental Health*, *5*, 45–75.

Angold, A., & Rutter, M. (1992). Effects of age and pubertal status on depression in a large clinical sample. *Developmental Psychopathology*, *4*, 5–28.

Angst, J., & Dobler-Mikola, A. (1984). The definition of depression. *Psychiatry Research*, *18*, 401–406.

Aro, H. (1994). Risk and protective factors in depression: a developmental perspective. *Acta Psychiatrica Scandinavica* (Suppl. 377), 59–64.

Bebbington, P.E. (Ed.) (1998). Editorial. Sex and depression. *Psychological Medicine*, *28*, 1–8.

Bebbington, P.E., Hurry, J., Tennant, C., & Wing, J.K. (1981). The epidemiology of mental disorders in Camberwell. *Psychological Medicine*, *11*, 561–579.

Bebbington, P.E., Brugha, T., MacCarthy, B., Potter, J., Sturt, E., Wykes, T., Katz, R., & McGuffin, P. (1998a). The Camberwell Collaborative Depression Study, I: depressed probands: adversity and the form of depression. *British Journal of Psychiatry, 152,* 754–765.

Bebbington, P.E., Dunn, G., Jenkins, R., Lewis, G., Brugha, T., Farrell, M., & Meltzer, H. (1998b). The influence of age and sex on the prevalence of depressive conditions: report from the National Survey of Psychiatric Morbidity. *Psychological Medicine, 28,* 9–19.

Bebbington, P.E., Tennant, C., & Hurry, J. (1991). Adversity in groups with an increased risk of minor affective disorder. *British Journal of Psychiatry, 158,* 33–40.

Birtchnell, J. (1988). Depression and family relationships. A study of young, married women on a London housing estate. *British Journal of Psychiatry, 153,* 758–769.

Bland, R.C., Newman, S.C., & Orn, H. (1988). Period prevalence of psychiatric disorders in Edmonton. *Acta Psychiatrica Scandinavica, 77*(Suppl. 338), 24–32.

Blazer, D.G., Kessler, R.C., McGonagle, K.A., & Swartz, M.S. (1994). The prevalence and distribution of major depression in a national community sample: the National Comorbidity Survey. *American Journal of Psychiatry, 151,* 979–986.

Boyce, P., & Mason, C. (1996). An overview of depression-prone personality traits and the role of interpersonal sensitivity. *Australian and New Zealand Journal of Psychiatry, 30,* 90–103.

Boyce, P., Parker, G., Barnett, B., Cooney, M., & Smith, F. (1991). Personality as a vulnerability factor to depression. *British Journal of Psychiatry, 159,* 106–114.

Boyce, P., Harris, M., Silove, D., Morgan, A., Wilhelm, K., & Hadzi-Pavlovic, D. (1998). Psychosocial factors associated with depression: a study of socially disadvantaged women with young children. *Journal of Nervous and Mental Disease, 186,* 3–11.

Brown, G.W., & Prudo, R. (1981). Psychiatric disorder in a rural and an urban population. 1. Aetiology of depression. *Psychological Medicine, II,* 581–599.

Brown, G.W., & Bifulco, A. (1990). Motherhood, employment and the development of depression: a replication of a finding? *British Journal of Psychiatry, 156,* 169–179.

Brown, G.W., Harris, T., & Bifulco, A. (1986). Long-term effects of early loss of parent. In Rutter, M., Izard, C., & Read, P. (Eds.), *Depression in Young People. Developmental and Clinical Perspectives* (pp.251–296). New York: Guilford Press.

Canino, G., Rubio-Stipec, M., Shrout, P., Bravo, M., Stolberg, R., & Bird, H. (1987). Sex differences and depression in Puerto Rico. *Psychological Women's Quarterly, 11,* 443–459.

Casper, R.C., Redmond, D.E. Jr, Katz, N.M., Schaffer, C.B., Davis, J.M., Koslow, S.H. (1985). Somatic symptoms in primary affective disorders: presence and relationship to the classification of depression. *Archives of General Psychiatry, 42*, 1098–1104.

Clancy, K., & Gove, W. (1974). Sex differences in mental illness: an analysis of response bias in self-reports. *American Journal of Sociology, 80*, 205–216.

Cohen, P., Cohen, J., & Brook, J. (1993). An epidemiological study of disorders in late childhood and adolescence. II. Persistence of disorders. *Journal of Child Psychology and Psychiatry, 34*, 869–877.

Commonwealth Fund (1993). *Survey of Women's Health.* New York: Commonwealth Fund.

Costello, E.J., Angold, A., Bums, B.J., Erkanli, A., Stangl, D.K., & Tweed, D.L. (1996). The Great Smoky Mountains Study of Youth: functional impairment and severe emotional disturbance. *Archives of General Psychiatry, 53*, 1137–1143.

Culbertson, F.M. (1997). Depression and gender. An international review. *American Psychologist, 52*, 25–31.

Davidson, J., & Pelton, S. (1986). Forms of atypical depression and their response to antidepressant drugs. *Psychiatry Research, 17*, 87–95.

Dawkins, K., & Potter, W.Z. (1991). Gender differences in pharmacokinetics and pharmacodynamics of psychotropics: focus on women. *Psychopharmacology Bulletin, 27*, 417–426.

Dew, M.A., Dunn, L.O., Bromet, E.J., & Shulberg, H.C. (1988). Factors affecting help-seeking during depression in a community sample. *Journal of Affective Disorders, 14*, 223–234.

Endicott, J. (1993). The menstrual cycle and mood disorders. *Journal of Affective Disorders, 29*, 193–200.

Ernst, C., & Angst, J. (1992). The Zurich study XII. Sex difference in depression. Evidence from longitudinal epidemiological data. *European Archives of Psychiatry and Clinical Neuroscience, 241*, 222–230.

Fava, G.A., & Molnar, G. (1987). Criteria for diagnosing depression in the setting of medical disease. *Psychotherapy and Psychosomatics, 48*, 21–25.

Fava, M., Abraham, M., Alpert, J., Nierenberg, A.A., Pava, J., & Rosenbaum, J.F. (1996). Gender differences in asix I comorbidity among depressed outpatients. *Journal of Affective Disorders, 38*, 129–133.

Fennig, S., Schwartz, J.E., & Bromet, E.J. (1994). Are diagnostic criteria, time of episode and occupational impairment important determinants of the female:male ratio for major depression? *Journal of Affective Disorder, 30*, 147–154.

Floyd, B.J. (1997). Problems in accurate medical diagnosis of depression in female patients. *Social Science and Medicine, 44*, 403–412.

Fombonne, E. (1995). Depressive disorders: time trends and possible explanatory mechanisms. In Rutter, M., & Smith, D.J. (Eds.), *Psychosocial Disorders in Young People: Time Trends and their Causes* (pp.549–615). Chichester: John Wiley & Sons.

Frank, E., Kupfer, D.J., Jacob, M., Blumenthal, S.J., & Jarrett, D.B. (1987). Pregnancy-related affective episodes among women with recurrent depression. *American Journal of Psychiatry, 144*, 288–293.

Frank, E., Carpenter, L.L., & Kupfer, D.J. (1988). Sex differences in recurrent depression: are there any that are significant? *American Journal of Psychiatry, 145*, 41–45.

Friedlander, M.L., & Phillips, S.D. (1984). Preventing anchoring errors in clinical judgment. *Journal of Consulting Clinical Psychology, 52*, 366.

Garmezy, N. (1985). Stress-resistant children: the search for protective factors. In Stevenson, J.E. (Ed.), *Recent Research in Developmental Psychopathology* (pp.213–233). Oxford: Pergamon Press.

Gater, R., Tansella, M., Korten, A., Tiemens, B.G., Mavreas, V.G., & Olatawura, M.O. (1998). Sex differences in the prevalence and detection of depressive and anxiety disorders in general health care settings. *Archives of General Psychiatry, 55*, 405–413.

Gater, R.A., Dean, C., & Morris, J. (1989). The contribution of childbearing to the sex difference in first admission rates for affective psychosis. *Psychological Medicine, 19*, 719–724.

Ginsberg, S.M., & Brown, G.W. (1982). No time for depression: a study of help-seeking among mothers of preschool children. In Mechanic, D. (Ed.), *Symptoms, Illness Behavior, and Help-seeking* (pp.87–114). New York: Prodist.

Glassman, A.H., Perel, J.M., & Shostak, M. (1977). Clinical implications of imipramine plasma levels for depressive illness. *Archives of General Psychiatry, 34*, 197–204.

Golomb, M., Fava, M., Abraham, M., & Rosenbaum, J.F. (1995). Gender differences in personality disorders. *American Journal of Psychiatry, 152*, 579–582.

Gonen, J. (1997). Managed care and women's mental health: a focus on depression. *Women's Health Issues* (Suppl. Insights), *5*, 1–11.

Gotlib, I.H., Whiffen, V.E., Mount, J.H., Milne, J., & Cordy, N.I. (1989). Prevalence rates and demographic characteristics associated with depression in pregnancy and the postpartum. *Journal of Consulting and Clinical Psychology, 57*, 269–281.

Hamilton, J.A., Grant, M., & Jensvold, M.E. (1996). Sex and treatment of depression: when does it matter? In Jensvold, M.F., Halbreich, U., Hamilton, J.A. (Eds.), *Psychopharmacology and Women: Sex, Gender, and Hormones* (pp.241–257). Washington DC: American Psychiatric Press.

Hawkins, D.R., Taub, J.M., & Van de Castle, R.L. (1985). Extended sleep (hypersomnia) in young depressed patients. *American Journal of Psychiatry, 142*, 905–910.

Heller, W. (1993). Gender differences in depression: perspectives from neuropsychology. *Journal of Affective Disorders, 29*, 129–143.

Hoffman, E. (1996). Psychosocial and behavioral factors in women's health: research, prevention, treatment, and service delivery in clinical and community settings. Paper presented at the meeting of the American Psychological Association, Washington, D.C.

Jarrett, R.B., Eaves, G.G., & Grannemann, B.D. (1991). Clinical, cognitive, and demographic predictors of response to cognitive therapy for depression: a preliminary report. *Psychiatry Research, 37*, 245–260.

Jensvold, M.F., Reed, K., & Jarrett, D.B. (1992). Menstrual cycle-related depressive symptoms treated with variable antidepressant dosage. *Journal of Women's Health, 1*, 109–115.

Jiménez, A.L., Alegría, M., Peña, M., & Vera, M. (1997). Mental health utilization in women with symptoms of depression. *Women Health, 25*, 1–21.

Kaufert, P.A., Gilbert, P., & Hassaret, T. (1988). Researching the symptoms of menopause: an exercise in methodology. *Maturitas, 10*, 117–131.

Keitner, G.I., Ryan, C.E., Miller, I.W., Kohn, R., & Epstein, N.B. (1991). 12-month outcome of patients with major depression and comorbid psychiatric or medical illness (compound depression). *American Journal of Psychiatry, 148*, 345–350.

Kendell, R.E., Chalmers, J.C., & Platz, C. (1987). Epidemiology of puerperal psychoses. *British Journal of Psychiatry, 150*, 662–673.

Kessler, R.C., McGonagle, K.A., Swartz, M., Blazer, D.G., & Nelson, C.B. (1993). Sex and depression in the National Comorbidity Survey I: lifetime prevalence, chronicity and recurrence. *Journal of Affective Disorders, 29*, 85–96.

Kessler, R.C., McGonagle, K.A., Nelson, C.B., Hughes, M., Swatz, M., & Blazer, D.G. (1994). Sex and depression in the National Comorbidity Survey II: cohort effects. *Journal of Affective Disorders, 30*, 15–16.

Kornstein, S.G. (1997). Gender differences in depression: implications for treatment. *Journal of Clinical Psychiatry, 58* (Suppl.), 12–8.

Kornstein, S.G., Schatzberg, A.F., Yonkers, K.A., Thase, M.E., Keitner, G.I., Ryan, C.E., & Schlager, D. (1995). Gender differences in presentation of chronic major depression. *Psychopharmacology Bulletin, 31*, 711–718.

Lawson, J.S. (1996). Gender issues in electroconvulsive therapy. *Psych Ann, 26*, 717–720.

Lehtinen, V., & Joukamaa, M. (1994). Epidemiology of depression: prevalence, risk factors and treatment situation. *Acta Psychiatrica Scandinavica, 377* (Suppl.), 7–10.

Leibenluft, E., Hardin, T.A., & Rosenthal, N.E. (1995). Gender differences in seasonal affective disorder. *Depression, 3*, 13–19.

Leiman, J.M. (1995). Foreword. In Glied, S., & Kofman, S. (Eds.), *Women and Mental Health: Issues for Health Care Reform*. New York: The Commonwealth Fund.

Leon, A.C., Klerman, G.L., & Wickramaratne, P. (1993). Continuing female predominance in depressive illness. *American Journal of Public Health, 83*, 754–757.

Levy, J., & Heller, W. (1992). Gender differences in human neuropsychological function. In Gerall, A.A., Moltz, H., & Ward, I.L. (Eds.),

Sexual Differentiation, Vol. 11 (pp.245–274), *Handbook of Behavioral Neurology*. New York: Plenum Press.

Lewinshon, P.M., Seeley, J.R., & Rohde, P. (1994). Major depression in community adolescents: age at onset, episode duration, and time to recurrence. *Journal of the American Academy of Child and Adolescent Psychiatry*, *33*, 809–818.

Magos, A.L., Brewster, E., Singh, R., O'Dowd, T., Brincat, M., & Studd, J.W. (1986). The effects of norethisterone in post-menopausal women on oestrogen replacement therapy: a model for the premenstrual syndrome. *British Journal of Obstetrics and Gynaecology*, *93*, 1290–1296.

McCall, W.V., Shelp, F.E., Weiner, R.D., Austin, S., & Norris, J. (1993). Convulsive threshold differences in right unilateral and bilateral ECT. *Biological Psychiatry*, *34*, 606–611.

McGrath, E., Keita, G.P., Strickland, B.R., & Russo, N.F. (1990). *Women and Depression: Risk Factors and Treatment Issues*. Washington DC: American Psychological Association.

Merikangas, K.R., Weissman, M.M., & Pauls, D.L. (1985). Genetic factors in the sex ratio of major depression. *Psychological Medicine*, *15*, 63–69.

Miranda, J., & Muñoz, R. (1994). Intervention for minor depression in primary care patients. *Psychosomatic Medicine*, *56*, 136–142.

Monroe, S.M., & Steiner, S.C. (1986). Social support and psychopathology: interrelations with preexisting disorder, stress, and personality. *Journal of Abnormal Psychology*, *95*, 29–39.

Monroe, S.M., Simons, A.D., & Thase, M.E. (1991). Onset of depression and time to treatment entry: roles of life stress. *Journal of Consulting and Clinical Psychology*, *59*, 566–573.

Montano, C.B. (1994). Recognition and treatment of depression in a primary care setting. *Journal of Clinical Psychiatry*, *55*, 18–33.

Murphy, J.M. (1990). Depression in the community: findings from the Stirling County Study. *Canadian Journal of Psychiatry*, *35*, 390–396.

Murphy, J.M., Oliver, D.C., Sobol, A.M., Moson, R.R., & Leighton, A.H. (1986). Diagnosis and outcome: depression and anxiety in a general population. *Psychological Medicine*, *16*, 117–126.

Murphy, J.M., Monson, R.R., Oliver, D.C., Sobol, A.M., Moson, R.R., & Leighton, A.H. (1987). Affective disorders and mortality: a general population study. *Archives of General Psychiatry*, *44*, 473–480.

Murray, C.J.L., & López, A.D. (Eds.) (1996). *The Global Burden of Disease*. Geneva: World Heath Organization.

Nolen-Hoeksema, S., Girgus, J.S., & Seligman, M.E.P. (1986). Learned helplessness in children: a longitudinal study of depression, achievement, and explanatory style. *Journal of Personality and Social Psychology*, *51*, 435–442.

O'Hara, M.W., Schlechte, J.A., Lewis, D.A., & Varner, M.W. (1991). Controlled prospective study of postpartum mood disorders: psychological, environmental, and hormone variables. *Journal of Abnormal Psychiatry, 100*, 63–73.

Parry, B.L. (1989). Reproductive factors affecting the course of affective illness in women. *Psychiatric Clinics of North America, 12*, 207–220.

Pastuszack, A., Schick-Boschetto, B., Zuber, C., Feldcamp, M., Pinelli, M., Donnerfeld, A., Sihn, S., McCormack, M., Leon-Mitchell, M., Woodland, C., Gardner, A., Hom, M., & Kornen, G. (1993). Pregnancy outcome following first-trimester exposure to fluoxetine (Prozac). *Journal of the American Medical Association, 269*, 2246–2248.

Patton, G.C., Hibbert, M.E., Carlin, J., Shao, Q., Rossier, M., Caust, J., & Bowes, G. (1996). Menarche and the onset of depression and anxiety in Victoria, Australia. *Journal of Epidemiology and Community Health, 50*, 661–666.

Paykel, E.S. (1991). Depression in women. *British Journal of Psychiatry, 158* (Suppl. 10), 22–29.

Paykel, E.S., & Cooper, Z. (1991). Life events and social stress. In Paykel, E.S. (Ed.), *Handbook of Affective Disorders* (2nd Edition). Edinburgh: Churchill Livingstone.

Petersen, A.C., Sarigiani, P.A., & Kennedy, R.E. (1991). Adolescent depression: why more girls? *Journal of Youth and Adolescence, 20*, 247–271.

Pies, R.W. (1994). Medical "mimics" of depression. *Psychiatry Annals, 24*, 519–520.

Preskorn, S.H., & Mac, D.C. (1985). Plasma levels of amitriptyline: effects of age and sex. *Journal of Clinical Psychiatry, 46*, 276–277.

Raskin, A. (1974). Age-sex differences in response to antidepressant drugs. *Journal of Nervous and Mental Disorders, 159*, 120–130.

Regier, D.A., Burke, J.D., & Burke, K.C. (1990). Comorbidity of affective and anxiety disorders in the NIMH Epidemiologic Catchment Area Program. In Maser, J.D., & Cloninger, C.L. (Eds.), *Comorbidity of Mood and Anxiety Disorders* (pp.113–122). Washington DC: American Psychiatric Press.

Regier, D.A., Narrow, W.E., Rae, D.S., Manderscheid, R.W., Locke, B.Z., & Goodwin, F.K. (1993). The *de facto* US mental and addictive disorders service system: Epidemiologic Catchment Area prospective 1-year prevalence rates of disorders and services. *Archives of General Psychiatry, 50*, 85–94.

Rehm, L.P., & Tyndall, C.I. (1993). Mood disorders: unipolar and bipolar. In Sutker, P.B., & Adams, H.E. (Eds.), *Comprehensive Handbook of Psychopathology* (pp.235–261). New York: Plenum.

Sackeim, H.A., Decina, P., Prohovnik, I. (1987). Seizure threshold in electroconvulsive therapy: effects of sex, age, electrode placement, and number of treatments. *Archives of General Psychiatry, 44*, 355–360.

Sargeant, J.K., Bruce, M.L., Florio, L.P., & Weissman, M.N. (1990). Factors associated with 1-year outcome of major depression in the community. *Archives of General Psychiatry, 47*, 519–526.

Schatzberg, A.F., Cohen, L.S., Casper, R.C., & Parry B.L. (1999). Managing depression and related disorders during a woman's life cycle. *The Journal of Clinical Psychiatry, 2,* 2–20.

Schmidt, P.J., & Rubinow, D.R. (1991). Menopause-related affective disorders: a justification for further study. *American Journal of Psychiatry, 48,* 844–852.

Shea, M.T., Glass, D.R., & Pilkonis, P.A. (1987). Frequency and implication of personality disorders in a sample of depressed outpatients. *Journal of Personality Disorders, 1,* 27–42.

Slap, G.B. (1981). Oral contraceptives and depression: impact, prevalence, and cause. *Journal of Adolescent Health, 2,* 53–64.

Stewart, D.E., & Boydell, K.M. (1993). Psychologic distress during menopause: associations across the reproductive cycle. *International Journal of Psychiatry Medicine, 23,* 157–162.

Stowe, Z.N., Casarella, J., & Landry, J. (1995). Sertraline in the treatment of women with postpartum major depression. *Depression, 3,* 49–55.

Teasdale, J.D. (1988). Cognitive vulnerability to persistent depression. *Cognition and Emotion, 2,* 247–274.

Thase, M.E., Reynolds, C.F. 3rd, Frank, E., Simons, A.D., McGeary, J., Fasiczka, A.L., Garamoni, G.G., Jennings, J.R., & Kupfer, D.J. (1994). Do depressed men and women respond similarly to cognitive behavior therapy? *American Journal of Psychiatry, 151,* 500–505.

Veijola, J., Puukka, P., Lehtinen, V., Moring, J., & Lindholm, T. (1998). Sex differences in the association between childhood experiences and adult depression. *Psychological Medicine, 28,* 21–27.

Wagner, K.D., & Berenson, A.B. (1994). Norplant-associated major depression and panic disorder. *Journal of Clinical Psychiatry, 55,* 478–480.

Weissman, M.M. (1987). Advances in psychiatric epidemiology: rates and risks for major depression. *American Journal of Public Health, 77,* 445–451.

Weissman, M.M., & Klerman, G.L. (1977). Sex differences and the epidemiology of depression. *Archives of General Psychiatry, 34,* 98–111.

Weissman, M.M., & Klerman, J.K. (1985). Gender and depression. *Trends in Neuroscience, 8,* 416–420.

Weissman, M.M., & Myers, J.K. (1978). Affective disorders in a U.S. urban community. *Archives of General Psychiatry, 35,* 1304–1311.

Weissman, M.M., Leaf, P.J., Holzer, C.E., Myers, J.K., & Tischler, G.L. (1984). The epidemiology of depression: an update on sex differences in rates. *Journal of Affective Disorders, 7,* 179–188.

Weissman, M.M., Bruce, M.L., Leaf, P.J., Florio, L.P., & Holzer, C. (1991). Affective disorders. In Robins, L.N., & Regier, D.A. (Eds.), *Psychiatric Disorders in America.* New York: Free Press.

Weissman, M.M., Bland, R., Canino, G., Faravelli, C., Greenwald, S., Hwu, H.G., Joyce, P.R., Karam, E.G., Lee, C.K., Lellouch, J., Lépine, J.P., Newman, S., Rubio-Stipec, M., Wells, J.E., Wickramaratne, P.,

Wittchen, H.U., & Yeh, E.K. (1992). The changing rate of major depression: cross-national comparisons. *Journal of the American Medical Association*, 268, 3098–3105.

Weissman, M.M, Bland, R., Joyce, P.R., Newman, S., Wells, J.E., & Wittchen, H.U. (1993). Sex differences in rates of depression: cross-national perspectives. *Journal of Affective Disorders*, 29, 77–84.

Weissman, M.M., Bland, R., Canino, G., Faravelli, C., & Greenwald, S. (1994). Women's increased vulnerability to major depression: cross-national perspectives. *Facing Depression*, 1, 1–3.

Wells, J.E., Bushnell, J.A., Hornblow, A.R., Joyce, P.R., & Oakley-Browne, M.A. (1989a). Christchurch Psychiatric Epidemiology Study, Part. I: methodology and lifetime prevalence for specific psychiatric disorders. *Australian and New Zealand Journal of Psychiatry*, 23, 315–326.

Wells, K.B., Golding, J.M., & Burnam, M.A. (1989b). Affective, substance use, and anxiety disorders in persons with arthritis, diabetes, heart disease, high blood pressure, or chronic lung conditions. *General Hospital Psychiatry*, 11, 320–327.

Wells, K.B., Stewart, A., Hays, R.D., Burnam, M.A., Roger, W., Daniels, M., Berry, S., Greenfield, S., & Ware, J. (1989c). The functioning and well-being of depressed patients: results from the medical outcomes study. *Journal of the American Medical Association*, 262, 914–919.

Wickramaratne, P.J., Weissman, M.M., Leaf, P.J., & Holford, T.R. (1989). Age, period and cohort effects on the risk of major depression: results from five United States communities. *Journal of Clinical Epidemiology*, 42, 333–344.

Wilhelm, K., & Parker, G. (1994). Sex differences in lifetime depression rates: fact or artefact? *Psychological Medicine*, 24, 97–111.

Wilhelm, K., Parker, G., & Asghari, A. (1998). Sex differences in the experience of depressed mood state over fifteen years. *Social Psychiatry and Psychiatric Epidemiology*, 33, 16–20.

Winokur, G., Coryell, W., Keller, M., Endicott, J., & Akistal, H. (1993). A prospective follow-up of patients with bipolar and primary unipolar affective disorder. *Archives of General Psychiatry*, 50, 457–465.

Wisner, K.L., Perel, J.M., & Wheeler, S.B. (1993). Tricyclic dose requirements across pregnancy. *American Journal of Psychiatry*, 150, 1541–1542.

Wittchen, H.U., Burke, J.D., Semler, G., & Pfister, H. (1989). Recall and dating of psychiatric symptoms: test–re-test reliability of related symptom questions in a standardized psychiatric interview. *Archives of General Psychiatry*, 46, 437–443.

Wittchen, H.U., Essau, C.A., von Zerssen, D., Krieg, J.C., & Zaudig, M. (1992). Lifetime and six-month prevalence of mental disorders in the Munich follow-up study. *European Archives of Psychiatry and Clinical Neuroscience*, 241, 247–258.

Yonkers, K.A., Kando, J.C., Cole, J.O., & Blumenthal, S. (1992). Gender differences in pharmacokinetics and pharmacodynamics of psychotropic medication. *American Journal of Psychiatry, 149*, 587–595.

Young, M.A., Fogg, L.F., Scheftner, W.A., Keller, M.B., & Fawcett, J.A. (1990). Sex differences in the lifetime prevalence of depression: does varying the diagnostic criteria reduce the female/male ratio? *Journal of Affective Disorder, 18(3)*, 187–192.

Section 3

WOMEN AND REPRODUCTIVE HEALTH

Chapter 13

The Post-Modernisation of Motherhood

Rosemary Gillespie

University of Portsmouth, United Kingdom

Historically, feminine identity and women's social roles have been constructed around the practice and symbolism surrounding motherhood. For women, motherhood has been seen to be universal, and ubiquitous; the desire for it or "maternal instinct", inevitable and central to "normal" feminine identity (Erikson, 1964; Russo, 1976; Stone, 1977). Consequently, the nurturing of children has universally been seen to be what women do and traditionally mothers are seen to be what women are. Women who are not mothers have frequently been pitied or vilified, as unfulfilled, deviant and unfeminine (Ireland, 1993).

To what extent is motherhood really a universal, unchanging, "pre-social" monolith? Is the current experience of motherhood really the same as women experienced in the past? Can we expect it to be the same in the future? Might motherhood be understood as integral and contextualised within the society in which it arises? The first part of this chapter will critically assess normative discourses that have come to be associated with motherhood and that define motherhood as central to the "essence" of feminine identity. It will then consider the extent to which motherhood might better be understood as a social and historical construction, comprised of and contained within the society in which it arises, and as diverse as the women who experience it. The second part of the chapter will assess the impact of social and technological change

Women, Health and the Mind
Edited by L. Sherr and J.S. St Lawrence. © 2000 John Wiley & Sons, Ltd

that occurred during the latter half of the twentieth century. It will suggest that social change and technological development within the contemporary period has resulted in motherhood changing at a faster rate and in more profound ways than ever before. The effects of this have been to significantly and dramatically transform the meanings and experiences of motherhood and mothering. It has had the effect of creating new possibilities and opportunities for human reproduction. In the contemporary era, we have come to experience a "post-modernisation of motherhood", whereby through these processes of transformation the meanings of motherhood have become disrupted and recast. Finally, although the process of the post-modernisation of motherhood potentiates exciting and radical new reproductive possibilities for women, it also creates risks never before encountered. These risks have the capacity to impact upon human reproduction in potentially catastrophic ways.

MOTHERHOOD DISCOURSES

Ideas both essentialist and determinist, that motherhood is fixed, unchanging, natural, fulfilling and central to feminine identity, are entrenched in western culture (Russo, 1976; Stone, 1977). Cultural discourses associated with motherhood have been drawn from ideological standpoints that inform everyday understandings of the meanings of motherhood and its relationship with feminine identity. For example, Judeo-Christian attitudes to sexuality and reproduction emphasise how bearing children, and the pain associated with childbirth, was God's curse on Eve for her sins. Mary is upheld as a symbol of perfect womanhood, passive, obedient and a recipient of God's will. Yet as both a virgin and a mother, she represents an impossible ideal for women (Gittens, 1985). The Christian marriage service defines motherhood for the woman within marriage as normal and desirable. It was not until 1958 that the Church of England yielded to the use of contraception within marriage, having discouraged its use through the early part of the century (Holdsworth, 1988). The Roman Catholic Church, however, remains wholly opposed to what it terms "unnatural" methods of birth control.

Motherhood discourses have also drawn on a legacy of modern science. Darwin's (1896) theory of sexual selection, explained what he saw to be "natural" evolutionary physical differences and social roles between males and females. More recently, this has been re-invented by Richard Dawkins (1989). He argues, in his book *The Selfish Gene*, that for women to fulfil the biological imperative of the "gene machine" by successful progenation, they must make an investment of years. Thus, sociobiology perpetuates discourses of femininity based upon motherhood as women's biological destiny and primary social role.

Psychoanalytical theory and medicine have also significantly influenced the ways in which motherhood is conceptualised. Freud developed an analysis of gender difference based on cognitive processes grounded in genital differences that emphasised the centrality of motherhood to feminine identity. His theories formed the basis of the "popularisation of psychology" that led to the production of child-rearing manuals by predominantly male experts such as Truby King and Donald Winnicot. Throughout the early part of the twentieth century, these emphasised the importance of the mother in child development. Similarly, drawing on expert knowledge, control over women's bodies is accessible only to a relatively small, male dominated group of medical experts (Faulkner & Arnold, 1985). Reproductive medicine provided an explanatory model whose normative scientific discourses and practices pervaded women's mothering experiences, as medical technologies associated with conception, pregnancy and birth became widespread. As a result of these psychological and medical discourses, feminine identity has become constructed around notions of motherhood and mothering.

Key political perspectives, especially those of the political right, reinforced motherhood ideology. Conservatives and neo-liberals support what are seen to be traditional "family values", associated with kinship, "natural" social roles and the containment of sexual behaviour. Theodore Roosevelt in 1905 for example, championed motherhood as "the true calling for women, a sacred and civic duty". More recently, the Conservative Thatcher and Major governments of the 1980s and 1990s in the United Kingdom set out to reverse what they saw to be the decline in "traditional family values" by setting themselves up as the "party of the family", reinforcing traditional family ideologies with a "Back to Basics" campaign. Similarly, in the late 1990s, New Labour sparred with the Conservative Party to be seen as the "family" party. In the United States, "born again" Protestantism is a central element of the New Right coalition whose agenda includes preserving "traditional" family values and restricting reproductive rights for women. Consequently dominant, normative discourses associated with motherhood, drawn from religious, scientific and right-wing political ideologies, pass into popular discourse and everyday understanding. They become "truth" and "facts", that ultimately inform the understanding of women themselves (Nicolson, 1993).

MOTHERHOOD AS A SOCIAL AND HISTORICAL CONSTRUCTION

Yet to what extent do we adequately understand motherhood as a universal phenomenon, one that is experienced by women throughout different historical periods and different cultures? Are women bound together by motherhood as an essentialist, pre-social phenomenon? In the next section, the diversity of women's experiences of motherhood will be considered to suggest that a fuller understanding of motherhood might be better depicted as a social and historical construction.

Differences in the meaning of motherhood can be starkly contrasted across different cultures. For many poor women and women in the developing world, a combination of poverty and sexual disempowerment leave them in poor health and lead to high levels of maternal deaths. For example, in the poorer countries in Africa and Asia, maternal deaths remain a hundred times that of women in the West (Doyal, 1995). Maternal and infant mortality rates are high as mothers are frequently left damaged as they give birth in poverty, in poor social conditions and without basic medical assistance. In Niger, for instance, a combination of poverty, debt repayment, military rule and Islamic fundamentalism perpetuate the desperate plight of women who, without access to reproductive rights and basic medical care, endure a starkly different experience of reproduction and mothering than women in the developed world (O'Kane, 1998).

Cross-cultural differences include the ways in which biological and genetic parenthood in Western patrilineal societies is distinct from societies described as "matrilineal". In matrilineal societies, the line of descent is determined by, and people are "made" of, the care and nurturence of women (Katz Rothman, 1994). In matrilineal societies, relationships are usually connected by "lineage", but the line is through the "growing of children" by women, rather than impregnation by men (Peterson, 1982, p.141 quoted in Katz Rothman, 1994). One such society is that of the Ponapean matriliny, located in Micronesia's Eastern Caroline Islands in the Pacific (Peterson, 1982).

Differences in what it means to mother can also be seen within societies. Nicolson has argued that the social conditions of contemporary motherhood exist within a clearly defined social context that includes heterosexuality, marriage and child rearing that constitute the "patriarchal parcel of rules" that regulate sexual behaviour in western society (Nicolson, 1993). For example, cultural discourses of motherhood contained within the "nuclear" family have emerged principally amongst the white bourgeois in western Europe and North America following the Enlightenment, the rise of industrial capitalism, modern science and Western scientific medicine (Bleir, 1984; Nakano Glen, 1994; Harding, 1986; Keller, 1983). During this period, the nuclear family constituted a new social arrangement following the rise of industrial capitalism that required particular family arrangements to facilitate the transmission of wealth inter-generationally amongst kin (Nakano Glen, 1994). Nakano Glen further argued that this idealised form of motherhood, universalised, yet primarily derived from the experiences of white middle-class Western women, increasingly coexists amongst other distinct and submerged constructions of mothering. She has argued that whilst dominant models of motherhood within the nuclear family applied to a European and North American bourgeois of the nineteenth and twentieth centuries, differences and diversity surrounding mothering, such as single parenting or lesbian parenting, have become marginalised and denied (Nakano Glen, 1994). For the majority of single mothers, working class women, native Americans, immigrants, African Americans and other racial minorities, mothering within the nuclear family is irrelevant to their lives.

The meaning and experience of motherhood has changed throughout different historical periods. In the West over several centuries, "demographic transitions" (Meade et al., 1988) have seen population changes that progressed from a time of high birth and death rates to stable birth and death rates, resulting in an ageing population (Moon, 1995). In addition, although most women in the West continue to become mothers at some time in their lives, demographic and social changes since World War II have meant that they are having fewer children, later in their lives, in a variety of different family configurations. As a result of changes in understandings of what constitutes a family, differences in women's reproductive and mothering experiences have emerged. In Great Britain, lone parents and one-person households have increased significantly, while the traditional nuclear family declined from 38% of all households in 1961 to only 25% in 1993 (*Social Trends*, 1995). Divorces in Great Britain doubled between 1971 and 1992, with one divorce for every two marriages in 1992 (*Social Trends*, 1995).

Further social change that impacted upon women's mothering occurred in the area of paid work. During World Wars I and II, large numbers of women entered paid work, many for the first time (Lewis, 1992), with numbers escalating further after World War II. However, the conditions surrounding women's paid work have included part time work and low pay (Witz, 1992). Nevertheless, as a consequence of entry into the work force, smaller proportions of women's lives are now spent in the home bearing and rearing children.

A further factor in the changing face of motherhood followed the influences of second-wave feminism. As a result of women's demands for greater reproductive freedom, an increased number of women now have access to safe abortion and contraception. New technologies enabled women to exert greater control over their fertility in terms of when, whether and in what context they will mother. Modernity has given rise to an era in which women have been able to safely control their fertility in ways never before possible. As a result of this, perhaps the most significant trend in women's reproductive experiences is the increasing number of women who choose not to become mothers. In 1976 the British Family Formation Survey found that 1% of married women stated a preference for no children (Dunnell, 1976). In 1991 the Office of Population Census and Surveys forecast that 20% of the 1960s, 1970s and 1980s British cohorts would remain childless (*Social Trends*, 1993). Similarly twice as many women in 1991 stated that they expected to remain childless compared to 1986 (*Social Trends*, 1995). In summary, women have become less confined to roles associated with nurturing and caring and have increasingly combined multiple roles whereby motherhood may constitute *one* of the ways, rather than the *sole* or *primary* way, in which women establish and experience a feminine self-concept.

In addition to the changing social context of mothering within the family, significant changes have also impacted upon the processes associated with becoming a mother. For example, Nicky Leap and Billie Hunter (1993) provided a harrowing account of motherhood in the United Kingdom in the early part of the twentieth century, before the inception of the National Health Service (NHS). Drawing on oral histories of the early twentieth century, Leap & Hunter highlighted how fertility was often a burden for working class women, whose lives were often constrained by poverty, drudgery and exhaustion. Women without access to fertility control often resorted to illegal, self-induced and often fatal abortion in desperation in their attempts to control their fertility (Leap & Hunter, 1993). In addition, single parenthood often meant rejection and social isolation from family and community (Holdsworth, 1988).

Since the inception of the NHS in Britain, women's experiences of becoming a mother have been radically transformed. As the number of births that take place in hospitals in the United Kingdom increased to 98%, pregnancy, labour and delivery increasingly became medicalised (Campbell & Macfarlane, 1990).

Conceptualisations of motherhood as natural, fixed, universal and central to constructions of "normal" feminine identity, contained with the enduring and heterosexual union of the nuclear family with its gender roles, traditionally dominated understandings of what it meant to mother. Yet, there has never been a time when motherhood was unfettered by its social and historical context. Social divisions, cultural difference and social change have always had a key bearing on women's experiences of motherhood and mothering. Motherhood is experienced in a multitude of ways across societies, between societies as well as throughout different historical periods. Thus, rather than natural, ubiquitous and universal, motherhood might therefore be more fully understood as a social and historical construction, as diverse as the societies in which it occurs and as diverse as the women who experience it. The next section will further argue that in the contemporary era of late modernity (Giddens, 1991), human reproduction, and in particular motherhood, is changing at a faster pace and in a more profound manner than ever before.

THE POST-MODERNISATION OF MOTHERHOOD

In the contemporary era, social forces impact upon human social life in highly significant ways, never before possible. Many contemporary theorists argue that the current temporal era has resulted in an age of new sociological understandings, that of post-modernity (Bauman, 1989; Lyotard, 1984). The focus of post-modernism is on a society with an increasing and far reaching pace of change that gives rise to uncertainty. Features of post-modernity include fragmentation and turbulence, the absence of clear structures, and diversity of social institutions and identities. Increased opportunities as a result of mass consumption through the spread of modern technology and communication technologies dominate meaning. The human subject is considered profoundly unstable and identities fragmented and decentred. Motherhood provides an interesting example of how social conditions have come to be inscribed upon human social life. For example, the technological changes that impacted upon motherhood in the contemporary era have transformed and fragmented its meanings in ways that render motherhood an increasingly unstable category. Technological transformations further undermine the notion of motherhood as an "essential" phenomenon, as social forces impact more and more on the nature of reproduction and motherhood. For instance, Giddens argued that in the contemporary era, increased options made available to individuals in society mean that the natural world has "come to an end" (Giddens, 1991, p.165). The biological is seen to become increasingly social, as natural events become "pulled into systems" (Giddens, 1991, p.166). Motherhood provides an example of social processes increasingly "determined by socialised influences" (Giddens, 1991, p.166). The following section will consider the ways in which technological change, brought about by contemporary conditions, alter and transform understandings, meanings and experiences of motherhood, in the context of "post-modernisation of motherhood". Thus as a new century dawns, new distinct radical possibilities for human reproduction are emerging.

In the contemporary period, social and technological changes associated with motherhood are occurring at a more rapid pace than in any previous historical period. Consequently, the social influences on motherhood have become increasingly profound, further rendering problematic and fragmenting what it means to be a mother. In particular, medical technologies have impacted upon women's fertility and mothering in a variety of ways. These changes have enabled women to exert greater control over their fertility, in terms of when, whether and in what context they will mother. Nevertheless, this increased choice is accompanied by legislation, policy frameworks and professional practices that impact upon the circumstances within which women make choices such as abortion and fertility treatments. The contemporary era has given women an opportunity to safely control their fertility in ways never before possible.

First, there has been a growth in contraceptive technologies designed to control fertility by interrupting the processes of reproduction. Modern techniques focus on the prevention of conception, implantation of an embryo or termination. They include barrier methods such as the diaphragm or condom, hormonal medications, intra-uterine devices, sterilisation and abortion as well as post-coital medication, such as the "morning after pill". Their availability has meant that wider reproductive choice has increasingly come to be available to a large number of women.

Second, modernity has given rise to a range of pre-natal and birth technologies and an increased medicalisation of pregnancy, labour and delivery. Human reproduction has never been "natural" or unfettered by its social context. Nevertheless, during the last century the place of birth, those who attended women and the techniques deployed to manage birth, changed in ways that have impacted upon becoming a mother in highly specific ways (Arney, 1985; Garcia et al, 1990; Oakley, 1984), in particular, increased hospital delivery and the technological management of reproduction, through for example, fetal heart monitoring, monitoring of uterine contractions, epidural anaesthesia, forceps or vacuum delivery, and caesarean section. The increased medicalisation of childbirth has generally been represented by the medical profession as being beneficial for women and contributing to reduce infant and maternal mortality in the developed world. However during the 1970s and 1980s, a critical account of technologies, founded in the concepts of oppression and colonialism, emerged whereby women were seen to lose control and autonomy over their bodies in the context of reproduction and mothering (Martin, 1989; Oakley, 1976, 1984, 1993).

The final aspect of medical technology to have a key impact on women's reproductive choices is conceptive and genetic technologies. Many who experience "involuntary infertility", now have at their disposal a range of experts, treatments and technologies that may enable them to produce a child. Examples include artificial insemination by donor (AID) and in vitro fertilisation (IVF).

Through the use of conceptive technologies, a child may now be produced using a woman's own eggs or those of another woman, the sperm of her male partner, if she has one, or that of a donor. Surrogacy and egg donation may mean that women are involved in reproductive processes that produce a child for other women. Eggs may be harvested from women at the height of their fertility and stored for use later in their lives, allowing them to reproduce in later years. In the future this process may be extended to embryos. An embryo may now be developed outside the body of a woman. Its production may involve more than two "parents". Conception may also take place after the death of a parent, such as the case of Diane Blood in the United Kingdom, who sought to become pregnant using her dead husband's sperm. In addition the cloning of human organisms and the availability of "artificial wombs" are estimated to be only a few years away.

Genetic technologies are a further example of medical technology that uses scientific techniques to control and change the genetic characteristics of the human organism through modifications to the DNA. Scientists are increasingly developing the knowledge and skills to isolate genes and to develop greater knowledge about congenital conditions in order to reduce genetic abnormalities. Examples include genetically transmitted diseases such as cystic fibrosis, severe combined immune deficiency (SCID) and forms of breast cancer.

The increasingly scientific and technological approaches to human reproduction have resulted in the experience and outcome of pregnancy becoming increasingly separated from the biological and the natural. This fragmentation of what it means to mother further problematises the notion of motherhood as a stable, natural and universal social category. The increasing use of conceptive, reproductive, genetic and conceptive technologies over human reproduction has had the effect of problematising, fragmenting and subverting the very meaning of parentage (Russell, 1994). For example artificial insemination, egg donation, sperm banks, in vitro fertilisation, embryo transfer and gestational surrogacy mean that women may gestate fetuses that carry none of their own genetic material. Reproductive technologies have the power not just to separate sex from reproduction but also to disengage and fragment biological, social and genetic parenthood (Lewis & Cannell, 1986).

This overwhelming pace of change and wide diversity in the possibilities for human reproduction has resulted in a "cafeteria approach" to human reproduction, whereby women may engage in a greater or lesser extent in the multiple and diverse activities associated with motherhood and mothering. Women may become mothers through a range of processes that may or may not involve sex with a man. They may be involved in reproductive processes that result in the fertilisation of other women. They may gestate a fetus for another woman through surrogacy. They may be involved in the gestation of a child that carries none of their genetic material. The freezing and storage of eggs until after a woman's egg production potential has passed, means that the "biological clock" may not limit women's reproductive opportunities as before. Women may engage in a wide diversity of procreative, parenting or mothering activities that may or may not result in a "child of their own", yet they may still consider themselves to have mothered in some way. In summary, the meaning of motherhood has significantly expanded to include a wealth of activities and processes that may or may not involve traditional mothering practices of birthing and nurturing.

MOTHERHOOD IN THE NEW MILLENNIUM: THE REAPPRAISAL OF RISK

The closing decades of the twentieth century saw important developments in reproductive medicine and these have, in turn, impacted upon the meanings and experiences of conception, pregnancy, labour and delivery, and mothering. Scientific developments and medical technology for example, have opened a multitude of choices for childbearing women that were not available to them until relatively recently. The future may expand the potential for this considerably further. The previous section assessed the ways technology makes it possible for women to prevent or terminate pregnancy, or to become mothers under circumstances never before imagined. However, the extent to which increased technological intervention in reproductive process has been a friend or foe to women has been the subject of much debate amongst feminists (Corea, 1985; Griffin, 1983; Oakley, 1976, 1984, 1993). These writers have suggested that technological intervention has been a two-edged sword for women. On the one hand, it has enabled women to control their fertility in ways never before possible, enabled women who otherwise may not have been able to produce a child to become mothers, and contributed to reduced maternal and infant mortality, morbidity and suffering. However, it has also limited choice by increased control over women's mothering by agencies such as the state and the medical profession. Thus, the "post-modernisation of mother-hood" has created a diversity of opportunities for women and transformed the meanings of motherhood in highly significant ways. It has also, however, created uncertainties and opened a Pandora's box of risks and additional burdens for women in relation to both the *nature* and *experience* of mothering.

Giddens (1991) argues that in late modernity the self becomes increasingly reflexive, making choices, taking opportunities and risks in an increasingly global arena. New ways of reproducing involve not simply new ways of enabling women to become pregnant and the technologies that facilitate this, they also involve re-conceptualising what it means to reproduce, to procreate and to mother. For example, they create possibilities whereby women who do not want a child of their own, who do not wish to be "biological" or "social" mothers by giving birth to and nurturing a child of their own, can participate in reproduction in other ways. It blurs the distinction between motherhood and childlessness, in ways that create a fragmented cafeteria approach to motherhood, whereby women can engage to a greater or lesser extent in reproduction and mothering. This transformative process signifies the emergence of a post-modernisation of motherhood.

Giddens (1991) emphasised that the conditions of contemporary society give rise to opportunities and risks never before encountered. In relation to reproduction and motherhood, tensions may also arise in relation to the *opportunities* as well as *hazards* associated with a post-modern model of reproduction. In particular, the ramifications of some of the technologies that are increasingly available are far reaching, and new fears concerning control over human reproduction emerge. Technologies Katz Rothman (1986, p.11) argues, may ultimately become a burden to women as they may, on the one hand open up choices for women, yet may also "close down others". New health risks, for instance, arise associated with increased fertility control. Examples include the contraceptive pill which has been associated with serious medical side-effects such as myocardial infarction, venous blood clots and hypertension (Khan, 1989). Similarly Norplant, a contraceptive implant that delivers a dose of the female hormone analogue, progestogen, has been associated with incorrect insertion and problems associated with its removal (Dyer, 1995). Health risks linked to clinical trials by drug companies on women in the developing world, as well as the non-consensual use of the contraceptive agents Depo-Provera (a long-lasting progestogen injection), intra-uterine devices and Norplant demonstrate the inequalities associated with fertility control (Doyal, 1995; Smyke, 1991). Similarly success rates for IVF are estimated to be as low as between 8% and 10%, potentiating psychological trauma for sub-fertile women (Medical Research Council/Royal College of Obstetrics and Gynaecology, 1989). Health problems have also been linked to some of the drugs used in hyperovulation, for example ovarian cysts, ovarian cancer and coagulation abnormalities (Carter & Joyce, 1987; Marsden & St Clair, 1989).

Other risks include threats to women's reproductive autonomy as increased human control over reproduction means state, medical and ultimately male control over reproductive decisions (Arditti, 1984; Berer, 1986; Corea, 1985). For example, backlash discourses emerge that reposition women in traditional family arrangements that others control. In the United Kingdom the *Warnock Report* (Committee of Enquiry into Human Fertilisation and Embryology, 1984), although in favour of semen and egg donation, articulated a staunch preference against donation of both gametes, whereby neither parent would be the biological or genetic parent (Lewis & Cannell, 1986). In addition, the greater availability of technologies for middle-class women and women in heterosexual partnerships, than for single women, poor women and lesbians, reinforces traditional ideologies associated with motherhood and the family (DiLapi, 1989). Lewis & Cannell (1986) argued that concerns regarding family relationships have led to a "hierarchy" of assisted reproduction methods. The most preferred method is either using the sperm of the husband or embryo replacement using IVF and the gametes of both husband and wife, therefore leaving intact, as closely as possible, the "natural" relationships of biological parenthood and adhering to traditional models of the family.

Further potential loss of autonomy for women might also include increased control by others over access to women's bodies and legislation governing what women may choose to do with their bodies. One example is the introduction of legislation to control the amount of money to be paid to women prepared to act as surrogates. Further examples might include the threat to women's physical autonomy, right to privacy and even human rights through forced intervention in pregnancy. One example of this is the case of Ms S. in the United Kingdom, who was detained in hospital against her will, held under powers governed by the Mental Health Act and subsequently forced to undergo a caesarean section, to which she had refused to consent.

Finally, genetic technologies have given rise to anxieties regarding the ways scientific developments may be underpinned by eugenics and regarding the implications that such knowledge may be used for population control, designer babies made to order, or "genetic discrimination". One such example is the availability of amniocentesis and chromosomal analysis to enable pre-natal diagnosis to take place for the detection of abnormalities such as Down's syndrome (Katz Rothman, 1986). However, some have expressed fears concerning the implications of how genetic technologies, in the future, may be used. For example, it may become possible, in the future, to create babies with specifications on demand. These might include hair or eye colour. More radically, it may also become possible to alter the intellect or character of the unborn. This might include the belief in the potential uncovering of a "gay gene", and other elements associated with the human personality, such as criminality or alcohol abuse. The belief that such factors can be uncovered by science may ultimately lead to seeking to eradicate them through gene manipulation, and the "manufacture of human beings to desired specification" (Katz Rothman, 1986, p.133).

Consequently new opportunities associated with the post-modernisation of motherhood widen opportunity and choice for women, but take place against additional risks. These include risks to their health; autonomy, control over their bodies, life-styles and practices, and finally risks to humanity associated with eugenics, as new forms of discrimination and the manipulation of human characteristics become possible. Technological developments in the contemporary era, as Giddens suggests, takes place amongst an increased "backdrop of risk" (Giddens, 1991, p.114). Although the potential gains for humanity in a post-modern model of motherhood may be significant, the possible losses include the potential for humanitarian catastrophe.

CONCLUSION

This chapter has examined the meanings of motherhood in the contemporary period and challenged dominant understandings of motherhood drawn from religious, scientific and political discourses that represent motherhood as natural and pre-social. It has argued that motherhood is better understood as a social and historical construction. The contemporary era has seen particularly rapid transformations in the meaning and experiences of motherhood. In particular, demographic change has transformed the experience and context of motherhood; women's increased participation in the paid work force has widened women's social role and determined that motherhood is one of a range of choices and options in women's lives. Technologies associated with reproduction have fundamentally transformed the experience of becoming a mother for many women.

Importantly, social and technological changes have given rise to a huge range of options and choices for women, creating a cafeteria approach to motherhood whereby women can engage to a greater or lesser extent in the production and/or nurturing of a child, whilst others can choose to remain childless. Humanity now exerts greater control over when, how and whether women mother than in any previous historical period. This post-modernisation of motherhood has created a whole new set of constraints, inequalities and uncertainties and gains, as well as risks coexisting with increasing technological approaches to reproduction. In particular, unresolved dilemmas remain as to who ultimately wields power and control over reproduction. As a result, the future for motherhood and the implications of this for human reproduction generally is uncertain and the risks that accompany the transformation cannot easily be predicted or quantified.

Finally, erosion of traditional meanings and the expansion of new meanings associated with motherhood result in the social category of motherhood becoming increasingly uncertain. Just as post-structuralism feminists projected that universal categories such as "male" and "female" may ultimately be subsumed under the need to celebrate diversity and difference (Alcoff, 1988; Butler, 1990), in the contemporary era the usefulness of the broad category "mother" as a universal and ahistorical construct can increasingly be questioned. The post-modernisation of motherhood has meant that no singular, unified definition or experience of motherhood exists. Rather it is better understood as one of a range of choices and options that women experience in their lives. Motherhood, childlessness and the multiplicity of possibilities between should therefore be understood as a broad continuum of diverse, legitimate, yet potentially fulfilling options impacting on the experience and identities of women in the new millennium.

REFERENCES

Alcoff, L. (1988). Cultural feminism versus post-structuralism: the identity crisis in feminist theory. *Signs, 13*, 405–436.

Arditti, R. (1984). *Test Tube Women*. London: Pandora.

Arney, W.R. (1985). *Power and the Profession of Obstetrics*. Chicago: University of Chicago Press.

Bauman, Z. (1989). *Modernity and the Holocaust*. Cambridge: Polity.

Berer, M. (1986). Breeding conspiracies: feminism and the new reproductive technologies. *Trouble and Strife, 9*, 33.

Bleir, R. (1984). *Science and Gender: A Critique of Biology and its Theories on Women*. New York: Pergamon Press.

Butler, J. (1990). *Gender Trouble: Feminism and the Subversion of Identity*. London: Routledge.

Campbell, R., & Macfarlane, A. (1990). Recent debate on the place of birth. In Garcia, J., Kilpatric, R., & Richards, M. (Eds.), *The Politics of Maternity Care: Services For Childbearing Women in Twentieth Century Britain*. Oxford: Clarendon Press.

Carter, M.E., & Joyce, D.N. (1987). Ovarian carcinoma in a patient hyper-stimulated by gonadotrophin therapy for IVF: a case report. *Journal of IVF and Embryo Transfer*, 4(2), 126–128.

Committee of Enquiry into Human Fertilisation and Embryology (1984). *Warnock Report*, Report of the Committee of Enquiry into Human Fertilisation and Embryology. London: HMSO.

Corea, G. (1985). *The Mother Machine*. New York: Harper Row.

Darwin, C. (1896). *The Descent of Man and Selection in Relation to Sex*. New York: Appleton.

Dawkins, R. (1989). *The Selfish Gene*. Oxford: Oxford University Press.

DiLapi, E.M. (1989). Lesbian mothers and the motherhood hierarchy. *Journal of Homosexuality*, 18(1/2), 101–121.

Doyal, L. (1995). *What Makes Women Sick: Gender and the Political Economy of Health*. London: Macmillan.

Dunnell, K. (1976). *Family Formation Survey*. London: OPCS.

Dyer, C. (1995). Women scarred by contraceptives. *Guardian Newspaper*, 11 August 1995.

Erikson, E.M. (1964) Inner and Outer Space Reflections on Womanhood. Daedalus, p. 590.

Faulkner, W., & Arnold, E., (1985). *Smothered by Invention*. London: Pluto Press.

Garcia, J., Kilpatrick, R., & Richards, M. (1990). *The Politics of Maternity Care: Services For Childbearing Women*. Oxford: Clarendon Press.

Giddens, A. (1991). *Modernity and Self-identity: Self and Society in the Late Modern Age*. Cambridge: Polity.

Gittens, D. (1985). *The Family in Question*. London: Macmillan.

Griffin, S. (1983). Foreword. In Caldecott, L., & Leland, S. (Eds.), *Reclaim the Earth*. London: The Women's Press.

Harding, S. (1986). *The Science Question in Feminism*. Milton Keynes: Open University Press.

Holdsworth, A. (1988). *Out of the Doll's House: The Story of Women in the Twentieth Century*. London: BBC Books.

Ireland, M. (1993). *Reconceiving Women: Separating Motherhood from Female Identity*. New York: Guilford Press.

Katz Rothman, B. (1986). *The Tentative Pregnancy: Prenatal Diagnosis and the Future of Motherhood*. New York: Viking.

Katz Rothman, B. (1994). Beyond mothers and fathers: ideology in a patriarchal society. In Nakano Glen, E., Chang, G. & Forcey, L.R. (Eds.), *Mothering Ideology, Experience and Agency*. London: Routledge.

Keller, E.F. (1983). Feminism and science. In Abel, E., & Abel, E.K. (Eds.), *Women, Gender and Scholarship: The Signs Reader*. Chicago: University of Chicago Press.

Khan, T. (1989). Recent developments in contraceptive technology: risks and benefits. In Kessel, E., & Awan, A. (Eds.), *Maternal and Child Care in Developing Countries*. Switzerland: Ott Publishers.

Leap, N., & Hunter, B. (1993). *The Midwife's Tale: An Oral History From Handywoman to Professional Midwife*. London: Scarlett Press.

Lewis, J. (1992). *Women in Britain Since 1945*. Oxford: Blackwell.

Lewis, J., & Cannell, F. (1986). The politics of motherhood in the 1980s: Warnock, Gillick and feminists. *Journal of Law and Society, 13(3)*, 321–342.

Lyotard, J.F. (1984). *The Postmodern Condition: A Report Knowledge*. Manchester: Manchester University Press.

Marsden, W., & St Clair, P. (1989). Are in vitro fertilization and embryo transfer of benefit to all? *The Lancet, 2(8670)*, 1027–1329.

Martin, E. (1989). *The Woman in the Body*. Milton Keynes: Open University Press.

Meade, M., Florin, J., & Gesler, W. (1988). *Medical Geography*. New York: Guilford.

Medical Research Council/Royal College of Obstetrics and Gynaecology (1989). *Fourth Report of the VLA*. London: Medical Research Council.

Moon, G. (1995). Demographic and epidemiological change. In Moon, G., & Gillespie, R. (Eds.), *Society and Health: An Introduction for Health Professionals*. London: Routledge.

Nakano Glen, E. (1994). Social constructions of mothering: a thematic overview. In Nakano Glen, E., Chang, G., & Forcey, L.R. (Eds), *Mothering Ideology, Experience and Agency*. London: Routledge.

Nicolson, P. (1993). Motherhood and women's lives. In Richardson, D., & Robinson, V. (Eds.), *Introducing Women's Studies*. London: Macmillan.

Oakley, A. (1976). Wise woman and medicine man: changes in the management of childbirth. In Mitchel, J., & Oakley, A. (Eds.), *The Rights and Wrongs of Women*. London: Harmondsworth.

Oakley, A. (1984). *The Captured Womb: A History of the Medical Care of Pregnant Women*. Oxford: Blackwell.

Oakley, A. (1993). *Essays on Women, Medicine and Health*. Edinburgh: Edinburgh University Press.

O'Kane, M. (1998). *The Guardian*, 23 June 1998.

Peterson, G. (1982). The Ponpean matriliny: production, exchange and the ties that bind. *American Ethnologist, 9(1)*, 129–144.

Russell, K. (1994). A value theoretic approach to reproductive engineering. *Science and Society, 58(3)*, 287–314.

Russo, N. (1976). *Journal of Social Issues, 32(3)*, 143–153.

Smyke, P. (1991). *Women and Health*. London: Zed Books.

Social Trends 23, (1993). Central Statistical Office (CSO). London: HMSO.

Social Trends 25, (1995). Central Statistical Office (CSO). London: HMSO.

Stone, L. (1977). *The Family, Sex and Marriage in England 1500–1800*. London: Weidenfeld and Nicolson.

Strickler, J. (1992). The new reproductive technologies: problem or solution? *Sociology of Health and Illness, 14(1)*, 111–132.

Weedon, C. (1987). *Feminist Practice and Poststructural Theory*. New York: Blackwell.

Witz, A. (1992). *Professions and Patriarchy*. London: Routledge.

Chapter 14

Older Mothers and Later Motherhood

Julia C. Berryman

University of Leicester, United Kingdom

This chapter reviews research on one particular group of older mothers. Whilst most women who become mothers do with time become older mothers, the older mothers considered here are those who give birth later in life. Today, in England and Wales, the average age for women at childbirth is 28.6 years (Birth Statistics, 1998). This is the highest average age for childbirth for over 40 years.

At one time, gynaecologists considered the ideal age for childbirth was between the ages of 20 to 25 years (Cunningham & Leveno, 1995) and a first-time mother aged 30 or more was termed an elderly primigravida. Thus by these standards the current norm for childbirth is old. Kitzinger's book *Birth Over Thirty* (1982) was published at a time when birth at this age was considered old or "elderly". In the 1990s, women aged 35 and over are more likely to be considered "older" and at risk, but attitudes to such mothers are much more positive than a few decades ago. This change in attitude has come about, in part, because there is now a trend in the Western World to delay childbirth that has led to more research on "older mothers". In recent years there also has been recognition that the label "elderly" was somewhat insulting to a woman of 30 or so (Llewellyn-Jones, 1982). Recent birth statistics for England and Wales show that whilst the majority of babies are born to women in their twenties (52%), 41% are now born to women

Women, Health and the Mind
Edited by L. Sherr and J.S. St Lawrence. © 2000 John Wiley & Sons, Ltd

aged 30 and over. Births to younger women are declining, and since 1992, the fertility of women aged 30–34 has exceeded that of women aged 20–24, whilst the fastest growing age-groups for births is women aged 35–39 and 40 and over (Birth Statistics, 1998).

The trend to delayed motherhood is not confined to England and Wales and is now common in much of the developed world including the United States and Australia (Department for Economic and Social Information and Policy Analysis, 1994; US Department of Commerce, 1997).

HOW LATE IS LATER MOTHERHOOD?

There are biological limits to the ages at which women can bear children, but in recent years these limits have become blurred by techniques such as in vitro fertilisation and egg donation. The latter has enabled postmenopausal women to bear children. In general, conception and birth are possible in the years between menarche and menopause from around 12–13 years of age to 50 or 51 years (Gray, 1976; Khaw, 1992; Tanner, 1978). In populations in which there is no attempt to control births, childbirth continues for most of a woman's reproductive life. Research on one interesting group, the North American Hutterites, reveals that women can expect at age 20 that they will have 10.82 live births ahead of them, by 30 5.46 live births, at 40 1.24 live births and at 50 years another 0.2 live births (Eaton & Mayor, 1953). Fertility declines with age and, as is evident from these figures, it appears to drop sharply for women by their forties. Although fertility in the Hutterites appears to decline markedly over 40, Maroulis (1992) warned that these figures may underestimate the capacity of women to bear children later in life, since older women, with an already large family, may be less eager to get pregnant and typically the frequency of intercourse diminished in older couples. Estimates of changes in fertility with age from other sources reveal varied findings. Henry's (1961) paper on sterility by age records a figure of 3% in married women at 20 years, 10% at 30 years, and 31% at 40 years. Studies of the success of artificial insemination by donor (AID) produce a more pessimistic picture. These show a cumulative percentage success rate of achieving a pregnancy of 73% at age under 25, 61.5% for age 31–35 and 53.6% over 35 years (Schwartz & Mayaux, 1982). The AID success figures may be low because of the stress generally surrounding this procedure. Gosden & Rutherford (1995) warned against women delaying starting a family for too long: women planning to start a family late do well to weigh the biological consequences, because oocytes disappear faster from the ovary after the age of 37 and, in their view, fertility "is almost gone by 40".

Today women may not rely on their natural potential to bear children. Assisted reproduction is widely available and has led to a number of well-reported late births. Mrs Liz Buttle in Britain had a baby boy on 20 November 1997 at the age of 60 (O'Neill, 1998) and, in Italy, Mrs Rosanna Della Corte gave birth to a baby boy on 18 July 1994 at the age of 62 (Phillip, 1994). The technique for such conceptions involves use of an egg from a younger woman that is fertilised and inserted into the uterus of an older woman who is stimulated hormonally so that she can receive it (for a discussion see Berryman et al., 1995; Sauer et al., 1992). Theoretically a woman of almost any age could receive such treatment providing she has a uterus and is in good health. Much later motherhood is a controversial issue; some believe that very late motherhood is "inherently wrong and offensive" (Warnock, 1993), whilst others argue forcefully for the right for older women to reproduce (van den Akker, 1994).

There does seem to be a prejudice against older women giving birth and yet none is evident where older fathers are concerned. In England and Wales, the most recent statistics show that 29% of births in marriage are registered with fathers aged 35 and over, including 4035 births registered to fathers aged 50 and 171 to fathers who were at least 65 years. Only 44 births were registered to married women at age 50 and above (Birth Statistics, 1998).

THE CHARACTERISTICS OF WOMEN WHO BECOME MOTHERS LATER

Wilkie (1981) observed that delaying motherhood "is a recent strategy adopted by women interested in careers, especially those in higher education." Rindfuss (1992) suggested that each additional year of schooling results in a delay of about nine months until the first birth. A more recent review (Santos & Beral, 1997) confirmed these findings using data from World Fertility Surveys, the Demographic and Health Surveys, and other national surveys. Overall, women of higher socio-economic status and with more education had later age at childbirth and lower fertility. However, the authors of this review also found wide variations from country to country. Women's reasons for post-poning motherhood also varied from culture to culture. Welles-Nystrom (1997) found that feminist ideology was an evident factor in the timing of first births in American women who postponed motherhood, but this was less evident in a sample of Swedish women who had delayed.

Family planning or the use of contraception is something that varies with the age of women. Planning a pregnancy is most prevalent in women who are in their thirties. In England and Wales, research suggests that about one-third of pregnancies are unintended. In pregnancies that lead to babies (i.e. pregnancies that are terminated are excluded from this figure), this figure varies from 25% in women aged 30 and over to as high as 57% in the under 20s (Fleissig, 1991). Research by Berryman & Windridge (1991a) indicates that, for women in their forties, planning is also not particularly evident. In their sample of 100 first-time mothers, fewer than half the babies were planned. Many women in this study had fertility problems and thus "planning" was hard to gauge because some women had wanted a child but waited many years to realise this goal.

Later babies, particularly those who are not first-borns, may also be the result of a second marriage or partnership. Over one-third of marriages in Britain are second marriages for at least one partner (*Social Trends*, 1994). In the Leicester Motherhood Project, nearly 30% of the older mothers who had had a baby at age 35 or over had been married before, whereas only one in 20 of the younger women aged 20–29 who were of a similar background had been married previously (Berryman & Windridge, 1995).

Another aspect of the older first-time mother that was an unexpected finding in two studies by the author and Windridge was the tendency for older primiparae to be women who were in a relationship with a younger partner. In a British study of 40-plus mothers, mothers of first-borns had partners who were on average 3 years younger than they were (Berryman & Windridge, 1991a). The Leicester Motherhood Project revealed a similar but non-significant trend in first-time mothers aged 35 and over (Berryman & Windridge, 1995).

Older first-time mothers are also more likely to be women who conceived before, relative to younger first-time mothers. In the Leicester Mother and Child Project (Berryman & Windridge, 1998), women whose first live birth was at age 35 or over had a one in three chance of having had a previous pregnancy compared to less than one in 10 in the sample of younger primiparae (women in their twenties). Such pregnancies had ended in a miscarriage, termination or stillbirth. This history of previous pregnancy loss may influence the women's feelings about a subsequent pregnancy.

PREGNANCY, BIRTH AND LATER MOTHERHOOD

It has already been noted that older mothers of first-borns are more likely to have experienced previous pregnancy loss than younger mothers. Although not all of these losses are spontaneous abortions there is plenty of evidence to link raised maternal age to an increased miscarriage rate. Estimates of the incidence of miscarriage vary. Warburton & Fraser (1964) report a rate of 12.2% for women under the age of 20, 18.7% at ages 35–39, and 25.5% at age 40. Hansen (1986) reports an incidence of 7.2–15% for women in their twenties, with a rate of increase of about 50% from the twenties to thirties and, compared with those in their twenties, a two- to four-fold increase in women above 40. When multiparous mothers aged 35 and over were compared with women in their twenties, the miscarriage rate was more than twice that of the younger women (Berryman & Windridge, 1998). Clearly miscarriage is a more common occurrence as women get older.

What other risks are associated with pregnancy in the older mother? Mansfield (1988), in a review of the research, identified eight pregnancy outcomes that had been commonly associated with "mid-life child-bearing". These were: pregnancy-induced hypertension (toxaemia), placental complications, prolonged labour, delivery by caesarean section, prenatal mortality, maternal mortality and low birth weight. Down's syndrome was excluded because of its well-established association with raised maternal age (see Nortman, 1974). Mansfield argued that the majority of the studies she reviewed were methodologically flawed. Often these studies did not take into account the many variables that are confounded with age: such as socio-economic status, income, occupation, health behaviour and others. These variables may vary with age but are not necessarily caused by it. She went on to claim that only caesarean sections were found to be more common in older mothers, and this will be discussed below.

In a review by the author, Thorpe & Windridge (1995) cited evidence that older women may be slightly at risk of hypertension (although the evidence is not conclusive). The evidence for placental complications is not clear-cut, women with more than two children are at increased risk but in the more recent studies, middle-class women over age 35 having a first or second child were not at greater risk of placental complications.

Prolonged labour has been linked to maternal age in some studies (Berkowitz et al., 1990; Cohen et al., 1980; Friedman, 1965; Morrison 1975; Piepert & Bracken, 1993; Stanton, 1956), but not in others (Biggs, 1973; Horgen & Smythe, 1997; Koren, 1963; Spellacy et al., 1986; Stein, 1983). Current evidence concerning the relationship between maternal age and duration of labour is inconclusive. For example, a Scandinavian study found that the second stage of labour was longer in older women, but not the first stage, in both primiparous and multiparous mothers (Rasmussen et al., 1994). Research by Berryman & Windridge (1995), on the other hand, only found this to be true for multiparae. No relationship was found for primiparae as a function of age. Duration of labour is linked to the use of anaesthesia, and induction of labour (Kirz et al., 1985; Morrison, 1975) and both of these are more frequent for older women. The reason for this is unclear and it may have less to do with the mother's physical capacities and more to do with the concern felt by mothers and obstetricians about the woman's age.

The type of pain relief used by women may also differ for women of different ages (Berryman & Windridge, 1995; Prysak et al., 1995; Roberts et al., 1994). For example: younger women were more likely to have used pethidine than older women (Berryman & Windridge, 1995).

Mansfield (1988) claims that only caesarean sections, out of the eight pregnancy outcomes she followed, were found to be more common in older mothers. She argued that they might reflect a concern about the mother's age, on the part of the physician and the woman herself, rather than any real evidence of complications due to age. Others (Newcomb et al., 1991) have echoed this point. Women of different ages are also found to differ in terms of their likelihood of having a pre-term delivery or breech presentation (Roberts et al., 1994).

To summarise, some birth complications have been linked to maternal age, but there is no simple relationship and many factors appear to play a role, other than the age of the mother *per se*.

Turning to maternal mortality, prenatal mortality, and low birth weight, in a review Berryman et al. (1995) found no clear evidence in relation to maternal age. On maternal mortality, there is some evidence for increased risk, especially in women over 40 years of age (Department of Health, 1991), which was not conclusively shown in several earlier reports (Kane, 1967; Kessler et al., 1980; MacDonald & Maclennon, 1960). It should be kept in mind that this is an extremely rare event. Increases in prenatal mortality are not found in all studies, and are more likely to be linked to maternal illness than age alone. Berkowitz et al. (1990) found no increase in mortality in a group of older women who were private patients, college educated, married and predominantly white.

There are two areas that have been linked to later motherhood and are associated with the mother's long-term health: these are breast cancer and uterine cancer. The incidence of breast cancer is higher for women who have not borne children than for those who have but the exact relationship between maternal age at childbirth and breast cancer is not fully understood. One large study (MacMahon et al., 1970) suggested that age at first pregnancy was important and found that women having children after the age of 30 were at increased risk of breast cancer. However, Cummings et al. (1994) argued that age at last pregnancy may be an important predictor of breast cancer and that having a larger family may protect against breast cancer. These authors believe that the increased incidence of breast cancer in the general population is explained by reductions in family size. The precise role of maternal age at childbirth is not clearly established.

Finally, on a more positive note, women having children later are found to be at decreased risk of uterine cancer (Kvale et al., 1992; Lesko et al., 1991). Apparently this is due to exfoliation of the uterus at delivery, which removes any harmful cells.

PSYCHOLOGICAL ASPECTS OF PREGNANCY

A number of studies suggest that older mothers' experiences of pregnancy may be different to those of younger women. Welles-Nystrom & de Chateau (1987) found evidence that women in their thirties are more anxious during pregnancy than women in their twenties and are more likely to regard their transition to motherhood as problematic. A number of studies draw attention to the anxieties that may be aroused by antenatal screening procedures (see Green's review, 1990) despite the fact that such procedures are generally reassuring for most women. Women aged 35 or over are more likely to be offered procedures such as amniocentesis. Because most women are well aware of the association between increased risk of chromosomal abnormality and raised maternal age, this knowledge can be "... a major pre-occupation ..." of the older pregnant woman (Berryman & Windridge, 1991a).

Research by the present author and Windridge (Berryman & Windridge, 1993, 1996) using the Maternal Fetal Attachment Scale (Cranley, 1981) examined women's feelings about their pregnancy and the unborn child in mothers aged 35 and over and in a younger sample of similar background (as far as education, occupational status and marital status were concerned). Older women in the study were assessed in mid and late pregnancy and it was found that such women experienced fewer feelings of attachment for their unborn child than did younger women in mid but not late pregnancy.

Close inspection of the sub-scales showed that the scales concerned with the well-being of the baby were not affected by maternal age. The scales that measured the extent to which the mother thought about her role as a mother, and saw the fetus as a separate being from herself, were affected by age. It was suggested that because older mothers are more anxious about the risks of chromosomal abnormalities and thus the possible loss of the fetus, they might view their pregnancy more tentatively in the early months than younger women. The authors suggested that it is not until the older women are reassured by the results of the various screening tests that they allow themselves to "believe" in their pregnancy. It is interesting to note that the preference *not* to have an amniocentesis increases with maternal age (Beekhuis et al., 1994).

Depression in pregnancy is correlated with depression after birth (Radke-Yarrow et al., 1993) and the evidence from a number of studies indicates that older mothers, particularly primiparous mothers, are not at increased risk of depression. Indeed, they may be at less risk than mothers of average age (see Berryman et al., 1995).

Thus pregnancy may be a time of anxiety for the older mother, particularly in the early months when she may be concerned about the risks to her and her baby because of her greater age, but as time passes older women show no greater concern than younger women. Older mothers do not appear to be at greater risk of depression.

RECOVERY FROM PREGNANCY AND BIRTH: PHYSICAL AND EMOTIONAL

Are the physical demands of being a new mother harder for the older woman to deal with or does her greater maturity help her to cope better than younger mothers? A major study entitled *Health After Childbirth* by MacArthur et al. (1991) investigated this topic in a sample of over 11 000 women. Whilst the focus of this study was not specifically maternal age, it was one of the variables that was examined. Several symptoms showed age effects in their analysis. Backache was a common problem for nearly one-quarter of the sample whatever their age, but younger women were more likely to say that they were suffering this problem for the first time. Headaches unaccompanied by backache, or unassociated with epidural anaesthesia, occurred most frequently in younger multiparaous women (women aged under 25).

Stress incontinence occurring within 3 months of delivery was found in more than one-fifth of the sample and was most likely to be found in older women (independent of parity) following both caesarean section and vaginal delivery (in spite of the fact that the former is slightly protective against the problem). Extreme tiredness was also found more frequently in older mothers and this finding has been replicated in a number of studies (Berryman & Windridge, 1995; Kern, 1982).

MacArthur et al. (1991) believe that health problems experienced following childbirth are much greater than was previously thought and noted that many women had not sought help with their problems. However, the number of problems that were notably greater in older mothers was reassuringly small. In the present author's study (Berryman & Windridge, 1995) of over 100 older mothers a similar picture emerged. In this research the same 25 symptoms assessed by MacArthur et al. were used and only four symptoms varied with maternal age: extreme tiredness, stress incontinence, leg pain and headaches. The first three were more prevalent in older mothers and the latter was found more frequently in younger primiparae (Berryman & Windridge, 1995). As with the research of MacArthur et al., Berryman & Windridge found quite a high percentage of women reporting a number of the 25 symptoms. For example, 68% of the sample reported extreme tiredness (of whom 61% were older women). Thus health problems after childbirth are undoubtedly a common feature of life.

The older mothers in the study above were women aged 35 and over at childbirth. How does the mother in her forties cope? A retrospective study by the author and Windridge examined this issue (Berryman & Windridge, 1991a,b). Women were asked how long it took them to get physically back to normal after childbirth. Forty-plus first-time mothers recorded a mean of over 11 months, compared to 7 months for multiparae at this age. Multiparae in this sample had their first birth at a mean age of 26.3 years and recalled a quicker recovery time after their first child, of around 5.5 months. Whilst these retrospective estimates must be treated with caution, they do give some idea of the possible recovery times for older women relative to those in their twenties.

PARENTING PRACTICES AND CHILD CARE

The medical literature concerned with later motherhood has been problem-centred and it is only in the last few years that the message is "cautiously optimistic" so far as later child bearing is concerned (Cunningham & Leveno, 1995). The results of research on older mothers as parents have been much more positive.

Ragozin et al. (1982) found that increased maternal age was associated with greater satisfaction with parenting (this study included women aged 16–38 years). Eichholz & Offerman-Zuckenberg (1980) suggested that mothers over the age of 35 (especially primiparae) were more likely to have fulfilled themselves prior to the birth and thus less likely to expect their children to do this for them. Frankel & Wise (1982) saw older mothers (women aged 33 and over) as more accepting and less conflicted than younger mothers. In this study the younger mothers stressed the "enormous sacrifices" of motherhood; isolation, financial stress and feelings of restlessness were particularly noted in this group. The experiences of women who become mothers later in life have not been widely researched, although more recent studies echo those from the early 1980s mentioned above.

Breastfeeding varies with maternal age. Not only does the incidence of breastfeeding increase with maternal age, but older mothers who breastfeed tend to do so for longer than younger mothers. There is also a correlation between being older, breastfeeding longer, and having higher educational and occupational status (Berryman & Windridge, 1995; Ever-Hadani et al., 1994; Kern, 1982; Peterson & Da Vanzo, 1992; Vestermark et al., 1991). The advantages to breastfeeding need not be enumerated here but de Man (1989) asserts that the women who breastfeed for longer durations tend to be less hostile, controlling and rejecting in their treatment of children later on. Another area where maternal age appears to make a difference is sleeping patterns. Women aged 35 and over were found to be more likely than those in their twenties to have their infant sleeping with them for all or part of the night (Berryman & Windridge, 1995). The reason for this difference is not clear, but it could be related to the higher breastfeeding duration of this older group.

A number of researchers have looked at parenting practices and maternal age. Thorpe & Cinnamon (1992) reported that older mothers were more responsive to their infants when they cried and found that such infants were taken out for more organised activities relative to those of younger mothers. Other researchers have reported similar findings (Broom, 1994; Lojkasek et al., 1990). Froman & Owen (1990) found that mothers' age (in sample aged 15–43 years) was correlated with overall self-efficacy (having confidence in the ability to succeed at a task) on the Infant Care Scale (Froman & Owen, 1989). Fox et al. (1995) studied parenting practices in over 1000 urban mothers. Maternal age (29 or less and 30 years or more) was one of seven variables they examined. Their results showed that younger mothers had higher discipline scores, lower nurturing scores and reported more child behaviour problems than did older mothers. However, a number of significant interactions between variables were found such as maternal age and "number of children living at home". Thus some caution is required in interpreting their findings. Younger mothers are generally more likely to be single, have lower incomes and less education, and it is important not to confound age with these variables.

The style of discipline has also been said to differ in older and younger mothers. Sears et al. (1957) suggested that older mothers were less likely to use physical punishment or ridicule to control their children. The mother's general attitude may also be different. Chatwin & MacArthur (1993) found, in a study of maternal perceptions of the pre-term infant, that older mothers (those aged 28 and above) were more optimistic about the future of their pre-term infant, and experienced greater confidence in their infants than did younger mothers.

MacDonald & Parke (1986) reported that older parents engage in less physical play with their children, and that fathers engage in physical play more than mothers. In view of the negative correlation between physical play and parental age, sons of older fathers may be perceived as disadvantaged relative to sons of younger fathers. Alternatively older adults may be viewed as providing less stereotypical gender-role training for their offspring. Research by Berryman & Windridge (1998) also found some differences in play as a function of maternal age. Whilst older mothers did not differ in the frequency of physical (energetic) play or sedentary play with their children relative to younger mothers, fathers in the families of older mothers did less energetic play than did fathers in younger mothers' families (according to mothers' reports). However, boys did less sedentary play with fathers in the younger maternal age group than did boys with fathers in the older maternal age group.

The research findings described above are those that found age-related differences. However, many studies find that age does not distinguish mothers' behaviour towards their children: some examples include Kemp et al. (1990) in looking at factors affecting maternal role attainment; Pridham's & Chang's (1991) research on the way new mothers view their own problem-solving competence; and Pascoe & Soloman's research (1994) on "spoiling" young infants.

THE GENERATION GAP

One comment that is often made about women who give birth later in life is the impact of the larger than usual generation gap between mother and child. Often this is viewed in negative terms because it is assumed that children naturally want younger parents and that this provides emotional closeness. Very little research has examined the issue in any systematic way, but the work that is available (often from anecdotal reports) will be considered.

In his book *Latecomers – Children of Parents Over 35*, Yarrow (1991) writes about children recalling their parents. He notes that "later born children often lamented that their parents were emotionally distant, serious, and formal". Informality and spontaneity were often reported to be lacking in the lives of these children and life seemed to be a more serious business. These comments are not widely reflected in the studies of older mothers in relation to younger children. Walter (1984) believes that the younger mother encounters difficulties in dealing with physical and emotional separation from her child because she herself is "struggling with separation and individualisation in her adult life". Other studies have found that older women who become mothers often view their maturity as an advantage for their children (Berryman & Windridge, 1991a,b; Kern, 1982). One mother encapsulated this view in Kern's study by pointing out that as the mother of a son she was far better able to accept him as himself (Kern, 1982). Mercer (1986) also found that women's approach as mothers varied with age; younger women saw motherhood as a gateway to maturity whereas those in their thirties saw it as a way of sharing their lives and a chance to foster new facets of themselves. One of the disadvantages of a younger parent may be their desire to compete with their children. One of Yarrow's respondents commented that "I was never in competition with my parents' ambitions and desires". This feeling that there is no competition may be a positive benefit for children.

It is not unusual for it to be said that a disadvantage of later motherhood is that a woman may be mistaken for the child's grandmother. Indeed in the 1980s, a free manual for expectant mothers published by the British Medical Association warns of this possibility in a section entitled "Mature Mothers" (Jeffries, 1985). Presumably looking like a grandmother is perceived by the author of this article as something that no-one would find desirable. In research by Berryman & Windridge (1991a,b), mothers who gave birth after 40 were asked if they had ever been mistaken in this way. Twenty-eight percent of first-time mothers and one-third of mothers with more than one child before they had a baby at 40+ had been so mistaken. Most had been amused by the mistake. Certainly in past times, when families were larger and often completed when a woman was in her forties, being a mother whilst also being a grandmother must have been a common occurrence (see Neugarten, 1972) and this ageist view of mothers may have been less prevalent. Not all children see youth in a parent as a virtue. Gutman (1985) found that children of early-timing parents sometimes wondered (as they reached adulthood) if their parents had been ready for them and thought that it might have been better for them if they had delayed. What can we conclude from these differing views?

Perhaps what most children want is a parent who does not stand out; one who reflects the average or norm. In England and Wales, in the 1960s, younger motherhood was the norm but today delaying parenthood occurs more frequently and mothers having babies over the age of 35 are on the increase. By virtue of the increased numbers of "older mothers", the norm for motherhood has shifted and hence the mother who could also be a grandmother is the subject of less comment than previously.

OUTCOMES FOR CHILDREN

Research on the outcomes for children of older mothers is sparse. In the past, maternal age has been linked with a wide range of problems including schizophrenia (Dalen, 1977), leukaemia (Gardner et al., 1990) anorexia and school phobia (Berg et al., 1972; Halmi, 1974). However the studies were not specifically designed to explore maternal age effects and it seems possible that these associations may be spurious.

A number of researches have linked positively the age of mother to the child's intellectual development (see Berryman & Windridge, 1998; Pollock, 1996; Ragozin et al., 1982; Wadsworth et al., 1984; Zybert et al., 1978). This relationship is evident even when potentially confounding variables such as education and social class are controlled. Pollock (1996), for example, carried out a longitudinal cohort study of first-born children born in one week in the United Kingdom (except Northern Ireland). Children were followed up at 5 and 10 years and a range of measures was used, including educational tests and questionnaires completed by the child's carer givers and teachers. Children born to mothers over 30 scored higher on a broad range of educational tests (the author notes that in eight of the nine separate educational tasks administered at age 10 these children were "significantly superior"; only in spelling was there no difference). Late primiparity was also associated with fewer adverse measures of behaviour in the child (e.g. fighting with other children, being often disobedient at age 5). The author suggested that one possible hypothesis to explain this association might be that mature mothers provide better care for their children, but he did not have details about their parenting styles and thus this remains to be tested.

It is possible to speculate on the causes of the relationship between improved performance on ability tests and raised maternal age. Perhaps the role of parental play is important (see Berryman & Windridge, 1998; MacDonald & Parke, 1986) in that older parents foster in their children behaviour that is advantageous for intellectual development.

CONCLUSIONS

In recent decades the trend towards later motherhood has become better established. Women are having babies later and the birth rate is increasing most rapidly in women over 35. Research on older motherhood has until recently focused on the problems and risks that women may experience in conceiving, in pregnancy and in childbirth. Less research has examined women's experiences of mothering children later in life and the outcomes for children. Many early studies of later motherhood confounded age with other variables, such as social class, and as a result their findings were questionable. Today it is clear that the negative effects of raised maternal age are often relatively small. There are slightly increased medical risks for a woman in her late thirties and older, in pregnancy and birth, but these risks should not be overstated. Indeed, today most women in the developed world are still young in their early 40s (Maroulis, 1992). Their chances of having a successful outcome to a pregnancy are better than at any time in history and certainly better than that of a younger women in a Third World country.

From a psychological perspective, older motherhood should not be viewed as a disadvantage for the woman or her child. Research studies reveal that older women often feel more ready to cope with the demands of motherhood and believe that their maturity is an advantage. From the child's point of view, there also appears to be benefits. A number of studies indicate that older and younger parents differ in the ways in which they relate to their children, and in their approach to parenthood. In several respects, children of older mothers seem to gain: for example in breastfeeding, parental responsiveness and discipline styles. One finding of particular interest is the better performance on ability tests by children of older mothers. It could be argued that the slightly increased medical risks of later child bearing are offset by the advantages in children's cognitive development. It would be wrong, however, to conclude that there is a right time for motherhood.

Becoming a parent is a decision that has to be made in the light of many factors of which age is only one. From the psychological perspective, the increased age of the parent does not appear to be the problem that it was once thought to be; it may have advantages, but the evidence should not be used to encourage individuals to delay. The results of research on parenthood and parenting are best used to promote better parenting in women and men whatever their age.

REFERENCES

Beekhuis, J.R., de Wolf, B.T.H.M., Mantingh, A., & Heringa, M.P. (1994). The influence of serum screening on the amniocentesis rate in women of advanced maternal age. *Prenatal Diagnosis, 14(3)*, 199–202.

Berg, I., Butler, A., & McGuire, R. (1972). Birth order and family size of school-phobic adolescents. *British Journal of Psychiatry, 121(564)*, 509–514.

Berkowitz, G.S., Skovron, M.L., Lapinski, R.H., & Berkowitz, R.L. (1990). Delayed childbearing and the outcome of pregnancy. *New England Journal of Medicine, 10(322)*, 659–664.

Berryman, J.C. & Windridge, K.C. (1991a). Having a baby after 40. I: A preliminary investigation of women's experience of pregnancy. *Journal of Reproductive and Infant Psychology, 9*, 3–18.

Berryman, J.C., & Windridge, K. (1991b). Having a baby after 40. II. A preliminary investigation of women's experience of motherhood. *Journal of Reproductive and Infant Psychology, 9,* 19–33.

Berryman, J.C., & Windridge, K. (1993). Pregnancy after 35: a preliminary report on maternal attachment to the foetus as a function of parity and maternal age. *Journal of Reproductive and Infant Psychology, 11,* 169–174.

Berryman, J.C., & Windridge, K.C. (1995). *Motherhood after 35: A report on the Leicester Motherhood Project.* Leicester: Leicester University and Nestle's UK Ltd.

Berryman, J.C., & Windridge, K.C. (1996). Pregnancy after 35 and attachment to the foetus. *Journal of Reproductive and Infant Psychology, 14,* 133–143.

Berryman, J.C., & Windridge, K.C. (1998). *Motherhood after 35: Mothers and Four-Year-Olds.* Leicester: Leicester University and Nestlés UK Ltd.

Berryman, J.C., Thorpe, K., & Windridge, K.C. (1995). *Older Mothers: Conception, Pregnancy and Birth after 35.* London: Pandora.

Biggs, I.S.C. (1973). Pregnancy at 40 years and over. *Medical Journal of Australia, 1,* 542.

Birth Statistics (1998). *Review of the Registrar General on Births and Patterns of Family Building in England and Wales,* 1996. *Office for National Statistics Series FM1 No. 25.* London: HMSO.

Broom, B.L. (1994). Impact of marital quality and psychological well-being on parental sensitivity. *Nursing Research, 43(3),* 138–143.

Chatwin, S.L., & MacArthur, B.A. (1993). Maternal perceptions of the preterm infant. *Early Child Development and Care, 87,* 69–82.

Cohen, W.R., Newman, L., & Friedman, E.A. (1980). Risk of labor abnormalities with advancing maternal age. *Obstetrics and Gynaecology, 55,* 414–416.

Cranley, M.S. (1981). Development of a tool for the measurement of maternal attachment during pregnancy. *Nursing Research, 30,* 281–284.

Cummings, P., Stanford, J.L., Daling, J.L., Weiss, N.S., & McKnight, B. (1994). Risk of breast cancer in relation to the interval since last full-term pregnancy. *British Medical Journal, 308,* 1672–1674.

Cunningham, F.C., & Leveno, K.L. (1995). Childbearing among older women – the message is cautiously optimistic. *The New England Journal of Medicine, 333(15),* 1002–1003.

Dalen, P. (1977). Maternal age and incidence of schizophrenia in the Republic of Ireland. *British Journal of Psychiatry, 131,* 301–305.

Department for Economic and Social Information and Policy Analysis (1994). *Demographic Yearbook 1992.* New York: United Nations.

Department of Health (1991). *Report of the Confidential Enquiry into Maternal Deaths in the United Kingdom, 1985–7.* London: HMSO.

Eaton, J.W., & Mayor, A.J. (1953). The social biology of very high fertility among the Hutterites: the demography of a unique population. *Human Biology, 25(3),* 20–64.

Eichholz, A., & Offerman-Zuckenberg, J. (1980). Later pregnancy. In Blum, B.L. (Ed.), *Psychological Aspects of Pregnancy, Birthing, and Bonding*. New York: Human Sciences Press.

Ever-Hadani, P., Seidman, D.S., Manor, O., & Harlap, S. (1994). Breastfeeding in Israel; maternal factors associated with choice and duration. *Journal of Epidemiology and Community Health, 48(3)*, 281–285.

Fleissig, A. (1991). Unintended pregnancies and the use of contraception: changes from 1984 to 1989. *British Medical Journal, 302*, 147.

Fox, R.A., Platz, D.L., & Bentley, K.S. (1995). Maternal factors related to parenting practices, developmental expectations, and perceptions of child behaviour problems. *Journal of Genetic Psychology, 156(4)*, 431–441.

Frankel, S.A., & Wise, M.J. (1982). A view of delayed parenting: some implications of a new trend. *Psychiatry, 45*, 220–225.

Friedman, E. (1965). Relation of maternal age to the course of labor. *American Journal of Obstetrics and Gynecology, 91*, 915–923.

Froman, R.D., & Owen, S.V. (1989). Infant care self-efficacy. *Scholarly Inquiry for Nursing Practice, 3*, 199–211.

Froman, R.D., & Owen, S.V. (1990). Mothers and nurses perceptions of infant care skills. *Research in Nursing and Health, 13*, 247–253.

Gardner, M.J., Shee, M.P., Hall, A.J., Powell, C.A., Downes, S., & Terrell, J.D. (1990). Results of case-control study of leukaemia and lymphoma among young people near Sellafield nuclear plant in West Cumbria. *British Medical Journal, 300*, 423–434.

Gosden, R.C., & Rutherford, A. (1995). Delayed childbearing: fertility declines at 30 and is almost gone by 40. *British Medical Journal, 311*, 1585.

Gray, R.H. (1976). The menopause epidemiological and demographic considerations. In Bearch, R.B. (Ed.), *The Menopause*. Lancaster: MTP Press.

Green, J.M. (1990). *Calming or Harming? A Critical Review of Psychological Effects of Fetal Diagnosis on Pregnant Women. Galton Institute Occasional Papers, Second Series, No.2*. London: Galton Institute.

Gutman, M.A. (1985). Fertility management: infertility, delayed childbearing and voluntary childlessness. In Goldberg, D.C. (Ed.), *Contemporary Marriage: Special Issues in Couples Therapy*. Illinois: Dorsey Press.

Halmi, K.A. (1974). Anorexia nervosa: demographic and clinical features in 94 cases. *Psychosomatic Medicine, 36(1)*, 18–26.

Hansen, J. (1986). Older maternal age and pregnancy outcome: a review of literature. *Obstetrical and Gynecological Survey, 41(11)*, 726–734.

Henry, L. (1961). Some data on natural fertility. *Eugenics Quarterley, 8*, 81–91.

Horgen, F., & Smythe, A.R. (1977). Pregnancy in women over 40. *Obstetrics and Gynaecology, 49*, 257–261.

Jeffries, M. (Ed.) (1985). *You and Your Baby: Pregnancy to Infancy*. London: British Medical Association, Family Doctor Publication.

Kane, S. (1967). Advancing age and the primigravida. *Obstetrics and Gynaecology, 29*, 409–414.

Kemp, V.H., Sibley, D.E., & Pond, E.F. (1990). A comparison of adolescent and adult mothers on factors affecting maternal role attainment. *Maternal–Child Nursing Journal, 19(1)*, 63–75.

Kern, I. (1982). '. . . an endless joy', the culture of motherhood over 35. *Papers in the Social Sciences, 2*, 43–56.

Kessler, I., Lancet, N.I., Borenstein, R., & Steinmetz, A. (1980). The problem of the elderly primigravida. *Obstetrics and Gynaecology, 56*, 165–169.

Khaw, K.T. (1992). Epidemiology of the menopause. *British Medical Bulletin, 48(2)*, 249–261.

Kirz, D.S., Dorchester, W., & Freeman, R.K. (1985). Advanced maternal age: the mature primigravida. *American Journal of Obstetrics and Gynecology, 152*, 7–12.

Kitzinger, S. (1982). *Birth Over Thirty*. London: Sheldon Press.

Koren, Z. (1963). Pregnancy and birth over 40. *Obstetrics and Gynaecology, 21*, 165–169.

Kvale, G., Heuch, I., & Nilssen, S. (1992). Parity in relation to mortality and cancer incidence: a perspective study of Norwegian women. *International Journal of Epidemiology, 23*, 691–699.

Lesko, S.M., Rosenberg, L., Kaufman, D.W., Stolley, P., Warshauer, M.E., Lewis, J.L. Jr, & Shapiro, S. (1991). Endometrial cancer and age at last delivery: evidence for an association. *American Journal of Epidemiology, 133*, 554–559.

Llewellyn-Jones, D. (1982). *Everywoman: A Gynaecological Guide for Life*. London: Faber and Faber.

Lojkasek, M., Goldberg, S., Marcovitch, S., & MacGregor, D. (1990). Influences on maternal responsiveness to developmentally delayed preschoolers. Special issue: families. *Journal of Early Intervention, 14(3)*, 260–273.

MacArthur, C., Lewis, M., & Knox, E.C. (1991). *Health After Childbirth*. London: HMSO.

MacDonald, I.R., & Maclennon, H.R. (1960). A consideration of the treatment of the elderly primigravidae. *Journal of Obstetrics and Gynaecology of the British Empire, 67*, 443–450.

MacDonald, K., & Parke, R.D. (1986). Parent-child physical play: the effects of sex and age of children and parents. *Sex Roles, 15(78)*, 367–378.

MacMahon, B., Cole, P., Lin, T.M., Lowe, C.R., Mirra, A.P., & Ravinhar, B. (1970). Age at first birth and breast cancer risk. *Bulletin of the World Health Organization, 42*, 209–221.

de Man, A. (1989). Early feeding practices and subsequent childrearing attitudes of French Canadian women. *Perceptual and Motor Skills, 68(3 part 1)*, 879–882.

Mansfield, P.K. (1988). Midlife childbearing: strategies for informed decision making. Special issue: women's health: our minds, our bodies. *Psychology of Women Quarterly, 12(4)*, 445–460.

Maroulis, K.T. (1992). Epidemiology of the menopause. *British Medical Bulletin, 48(2)*, 249–261.

Mercer, R.T. (1986). *First-time Motherhood: Experiences from Teens to Forties*. New York: Springer.

Morrison, I. (1975). The elderly primigravida. *American Journal of Obstetrics and Gynaecology, 121*, 465–470.

Neugarten, B. (1972) Social Clocks. Paper presented at the American Psychoanalytic Association, New York, December. Quoted in Tuirini, P. (1980) Psychological crises in normal pregnancy. In Blum, B.L. (Ed.), *Psychological Aspects of Pregnancy, Birthing, and Bonding*. New York and London: Human Sciences Press.

Newcomb, W.W., Rodriquez, M., & Johnson, L.W.C. (1991). Reproduction in the older gravida. *The Journal of Reproductive Medicine, 36(12)*, 839–945.

Nortman, D. (1974). *Parental Age as a Factor in Pregnancy Outcome and Child Development. Reports of Population/Family Planning, No.16*. New York: Population Council.

O'Neill, S. (1998). Gran is amazing, say family of Britain's oldest mother. *The Daily Telegraph*, 11 January 1998.

Pascoe, A.M., & Soloman, R. (1994). Prenatal correlates of indigent mothers' attitudes about spoiling their young infants: a longitudinal study. *Developmental and Behavioural Pediatrics, 15(5)*, 367–369.

Peterson, C.E., & DaVanzo, J. (1992). Why are teenagers in the United States less likely to breast-feed than older women? *Demography, 29*, 431–550.

Phillip, I. (1994). Woman, 62, gives birth as "oldest mother in world!". *The Times*, 19 July 1994.

Piepert, J.F., & Bracken, M.B. (1993). Maternal age: an independent risk factor for caesarean section. *Obstetrics and Gynaecology, 81*, 200–205.

Pollock, J.I. (1996). Mature maternity: long term association in first children born to older mothers in 1970 in the UK. *Journal of Epidemiology and Community Health, 50*, 429–435.

Pridham, K.F., & Chang, A.S. (1991). Mothers' perceptions of problem-solving competence for infant care. *Western Journal of Nursing Research, 13(2)*, 164–180.

Prysak, M., Lorenz, R.P., & Kisly, A. (1995). Pregnancy outcome in nulliparous women 35 years and older. *Obstetrics and Gynaecology, 85(1)*, 65–70.

Radke-Yarrow, M., Nottelman, F., Martinez, P., Fox, M.B., & Belmont, B. (1993). Young children of affectively ill parents: a longitudinal study of psychosocial development. *Annual Progress in Child Psychiatry and Child Development, 31*, 191–212.

Ragozin, A.S., Basham, R.B., Crnic, K.A., Greenberg, M.T., & Robinson, N.M. (1982). Effects of maternal age on parenting role. *Developmental Psychology, 18*, 627–634.

Rasmussen, S., Bungum, L., & Hoie, K. (1994). Maternal age and duration of labor. *Acta Obstetrica et Gynecologia Scandinavica, 73(3)*, 231–234.

Rindfuss, R.R. (1991). The young adult years: diversity, structural change, and fertility. *Demography, 28(4)*, 493–512.

Roberts, C.L., Algert, C.S., & March, L.M. (1994). Delayed childbearing – are there any risks? *Medical Journal of Australia, 160(9)*, 539–544.

Santos, S.I., & Beral, V. (1997). Socioeconomic differences in reproductive behaviours. *Independent Assessment & Research Centre Scientific Publication, 138*, 285–308.

Sauer, M.V., Paulson, R.J., & Lobo, R.A. (1992). Reversing the natural decline in human fertility. An extended clinical trial of oocyte donation to women of advanced reproductive age. *Journal of the American Medical Association, 9(268)*, 1275–1279.

Schwartz, D., & Mayaux, M.J. (1982). Female fecundity as a function of age. *New England Journal of Medicine, 306(7)*, 404–406.

Sears, R.R., Maccoby, F., & Levin, H. (1957). *Patterns of Child Rearing.* Evanston, IL: Rowe Peterson.

Social Trends (1994). Great Britain Central Statistical Office, 24. London: HMSO.

Spellacy, W.N., Miller, S.J., & Winegar, A. (1986). Pregnancy after 40 years of age. *Obstetrics and Gynaecology, 68*, 452–454.

Stanton, E. (1956). Pregnancy after forty-four. *American Journal of Obstetrics and Gynecology, 71*, 270–284.

Stein, A. (1983). Pregnancy in gravidas over age 35 years. *Nurse Midwife, 28(1)*, 17–20.

Tanner, J.M. Cited in May, R.M. (1978). Human reproduction reconsidered. *Nature, 272*, 491–495.

Thorpe, K., & Cinnamon, J. (1992). The timing of motherhood. Unpublished Research Report. University of Queensland, Department of Psychology.

US Department of Commerce (1997). *Statistical Abstract of the United States 1997: The National Data Book.* Washington DC: Bureau of the Census.

van den Akker, O.B.A. (1994). Something old, something new, something borrowed, something taboo. *Journal of Reproductive and Infant Psychology, 12*, 179–188.

Vestermark, V., Hogdall, C.K., Plenov, G., Birch, M., & Toftager-Larsen, K. (1991). The duration of breastfeeding. A longitudinal prospective study in Denmark. *Scandinavian Journal of Social Medicine, 19(2)*, 105–109.

Wadsworth, J., Taylor, B., Osborn, A., & Butler, N. (1984). Teenage mothering: child development at five years. *Journal of Child Psychology and Psychiatry and Allied Disciplines, 25(2)*, 305–313.

Walter, C.A. (1984). *The Timing of Motherhood.* Lexington, Massachusetts: Lexington Books.

Warburton, D., & Fraser, F.C. (1964). Spontaneous abortion risks in man. Data from reproductive histories collected in a medical genetics unit. *American Journal of Human Genetics, 16*, 1–25.

Warnock, M. Cited in Neustatter, A. (1993). Pioneer in the laboratory of life. *The Independent*, 3 August 1993.

Welles-Nystrom, B.L. (1997). The meaning of postponing motherhood for women in the United States and Sweden: aspects of feminism and radical timing strategies. *Health Care for Women International*, *18(3)*, 279–299.

Welles-Nystrom, B.L., & de Chateau, P. (1987). Maternal age and transition to motherhood: prenatal and perinatal assessments. *Acta Psychiatrica Scandinavica*, *76(6)*, 719–725.

Wilkie, J.R. (1981). The trend towards delayed parenthood. *Journal of Marriage and the Family*, *43(3)*, 583–591.

Yarrow, A.L. (1991). *Latecomers – Children of Parents Over 35*. New York: Free Press.

Zybert, P., Stein, Z., & Belmont, L. (1978). Maternal age and children's ability. *Perceptual and Motor Skills*, *47*, 815–818.

Chapter 15

Sexual Victimisation of Girls: Implications for Women's Health and for Prevention

Judith Greenberg

Centers for Disease Control and Prevention, United States

Then there was the pain. A breaking and entering when even the senses are torn apart. The act of rape on an eight-year-old body is a matter of the needle giving because the camel can't. The child gives, because the body can, and the mind of the violator cannot. – Maya Angelou

When he would come home he would make me have sex with him and he would beat me and call me names just like my father did to my mother. Some times my son would cry outside the door and I would get angry 'cuz it would take Ricky longer to get off me. – HIV-seropositive woman whose sexual abuse began in childhood (quoted from Cuccinelli & De Groot, 1997, p.228)

Child sexual abuse (CSA) is a social and public health problem with enormous consequences for women throughout the life cycle. Apart from lingering physical and emotional injuries, a growing body of

Women, Health and the Mind
Edited by L. Sherr and J.S. St Lawrence. © 2000 John Wiley & Sons, Ltd

evidence indicates that sexual abuse in childhood or adolescence may be linked to some of the most persistent health issues of our time. Increased public awareness of the frequency of such sex crimes has resulted in school-based prevention programmes as "Good Touch, Bad Touch," the expansion of services by rape crisis centres to include violence against children, and specialised training for therapists and judges. It also has inspired innovative behavioural approaches to therapy for perpetrators. This chapter provides an overview of the sexual abuse of female children, its health consequences for girls and women, and prevention and intervention strategies. It examines the prevalence of CSA, focusing on girls, on risk factors for such abuse, on short- and longer term effects of CSA for girls and women, and on theoretical perspectives on the links between CSA and adult health problems. In particular, the focus on primary, secondary and tertiary prevention strategies suggested by the literature fills a major gap in the literature.

PREVALENCE OF THE SEXUAL ABUSE OF CHILDREN

Although several early studies of sexual behaviour, including Kinsey's landmark study of females' sexual behaviour, showed that child molestation was common in the lives of children in the United States (Kinsey et al., 1953), it is only recently that research has focused on CSA. As noted by Conte (1994, p.224), five landmark documents on child sexual abuse between 1978 and 1984 (Burgess et al., 1978; Butler, 1978; Finkelhor, 1979; Rush, 1980; Russell, 1984) ignited a media and a research explosion in the United States, with increased attention from professionals, parents, and policymakers. There has also been increased attention at the international level, with researchers documenting sexual abuse of girls in many different countries (Heise et al., 1995). Even so, it is difficult to estimate the exact prevalence of CSA because it is not known to what extent cases of abuse go unreported. For example, in a three-city intervention study of women at high risk for sexually transmitted diseases (STDs), half of whom reported CSA, 25% of those victimised had never mentioned this early abuse to anyone before the interview (Greenberg et al., 1999). By the time a repeat offender comes to the attention of authorities, he or she has possibly had extensive sexual involvement with children.

Problems with Definitions

To further complicate our understanding of prevalence, definitions of what actually constitutes CSA vary from study to study and from culture to culture, with no single operational definition. Finkelhor &

Browne (1986, pp.22–27) discuss three common dimensions of the definitions used by researchers in the United States that can affect prevalence rates. The first is the victim's age at the time the incident took place, with most studies setting an upper age limit to childhood at 15–17 years. A second dimension in defining CSA is the type of sexual behaviour involved. Definitions typically include both non-contact abuse (i.e. encounters with exhibitionists) and contact abuse (from fondling of the child's breasts and genitals to vaginal or anal penetration); some researchers report prevalence rates separately for the two categories, and some combine them. A third dimension that is sometimes used to define CSA is the age difference between the molester and the victim. While all definitions would consider sex between a little girl and an adult as abuse, at some point in adolescence, a girl acquires the ability to consent. Consequently, some definitions set an age discrepancy of at least 5 years between the victim and perpetrator, although others define any sexual activity with peers as abuse if the person alleging the abuse considered it to be so. District attorneys sometimes use the inconsistencies in and overlap of definitions related to sex crimes to assist in prosecutions. For example, in exchange for the state's dropping of child molestation and rape charges, four high school seniors in Georgia pled guilty to statutory rape of two 15-year-old girls (Simmons, 1998).

The lack of a common definition may also explain why there has been limited cross-cultural comparison of sexual abuse of children. As noted by Korbin (1987) in an exploratory survey of CSA from cross-cultural records, there is considerable variation on how societies define inappropriate sexual contact with children. For example, sexual contact between children and adults may occur in religious or ceremonial events (i.e. ritualised homosexuality as part of male initiation rites has been well documented in some New Guinea societies). And sexualised behaviours such as fondling or kissing a young child's genitals occur in some cultures (e.g. Turkey) as part of daily child rearing practices.

In addition to the lack of a common definition of CSA, there is a lack of agreement between researchers on terms for abusers. This chapter uses the definitions offered by Abel & Osborn (1995). It is important to clarify the distinction between the terms paedophile and child molester, as the terms are not interchangeable. A child molester is an individual who carries out a sexual interaction with a child regardless of the reasons, which could include lack of other sexual outlets, or the influence of drugs, or the perception that a young girl was actually older, or during an unusual opportunity. On the other hand, paedophilia is a specific psychiatric diagnosis that refers to the sexual preference of the patient (see Table 15.1). Paedophiles who do not act upon their urges cannot be labelled as child molesters, and child molesters who do not meet the diagnostic criteria are not paedophiles.

Table 15.1 Definitions and child molestation

Term	Definition
Child molester	An individual who carries out a sexual interaction with a child, regardless of the reason
Paedophile	An individual who has recurrent, intense sexual urges and sexually arousing fantasies involving sexual activity with a pre-pubescent child (13 years of age or younger) that persist for at least 6 months; the paedophile must be at least 16 years of age and at least 5 years older than the children to whom he is attracted; he or she may or may not have acted upon these urges
Sex offender	Any individual who carries out any type of sexual offence, including child molestation
Perpetrator	An individual who carries out the inappropriate sexual act (applies to all types of sex offenders)

Source: Adapted from Abel & Osborn (1995) and from American Psychiatric Association (1994).

The Repressed Memory Debate

Memory also clouds the prevalence issue. Recently a debate has surfaced around the issue of forgotten or repressed trauma of childhood abuse. Several studies suggest that adults in psychotherapy commonly report some period in their lives of which they had incomplete or no memory of CSA (Briere and Conte, 1993; Herman & Schatzow, 1987). Some theorists have argued that these forgotten traumas must be recovered in order for a person to address these memories and move on with their lives (Harber & Pennebaker, 1992; Harvey & Herman, 1994). Although many therapists have employed memory recovery techniques to assist clients in revisiting childhood traumas that may include CSA, such techniques may result in the actual creation of false childhood "memories", which can lead to both psychological distress and litigation that devastate families (Hyman & Loftus, 1997). By way of an example, in a sample of 30 crime victims registered with the State of Washington between 1991 and 1995 concerning repressed memories that surfaced primarily during therapy, those predominately female clients manifested drastic increases in suicide, self-mutilation, divorce or separation, loss of custody of children who were minors, or estrangement from extended families. Illustrative of the difficulties in "recovering" memory is that virtually all of the memories in this restricted sample were of abuse in satanic rituals, begun, on average, at age 7 months. None were corroborated by medical exams or other evidence (Loftus, 1997). Hyman & Loftus (1997) argued that the benefits of memory recovery have not been clearly demonstrated, and that, without corroborating evidence, distinguishing between true and false "memory" is virtually impossible.

Prevalence Results from Studies

In spite of definitional problems and memory constraints, prevalence studies of CSA suggest that at least one in five adult women in North America and 5–10% of North American men may have experienced either contact or non-contact sexual abuse during childhood, with a peak age of vulnerability between 7 and 13 years (Finkelhor, 1994). Of the episodes reported by women, 20–25% involved either vaginal penetration or oral–genital contact. Based on a national survey of adults and CSA, the majority of child molesters were men and were either family members or acquaintances, with girls more likely than boys to be abused by family members (29 versus 11%) (Finkelhor et al., 1990).

In the National Health and Social Life Survey, 17% of adult women and 12% of adult men reported that as children they had been sexually touched by adolescents or by adults; those who reported showed no significant differences by age group, race, or level of education (Laumann et al., 1994). Women were more likely than men (70 versus 45%) to respond to a question as to whether the experience had affected their lives, and nearly all who responded indicated that its effects were negative. In the National College Health Risk Behavior Survey (Centers for Disease Control and Prevention, 1997), 13.1% of college students reported that they had sexual intercourse against their will at some time. Female students (20.4%) were significantly more likely than male students (3.9%) to report ever having been forced to have sexual intercourse. This study concluded that, nationwide, 2.6% of students reported that they were younger than 13 the first time they had been forced to have sexual intercourse.

Cross-cultural research on child sexual abuse suggests the universality of this problem for women. During a 2-day seminar on sexual coercion and women's reproductive health sponsored by The Population Council and the Health and Development Policy Project, studies from around the world (including national random samples from Barbados, Canada, The Netherlands, New Zealand, Norway, and the United States) documented sexual abuse in childhood (Heise et al., 1995). For example, a hospital study in Lima, Peru, indicated that 90% of mothers aged 12–16 were victims of rape – the majority by a father, stepfather, or other male relative (Rosas, 1992). Abuse can also include forced prostitution, especially in countries with high levels of poverty where family members may be given an advance on a young girl's earnings. It can also include violent and traumatic sex on a girl's wedding night. For example, in countries where virginity is highly valued, girls are frequently married to much older men, with consummation being "as quick and as bloody as possible" to demonstrate virginity and defloration.

According to The New York Times (Daley, 1998), reported cases of sexual assault against children in South Africa have doubled in 4 years. In Soweto, a large South African township, police officers arrest child rapists in weekly round-ups. "On a recent night's sweep, each officer had more than 80 assigned cases, and the team picked up 10 men in 5 hours. One was accused of raping his 2-year-old daughter, and one was a teenager accused, with six classmates, of beating and raping his 12-year-old cousin and leaving her for dead, half-buried in a fresh grave. But most were neighbours of the victims" (Daley, 1998, p.32).

Daley offered numerous sociological reasons for this explosion of sexual assault, including a successful liberation movement that has left thousands of young, uneducated men without employment or purpose and accustomed to violence. The breakdown of apartheid laws also has encouraged widespread migration to squatter camps in the cities where privacy is non-existent and alcoholism is common. These conditions make it difficult to supervise children who are taught to be extremely submissive to adults. Also, concern about AIDS has made young girls attractive to predatory men (Daley, 1998).

The focus of this chapter on women as victims should not imply that sexual abuse of male children does not take place. Information from child molesters suggests that when only touching (as distinguished from no touching) is involved, the majority of victims are boys. Boys may be less likely to report CSA because of concerns that their molestation might be labelled homosexual activity, or, if the perpetrator is a female, because they may be embarrassed that they could not defend themselves against a woman (Abel & Osborn, 1995).

RISK FACTORS FOR ABUSE

Apart from cultural prescriptions and social upheavals, what places a girl at risk for sexual abuse? In a national United States survey of adults concerning history of sexual abuse, higher rates of abuse were found among both men and women who grew up in unhappy homes or who had lived without one of their natural parents (Finkelhor et al. 1990). Finkelhor suggested that not only may such children receive poorer supervision when out of the home but that they may also be more vulnerable to non-family perpetrators because of their needs for attention. The testimony of a convicted perpetrator echoes those associations:

> I used all the normal techniques used by paedophiles. I bribed my victims; I pleaded with them, but I also showed them affection and attention. Almost without exception, every child I molested was lonely and longing for attention. (cited in Arndt, 1991, p.225)

Similar findings were drawn from a study of 492 women in Britain. Mullen et al. concluded that CSA was more common in those from disturbed and disrupted families and "the unholy trio of physical abuse, emotional deprivation, and sexual abuse tend to be found together" (Mullen et al., 1994, p.43). A survey of more than 9000 adult members of a large health maintenance organisation in California found that 65% of those who reported childhood sexual abuse also reported other adverse childhood experiences, including psychological abuse; physical abuse; or living in a home where there was substance abuse, mental illness, violent treatment of a mother, or a member of the family who had been imprisoned (Felitti et al., 1998). A meta-analytical review of such findings has led Rind & Tromovitch (1997) to conclude that a causal link between CSA and later psychological maladjustment in the general population cannot be made because of the reliable presence of confounding variables such as emotional neglect, physical abuse, psychological abuse, and general family disruption. They note, however, that when CSA is accompanied by force or perpetrated by those with close family ties, it has the potential to produce significant harm in individual cases.

OUTCOMES OF SEXUAL ABUSE FOR CHILDREN

A review by Kendall-Tackett et al. (1993), of 45 studies, found that sexually abused children were more prone than their unabused counterparts to fear, nightmares, post-traumatic stress disorder (PTSD), withdrawn behaviour, delinquency, inappropriate sexual behaviour, regressive behaviour (e.g. bed wetting), running away, general behaviour problems, and self-injurious behaviour. The percentage of victims with any particular symptom averaged between 20 and 30%. However, when sexually abused children were compared with their unabused clinical counterparts, they appeared less symptomatic except with respect to sexualised behaviour and PTSD, lending support to the idea that other adverse family experiences contribute to the symptoms named here.

When these researchers analysed the 25 studies that examined characteristics of the abuse experience, they found that when CSA involved a closely related perpetrator (e.g. a father or stepfather), high frequency of sexual contact, a long duration over time, the use of force, or sex acts that included penetration (oral, anal, or vaginal) it seemed to lead to a greater number of symptoms in victims (Kendall-Tackett et al., 1993). Beitchman et al. (1992) noted similar findings in a review.

A later study of 775 women survivors who responded to a survey in a women's magazine found that the most important predictors of long-term psychological effects from CSA were the presence of violence, threats, or verbal coercion, followed by prolonged or repeated abuse (Ussher & Dewberry, 1995). Lack of maternal support at the time of disclosure has been identified as a key factor in adjustment. This last finding is supported by a survey of female college students in the United States for whom family environment (as measured by The Parental Support Scale) was a better predictor of later psychological adjustment than was the sexual abuse (Fromuth, 1986).

Not all sexually abused children have symptoms. For example, 21% of 369 abused children recruited from sex abuse treatment and evaluation appeared to have no symptoms at all in spite of using very broad terms to elicit problems such as "emotional upset" (Conte & Schuerman, 1987). Although it is possible that some children repress symptoms or have not yet processed their experiences, it is also possible that some asymptomatic children may be the most resilient children with the most inner resources.

LONG-TERM EFFECTS OF CSA

Of particular concern to women are the long-term effects of CSA. Summarising studies of clinical and non-clinical populations, Browne & Finkelhor (1986) found that from one-fifth to two-fifths of abused children seen by clinicians manifested pathological disturbance. When studied as adults and compared with non-abused adults, victims as a group demonstrated impairment, but less than 20% showed any serious psychopathology. However, Browne & Finkelhor, and many other researchers who have focused on the long-term effects of CSA have identified a number of associated health problems (see Table 15.2). These range from chronic headaches to eating disorders. Recently, Felitti et al. (1998) found that the leading causes of adult death (such as heart attack, cancer, stroke, chronic bronchitis, and emphysema) are associated with childhood exposure to physical, sexual, or psychological abuse or household dysfunction during childhood; to smoking, alcohol, or drug abuse; to overeating; or to risky sexual behaviours.

In the era of AIDS, a major concern is that sexual abuse of children has been linked with a variety of risky behaviours in adulthood that are associated with HIV infection. For example, women who exhibited at least one behaviour that placed them at risk for acquiring a STD and who volunteered for a group intervention in three cities in the United States reported sexual abuse in childhood at a rate considerably higher than the general population in national surveys. Sixty-six percent of women in Seattle, 46% in Baltimore, and 38% in New York reported CSA (see Table 15.3.) Abusers were usually friends or relatives. For example, one woman who had never told anyone about her abuse before, confided to an interviewer that when she baby-sat for relatives, they got her drunk so that the husband could abuse her. Study participants who acknowledged CSA reported less protected sex with main partners at the most recent sex encounter, higher use of drugs before sex in the preceding 30 days (see Table 15.4), higher numbers of lifetime male partners, and higher numbers of different STDs during a lifetime (see Table 15.5). Abused women also scored lower on scales measuring self-esteem and mastery, psychological resources considered to facilitate behaviours that can prevent STDs.

Table 15.2 Long-term health problems in women related to child sexual abuse[1]

Health problem	Researcher[2]
Chronic headaches	Felitti (1991)
Chronic gastrointestinal distress	Felitti (1991), Lechner et al. (1993)
Eating disorders	Briere & Elliott (1994), Dansky et al. (1997), Felitti (1991), Jeffrey & Jeffrey (1991), Jones & Emerson (1994), Weiner & Stephens (1993)
Gynaecological problems	Plichta and Abraham (1996)
High use of medical care	Felitti (1991)
Leading causes of adult death (heart attack, cancer, stroke, chronic bronchitis/emphysema)	Felitti et al. (1998)
Pregnancy including early, unintended, and terminated	Boyer & Fine (1992), Briere & Elliott (1994), Springs & Friedrich (1992), Stock et al. (1997)
Revictimisation (i.e. battering/rape)	Beitchman et al. (1992), Boyer & Fine (1992), Jeffrey & Jeffrey (1991), Urquiza & Goodlin-Jones (1994)
Risky sexual behaviours including early age at first intercourse, frequent short-term activity, multiple partners, prostitution, unprotected sex	Boyer & Fine (1992), Briere & Elliott (1994), Cunningham et al. (1994), Felitti et al. (1998), Jeffrey & Jeffrey (1991), Neumann (1994), Springs & Friedrich (1992), Stock et al. (1977), Thompson et al. (1997), Widom & Kuhns (1996), Wyatt (1988)
Self-mutilation	Briere & Elliott (1994)
Sexual dysfunction including difficulties experiencing arousal and orgasm, pain during intercourse, compulsive desire for sex, avoidance of sex, confusion about sexual orientation	Beitchman et al. (1992), Briere & Elliott (1994), Browne & Finkelhor (1986), Mullen et al. (1994), Neumann (1994)
Smoking, alcohol, or substance abuse	Briere & Elliott (1994), Browne & Finkelhor (1986), Felliti et al. (1998), Jeffrey & Jeffrey (1991)
STDs	Briere & Elliott (1994), Felitti et al. (1998), Gutman et al. (1991, 1994), Vermund et al. (1990)
Suicidal ideas and behaviour	Beitchman et al. (1992), Briere & Elliott (1994), Felitti et al. (1998), Jeffrey & Jeffrey (1991), Neumann (1994)

[1] The majority of studies referred to focused on women. Cunningham et al. (1994), Felitti et al. (1998), Vermund et al. (1990), and Widom & Kuhns (1996) included both men and women.
[2] Briere & Elliott (1994), Beitchman et al. (1992), Browne & Finkelhor (1986), Jeffrey & Jeffrey (1991), and Neumann et al. (1994) provide review articles.

Table 15.3 Demographics and responses to questions about childhood sexual abuse[1]

	Baltimore (n = 285)	New York (n = 277)	Seattle (n = 263)
Mean age (range)	34 (18–51)	19 (17–28)	33 (18–61)
Race/ethnicity (%)			
Black	93	44	30
Hispanic		52	2
White	6		47
Other[2]	1	4	21
Child sexual abuse (%)	46	38	66
Mean age (range)			
At first abuse[3]	10 (2–17)	10 (3–17)	9 (2–17)
At first voluntary sex	15 (10–22)	15 (10–21)	16 (10–26)
Relationship of first abuser (%)[3]			
Parent	13	6	14
Other relative	35	44	36
Family friend	28	21	24
Husband/boyfriend	6	5	7
Stranger	6	5	12
Supervisor/authority	5	7	2
Acquaintance/co-worker	1	7	3
Other	8	7	2
Repeated abuse by first abuser (%)[3]	65	59	67
Mean no. of months (range)			
that this abuse continued	27 (1–96)	21 (1–87)	38 (1–98)

[1] This table initially appeared in *AIDS and Behavior* (see Greenberg et al., 1999).
[2] Includes Asian, Pacific Islander, American Indian, Alaskan Native, mixed racial, and "unsure."
[3] Based on those who reported child sexual abuse.

Children who are abused are also at immediate risk for STD or HIV infection as well as for the long-term sequelae of such infections. Of 96 HIV-infected paediatric patients at Duke University, 14.6% were confirmed by Duke University researchers to have been sexually abused (Gutman et al., 1991). Four of the study children acquired HIV from the abuse, and in six, abuse was a suspected source. The abused children showed multiple risk factors for sexual abuse, including drug abuse and alcoholism in the home, prostitution of a parent, lack of parenting, poverty, and chronic illness of the child. In a subsequent study of 18 girls with external genital warts, eight had evidence of cervical–vaginal or intra-anal infection with the human papillomavirus, which has been related to cervical cancer in women. Sexual abuse was confirmed in seven of the girls and was probable in two others (Gutman et al., 1994). The long-term prognosis for children infected with human papillomavirus is unknown.

Table 15.4 Child sexual abuse as a predictor of adult risk behaviours for STDs or HIV infection – logistic regression analysis[1]

Categorical variable	Odds ratio[2] (confidence interval)[3]
Condom use at most recent sex (main partner)	0.61 (0.39–0.95)
Consistent condom use (main partner)	0.75 (0.44–1.29)
Consistent condom use (other partner)	0.57 (0.28–1.14)
Could refuse unprotected sex (main partner)	0.69 (0.61–1.46)
Could refuse unprotected sex (other partner)	0.49 (0.22–1.07)
Risky partner	1.12 (0.69–1.82)
Drugs/alcohol before sex in past 30 days	1.54 (1.02–2.32)
Illicit drug use in past 30 days	1.29 (0.85–1.95)

[1] Adapted from Greenberg et al. (1999).
[2] Adjusted for site (two dummy variables), respondent's age, ethnicity/race (three dummy variables), and age at first voluntary intercourse.
[3] Logistic regression confidence intervals based on overall 0.05 significance level at the equation level. OLS regression coefficients require a Z ratio of + or −2.75 to attain statistical significance.

REVICTIMISATION

A long-term consequence of CSA documented by research is adult sexual revictimisation (Briere & Runtz, 1988; Koss & Dinero, 1989; Urquiza & Goodlin-Jones, 1994; Wyatt et al., 1992). In a community sample of 248 African American and White American women, ages 18–36, Wyatt et al. (1992) found that women who were sexually abused during childhood were over twice as likely to experience adult sexual abuse as women who reported no CSA. Revictimised women also reported higher rates of unintended and aborted pregnancies than non-victimised women. Wyatt suggested that revictimisation may be a function of not knowing how to select appropriate partners and how to negotiate with them. In a study of 243 randomly selected community college students, Urquiza and Goodlin-Jones (1994) found that women with a history of CSA were three times more likely to be raped than adults who were not victimised as children.

Cuccinelli & De Groot (1997) provided an interesting case report on "Debi", whose quote opened this chapter. They described how early abuse can beget a dangerous life course that includes revictimisation and HIV infection. The physician treating Debi sees her story as just one variation on a tragic theme heard many times in the physician's prison clinic:

> childhood sexual abuse, early and frequent sex in exchange for temporary emotional support, drug use as self-medication, and drug use to make intimacy more tolerable and to diminish their emotional pain, drug dependency, abusive relationships, sex work, and eventually incarceration. (Cuccinelli & De Groot, 1997, p.237)

Table 15.5 Childhood sexual abuse as a predictor of adult risk behaviours for STDs and HIV infection – linear regression analyses[1]

Continuous variable	Parameter estimate[2]	Slope/*SE* ratio[3]
Log odds of protected sex (main partner)	−0.443	−2.46
	Equivalent odds ratio = 0.642 (0.39–1.053)	
Number of lifetime male partners	5.87	3.88
Number of different lifetime STDs	0.33	3.69
Mastery Scale score	−0.835	−3.09
Self-Esteem Scale score	−1.78	−4.08

[1] Adapted from Greenberg et al. (1999).
[2] Adjusted for site (two dummy variables), respondent's age, ethnicity/race (three dummy variables), and age at first voluntary intercourse.
[3] Logistic regression confidence intervals based on overall 0.05 significance level at the equation level. OLS regression coefficients require a *Z* ratio of plus or minus 2.75 to attain statistical significance.

LINKS BETWEEN CSA AND ADULT HEALTH PROBLEMS

While researchers have discovered considerable evidence that CSA is associated with a variety of long-term adverse health outcomes for women, they have been less able to provide a clear understanding of the links between CSA and those outcomes. One theoretical explanation sees adult–child sex as a traumatic event consisting of multiple factors that produce both psychological effects and their later behavioural manifestations. Using this approach, Finkelhor's & Browne's (1986) model suggested that CSA traumatises children through four dynamics:

• traumatic sexualisation, a process in which a girl's sexuality is shaped in a developmentally inappropriate way
• betrayal, in which a girl discovers that her trust and vulnerability have been manipulated
• powerlessness, or the process in which a girl's territory and body space are invaded
• stigmatisation, where a girl is ashamed and sees herself as different.

The amount and type of dynamic accounts for the variety of outcomes. Intervention from this perspective would involve an assessment to see which of the dynamics caused the greatest trauma and then targeting that area. For example, if stigmatisation was high for a girl, intervention might include involvement with a support group for others who had experienced CSA.

A competing explanation for long-term outcomes has been offered by Browning & Laumann (1997) who argue that focusing on the type and degree of trauma experienced during adult–child sex ignores the unfolding life course of a young woman. Browning & Laumann suggest that adult–child sex provides an inappropriate model of sexual behaviour that can promote early adolescent sexual activity. For example, girls who experience adult–child sex may have an increased interest in sexual activity or be less inclined to discourage the sexual advances of others. Much as the previous case study of Debi indicates, CSA sets the stage for a sexual career that includes teenage pregnancy, multiple sexual partners, and the accompanying risks of forced sex and sexually transmitted infections. These intervening variables, in turn, can account for the long-term outcomes. Using a national probability sample of men and women, Browning & Laumann provided evidence that when intervening sexual career variables (teenage childbirth and number of sex partners) and intervening adverse sexual experience variables (sexually transmitted infection and forced sex) are controlled, the direct effect of adult–child sex on long-term outcomes such as sexual dysfunction disappeared in most cases.

From a life course perspective, intervention would include helping young girls who have experienced adult–child sexual contact to rewrite their current risky sexual scripts by skill building for sexual negotiation and boundary setting. Findings from the study by Wyatt et al. (1992) of 176 abused women, in which there was little association between sexual revictimisation and psychological outcomes, lends support to this strategy. In their discussion of clinical implications, the researchers note:

> Given that they may have been the survivors of child sexual abuse, they may need to relearn strategies for expressing their needs in relationships and for selecting partners with whom they can share sexual decision making. In these instances, learning how to perceive themselves as sexual beings and not sexual objects, to communicate their sexual needs, to anticipate when contraceptive use is needed, and to negotiate with partners about the type and frequency of behaviours in which to participate may be central to efforts to prevent revictimization. (Wyatt et al., 1992, p.171)

Fellitti et al. have provided another perspective on the mechanisms linking childhood abuse and adult disease. In a study of adverse childhood experiences (ACE) based at Kaiser Permanente's San Diego Health Appraisal Clinic, Felitti et al. (1998) found a strong relationship between exposure to abuse and multiple risk factors for several of the leading causes of death of adults. Three categories of exposure to childhood abuse – psychological, physical, or sexual, and exposure to household dysfunction (substance abuse, mental illness, violent treatment of mother or stepmother, and criminal behaviour) – were measured. The clear majority of patients who had been subjected to one category of childhood abuse had been subjected to at least one other.

The linking mechanisms appear to arise from behaviours such as smoking, alcohol or drug abuse, overeating, or sexual behaviours that may be consciously or unconsciously used because they have an immediate pharmacological or psychological benefit in coping with the stress of abuse, domestic violence, or other forms of family dysfunction. These mediating behaviours may start early in the life cycle. A study of girls in grades 7–12 who had been sexually molested found that these girls had significantly higher rates of drug abuse for almost all drugs over a lifetime (Watts & Ellis, 1993).

These differing explanations suggest that there is no single link between being sexually abused as a child and experiencing a specific pattern of symptoms or problems as adults. Moreover, it is important to remind ourselves that many women who were sexually abused as children do not report adverse outcomes as adults and that many women who were not sexually abused do report these same outcomes. It may be the case that biological and genetic factors mediate for these subgroups. Consequently, it is unlikely that any one theoretical model will provide all the answers as to the nature of the link. It is likely that different aspects will play out differently for different women given the degree of trauma, the stability of the family, support services available, personal resiliency, socialisation, and genetically determined behavioural traits.

PREVENTION

While preventing child sexual abuse is certainly preferable to intervening in its short- and long-term consequences, there is almost no research that documents successful prevention programmes. A national telephone survey of youths aged 10–16 and of their caretakers was conducted in 1992 to determine whether victimisation prevention instruction in school has any effect on children's behaviour in threatening situations. Programmes were classified as comprehensive if they contained at least nine of the following 12 components recommended by prevention educators: information about sexual abuse, including incest and good and bad touch; bullies; confusing touch; screaming to attract attention when threatened by an adult and telling an adult about the abuse; reassurance that abuse is never the child's fault; a chance to practise avoidance skills; information to take home about the prevention training; a meeting for parents; and repetition of the material with the child over more than a single day. Exposure to a more comprehensive programme was not associated with reduced incidence of victimisation, injury, or upset. However, some of the exposure conditions were associated with an increased likelihood that children would disclose victimisation, see themselves as having successfully protected themselves, and a decreased likelihood that they would blame themselves for the episode (Finkelhor et al., 1995). Given the avoidance of sex education at the elementary school level, we do not know the implications of introducing sex in terms of abuse for pre-school or early elementary-age children. For example, some children could pick up negative attitudes about sex and could then carry those into adult relationships.

Because CSA has been related to other types of child abuse and to dysfunctional family situations, it would seem that a broader type of information programme would be important to prevention. One example is Educating Children for Parenting (ECP), founded in 1978 by a non-profit organisation of the same name, in response to increasing incidents of child abuse. As noted by Alvin Poussaint, clinical professor of psychiatry at Harvard, and member of the group's national advisory board:

> If we can reach our students about parenting, perhaps we can help them in their relationships with others and help them be better aunts, cousins, friends and baby sitters. They will understand the impact of their own behaviours on other people. They will learn not to abuse a child physically or psychologically. And they can learn how to discipline without using violence. That way, they can model non-violent behaviour. And perhaps their children will be less likely to adopt violence and more likely to adopt other methods of resolving conflict. ("Raising Cain?", *The Philadelphia Inquirer*, 10 June 1998)

The programme uses a monthly classroom visit by a local parent (or parents) and baby to help teach students life-long relationship skills in 61 schools around the country (Educating Children for Parenting, 1997). Preliminary evaluations suggested that children exposed to the programme chose significantly more positive caring and nurturing strategies for dealing with solutions to parent–child problems. Currently, Research for Action, an independent education research and evaluation firm, is conducting a 3-year study of ECP's effectiveness which will include student outcomes. Although the programme does not focus on sexual abuse, the format can help students talk about things they normally don't discuss such as "I don't live with my Dad". And these things may include abuse. The programme trains guidance counsellors or school social workers to support teachers in helping students get needed services. Delivering the programme within an institutional setting such as the school provides stability.

Shifting from parenting skills to the policy changes that are needed to strengthen the ability of parents to balance work and family responsibilities, Hewlett & West (1998) drew from their involvement with the Task Force on Parent Empowerment and from testimony of parents around the country. Citing the link between poverty and child abuse, including sexual abuse, documented in national studies (e.g. National Center on Child Abuse and Neglect, 1988), these advocates argued for legislative changes that would increase economic security for parents and give them more time for their children. As a case in point, they cited an interview with a widowed mother working two jobs to support her three children. She is desperately worried because her 14-year-old daughter is "hanging" with a 21-year-old man. In the mother's words: "I know what happens to neglected kids. I work with them nineteen hours a day" (p.59).

Hewlett's & West's (1998) proposed Parents' Bill of Rights would bolster economic security for parents and ease their time "crunch". For example, the Bill advocates tax incentives for companies that offer flexible hours, job sharing, part-time work with benefits, and home-based employment opportunities. The Bill also would address the sagging wages and mounting job insecurity of parents through government and private support for a living wage, tax relief, and help with housing.

Yet another prevention approach would address the broader category of abuse from an ecological perspective. Belsky (1980) argues that an appreciation of the various levels of forces at work in the individual, the family, the community, and the culture can contribute much to the design of primary prevention programmes. For example, a visiting nurse programme developed by Olds et al. (1997) can intervene at a number of levels. Nurses provide young, unmarried, or poor pregnant women with information regarding maternal and child health. Nurses recruit the support of family members or peers for such women to help them out by serving as substitute caregivers as the need arises. Nurses also endeavour to make the social service system more responsive and encourage expectant women and men to participate in childbirth education. A randomised trial of home visitation services for 400 women during pregnancy and through their child's second birthday indicated that women receiving these services were significantly less likely ($p < 0.001$) to be identified as perpetrators of child abuse and neglect during the child's first 15 years (Olds et al., 1997).

Moreover, insights from cognition and neuroscience research show that the human brain is significantly affected by early experience. The effects of enriched, compared with deprived, environments in the laboratory on brain development are unmistakable and are evident at both behavioural and neuronal levels of organisation (Weiss & Wagner, 1998). Because the brain is most receptive during the first few years of development, it is particularly important to prevent abuse and to provide positive experiences. Although the public health benefits of prevention and early intervention are enormous, these benefits do not translate into funding. As Weiss & Wagner noted,

> ... funding for research and intervention programs for young children as a percentage of federal and state support is far less than for any other period of life. It is tragic that during the period of development where we can do so much, we do so little; and during the period of development where the interventions of society can have the least long-term effect, we spend so much. (p.359)

SCREENING AND INTERVENTION

Intervention with Victims

Because many girls do not report CSA, screening by professionals appears critical for assessment and referral. However, the literature suggests that this may not be happening. Interviews with professionals (e.g. social workers, psychologists, and paediatricians) in The Netherlands indicated shortcomings in their own knowledge and skills in working with abused women. Survivors also were dissatisfied with the professionals' unwillingness to detect and discuss sexual abuse and with their ability to provide satisfactory therapeutic contact (Frenken & Van Stolk, 1990). Moreover, five of the women interviewed reported either actual sexual abuse by a professional or explicit attempts in that direction. Data collected through anonymous, multiple-choice questionnaires from 27 physicians and 164 patients at two New England hospitals suggested that while most patients favour inquiries about physical and sexual abuse and believe physicians can help with these problems, physicians frequently do not inquire (Friedman et al., 1992). A later study in Michigan found that only 5.1% of 136 patients who acknowledged a history of CSA on a questionnaire had ever revealed that history to a physician (Lechner et al., 1993).

Although it is common to recommend psychotherapy for sexually abused children who come to the attention of professionals, studies of sexually abused children have yet to prove the effectiveness of treatment through randomised trials (Finkelhor & Berliner, 1995). Finkelhor & Berliner's review of findings from 29 studies that featured a range of treatment modalities and theoretical perspectives (e.g. family, group, and individual therapies and reinforcement, abuse-specific, and cognitive–behavioural theories) did suggest positive outcomes. A subsequent study by Berliner & Saunders (1996) randomly assigned 80 children, aged 4–13, to 10 weeks of group therapy or group therapy plus the enhancement of stress inoculation training (SIT) and gradual exposure procedures that teach specific coping skills to reduce fear and anxiety. Both groups improved significantly over a 2-year time period on most outcome treatment measures, with no differences between the groups on fear and anxiety. The researchers provided several explanations for their results including the idea that a supportive, abuse-specific treatment may be sufficient for the moderate levels of fear and anxiety present in the children. They also suggested that greater attention should be paid to the small group of children in both groups whose symptoms got worse during the study period. Studies, however, have not included longitudinal follow-up to see whether early intervention can reduce the long-term effects of sexual abuse, in particular, delayed effects that may emerge with the awakening sexual concerns of adolescence.

Existing clinical articles on the topic of group therapy for adults who were sexually abused in childhood also are limited in their methods with respect to control conditions for comparing the effectiveness of the treatment format (Alexander and Follette, 1987; Bowers, 1992; Graziano 1992). One empirical study in the literature that compared two short-term group therapy formats and a control condition suggested that the group therapy was effective in reducing depression and distress. The interpersonal transaction format (in which therapists introduced issues common to the experience of incest, for women to discuss in pairs) proved more effective for women who had no previous therapy experience. The process format (in which members selected the topics and focused on new ways of relating with the group) proved more advantageous for women with experience of therapy (Alexander et al., 1991). A higher level of education and single marital status predicted more improvement regardless of the format. The findings from that study emphasised the need for varied modes of treatment, including the possibility of concurrent individual therapy or couples therapy.

Foa et al. (1999) conducted a comparison of four treatment conditions: prolonged exposure (PE) that allows the participant to recall the abuse and process the memory until it is no longer intensely painful, stress inoculation training (SIT) that gives the participant a sense of mastery over fears by teaching a variety of coping skills, a combination treatment (PE + SIT), and a wait-list control. Ninety-six female assault victims (both sexual and non-sexual assault) with chronic PTSD attended nine, twice-weekly, individual sessions. All three active treatments reduced the severity of PTSD through a 12-month follow-up period compared with the wait-list condition, but they did not differ significantly from one another. Brief interventions of this type may also be useful for women who have experienced CSA, especially since therapists can be trained to deliver exposure therapy.

In a review of current practices in the treatment of victims of child sexual abuse, Beutler et al. (1994) contended that current practices apply "a variety of treatments without benefit of either a guiding philosophy or a clear set of guidelines based on knowledge about which of these various treatments will be most successful with which patients." They also cautioned that experiencing sexual abuse does not, in and of itself, create a need for treatment. From a clinical perspective, these authors recommended implementing existing models of treatment for substance abuse, eating disorders, anxiety, and depression for sexually abused clients who have these symptoms. From a research perspective, they recommended controlled clinical trials that compare the effectiveness of adaptations of these models in the domain of CSA. It would also seem critical to implement existing models for promoting safer sex and to test these with abused women who continue to engage in high-risk sexual behaviour.

Legal Intervention

Human service professionals including psychologists, social workers, teachers, and psychiatrists, are required by law to report known or suspected child abuse in all 50 states of the United States. However, the issue of how to stop incest without losing the co-operation of young victims is a common one for professionals (Frenken & Van Stolk, 1990). In a comprehensive discussion of mandated reporting of suspected child abuse, including sexual abuse, Kalichman (1993) pointed to the need for reform of reporting laws that are vague and that set legal standards that do not translate well to the complexity of situations faced by professionals: for example, an adolescent client tells her therapist of prior sexual abuse by a cousin (now living outside the state) but threatens to leave therapy if the therapist discloses that information, or a grade school child implies sexual abuse in a survey of stressful life events during which children have been assured responses were confidential. Toward improving child protection policy, Kalichman (1993) noted the need for research that examines the effect of laws across professions.

Intervention with Offenders

Behaviour therapy for sex offenders is the obvious counterpart to interventions for victims. The more recent behaviour therapies and hormonal therapies, accompanied by an organised monitoring system, appear to be the most effective approach for reducing victimisation of children (Abel & Osborn, 1996). Such programmes now combine a variety of behaviour therapies into a unified treatment plan called cognitive–behaviour treatment. Current therapies include three innovative approaches: imaginal desensitisation, relapse prevention, and modified aversive rehearsal. Imaginal desensitisation has the offender developing a few imaginary scenes that typify his or her usual molesting behaviour, but rather than carrying these scenes out in actual, offensive acts, the offender is asked to imagine scenarios in which he or she overcomes urges. Relapse prevention combines skill-training procedures with cognitive techniques. For example, offenders learn to identify factors that trigger the urge to molest and how to cope with them, for example by avoiding risky situations. Modified aversive rehearsal provides the offender with the opportunity to carry out his or her typical molesting behaviour with a mannequin while verbalising his or her usual self-statements before, during, and after the actual molestation, including possible sequelae for the child. Subsequent replays of this video-taped activity are reviewed with the perpetrator, the therapist, and others who provide a critique of the perpetrator's self-statements, based on their own experience or knowledge of what child victims have typically reported regarding the effects of victimisation. Most perpetrators find it untenable to maintain their cognitive distortions in the face of repeated feedback. Persons assessing or treating sex offenders should have specialised clinical training and experience in the assessment and treatment of sex offenders' problems, as well as appropriate licensing as a psychiatrist, psychologist, or clinical therapist (Coleman et al., 1996).

As noted by Abel & Osborn (1996), one reason that professionals are reluctant to treat sex offenders is that, when relapse occurs, not only is there a sense of professional failure but, more importantly, others are victimised. Consequently, surveillance systems must be built into treatment. This involves feedback by the offender, therapist, and individuals from family, work, and social environments on observable behaviours and personality characteristics or stressors that have been antecedent to previous relapses, and incorporates probation and parole officers.

Treatment outcomes are difficult to assess for many reasons, including the fact that outcome is usually measured by recidivism. Perpetrators often commit many offences for which they are not caught and are reluctant to report such to therapists who are required by law to report sex crimes to authorities. Also, forming a control group is ethically impossible since it would deny treatment to potentially dangerous persons and open therapists to the potential for lawsuits. Given these constraints, rates of relapse after treatments that include victim empathy training and a relapse prevention model that uses close supervision by therapists and court officers suggest that recidivism rates can fall to less than 10%. Moreover, specialised cognitive–behavioural treatment in a group setting costs far less than incarceration without treatment.

Another intervention strategy is to use assessment tools for measuring sexual interest of those accused of or admitting to child molestation. One such tool, the Abel Assessment for Sexual Interest, has been used extensively by the criminal justice system and by therapists to evaluate who is more likely to recidivate, who is a sadist and who isn't, and the ages and sexes of those children who arouse the offender's sexual interest. Such assessment provides guidance for therapy as well as the degree of supervision needed (Abel et al., 1994, 1998). A screening tool for employers (especially organisations that serve children, such as the Boy Scouts of America, orphanages, residential programmes for emotionally disturbed youth, day care centres, and churches) is undergoing preliminary trials. This screening tool would identify those who are quite likely paedophiles. Its ability to sort out individuals who molest young boys is quite high, but further refinements are needed for identifying those who molest girls.

SUMMARY

Because CSA is common and has long-term associations with risk behaviours and problems for women over the life cycle, increased attention to prevention strategies is imperative.

1. *Primary prevention*: given that CSA appears so closely associated with dysfunctional families, primary prevention needs to address parenting. This would include teaching parenting skills to future generations of parents (both girls and boys), providing parenting support to already high-risk families headed by single mothers, and assisting parents in balancing work and family responsibilities through economic benefits and opportunities. Primary prevention also would include improved assessment tools for evaluating sex offenders.
2. *Secondary prevention*: for those who do experience CSA, preventing the adoption of behaviours that lead to negative health outcomes should also be a high priority. These prevention strategies would include training of physicians and other health professionals in screening for CSA and in providing appropriate referrals for children and families when warranted.
3. *Tertiary prevention*: because current practices in the treatment of girls and young women apply a variety of strategies (without the benefits of either a guiding philosophy or a clear set of guidelines based on knowledge about which treatment will be most successful), future studies are needed to better understand which components of therapy are associated with successful outcomes for which clients.

In conclusion, researchers, activists, and health practitioners are increasingly aware that sexual victimisation early in a child's life has a profound effect on the quality of her life as an adult. Implementing the necessary programmes, research, and training to end such victimisation is a complex and challenging task but offers a major opportunity to improve women's and girls' mental and physical well-being over the life cycle.

REFERENCES

Abel, G.G., & Osborn, C. (1995). Pedophilia. In Diamant, L., & McAnulty, R. (Eds.), *The Psychology of Sexual Orientation: A Handbook* (pp.270–281). Westport, CT: Greenwood Publishing Group.

Abel, G.G., & Osborn, C.A. (1996). Behavioural therapy treatment for sex-offenders. In Rosen, I. (Ed.), *Sexual Deviation*, 3rd Edition, (pp.382–398). London: Oxford University Press.

Abel, G.G., Lawry, S.S., Karlstrom, E., Osborn, C.A., & Gillespie, C.F. (1994). Screening tests for pedophilia. *Criminal Justice and Behavior*, 21, 115–131.

Abel, G.G., Huffman, J., Warberg, B., & Holland, C.L. (1998). Visual reaction time and plethysmography as measures of sexual interest in child molesters. *Sexual Abuse: A Journal of Research and Treatment*, 10, 81–95.

Alexander, P.C., & Follette, V.M. (1987). Personal constructs in the group treatment of incest. In Neimeyer, R.A., & Neimeyer, G.J. (Eds.), *Personal Construct Therapy Casebook* (pp. 211–229). New York: Springer.

Alexander, P.C., Neimeyer, R.A., & Follette, V.M. (1991). Group therapy for women sexually abused as children: a controlled study and investigation of individual differences. *Journal of Interpersonal Violence, 6,* 218–231.

American Psychiatric Association (1994). *Diagnostic and Statistical Manual of Mental Disorders,* 4th Edition. Washington DC: American Psychiatric Association.

Angelou, M. (1969). *I Know Why the Caged Bird Sings* (p.76). New York: Random House.

Arndt, W.B. (1991). *Gender Disorders and the Paraphilias.* Madison, WI: International Universities Press, Inc.

Beitchman, J.H., Zucker, K.J., Hood, J.E., DaCosta, G.A., Akman, D., & Cassavia, E. (1992). A review of the long-term effects of child sexual abuse. *Child Abuse and Neglect, 16,* 102–118.

Belsky, J. (1980). Child maltreatment: an ecological integration. *American Psychologist, 35,* 320–335.

Berliner, L., & Saunders, B.E. (1996). Treating fear and anxiety in sexually abused children: results of a controlled 2-year follow-up study. *Child Maltreatment, 1,* 294–309.

Beutler, L.E., Williams, R.E., & Zetzer, H.A. (1994). Efficacy of treatment for victims of child sexual abuse. *The Future of Children, 4,* 156–175.

Bowers, J. (1992). Therapy through art: facilitating treatment of sexual abuse. *Journal of Psychosocial Nursing, 30,* 15–23.

Boyer, D., & Fine, D. (1992). Sexual abuse as a factor in adolescent pregnancy and child maltreatment. *Family Planning Perspectives, 24,* 4–11, 19.

Briere, J., & Runtz, M. (1988). Symptomatology associated with childhood sexual victimization in a nonclinical adult sample. *Child Abuse and Neglect, 12,* 51–59.

Briere, J., & Conte, J. (1993). Self-reported amnesia for abuse in adults molested as children. *Journal of Traumatic Stress, 6,* 21–31.

Briere, J.N., & Elliott, D.M. (1994). Immediate and long-term impacts of child sexual abuse. *The Future of Children, 4,* 54–69.

Browne, A., & Finkelhor, D. (1986). Impact of child sexual abuse: a review of the research. *Psychological Bulletin, 99,* 66–77.

Browning, C.R., & Laumann, E.O. (1997). Sexual contact between children and adults: a life course perspective. *American Sociological Review, 62,* 540–560.

Burgess, A.W., Groth, A.N., Holmstrom, L.L., & Sgroi, S.M. (1978). *Sexual Assault of Children and Adolescents.* Lexington, MA: D.C. Heath.

Butler, S. (1978). *Conspiracy of Silence: The Trauma of Incest.* San Francisco: New Glide Publications.

Centers for Disease Control and Prevention (1997). Youth risk behavior surveillance. CDC Surveillance Summaries, 14 November 1997; *MMWR, 46 (No.SS-6).* Atlanta: Centers for Disease Control and Prevention.

Coleman, E., Dwyer, S.M., Abel, G., Berner, W., Breiling, J., Hindman, J., Knopp, F.H., Langevin, R., & Friedemann, P. (1996). Standards of care for the treatment of adult sex offenders. In Coleman, E. (Ed.), *Sex Offender Treatment: Biological Dysfunction, Intrapsychic Conflict, Interpersonal Violence* (pp.5–11). Binghamton, NY: Haworth Press, Inc.

Conte, J.R. (1994). Child sexual abuse: awareness and backlash. *The Future of Children, 4*, 224–232.

Conte, J., & Schuerman, J. (1987). The effects of sexual abuse on children: a multidimensional view. *Journal of Interpersonal Violence, 2*, 380–390.

Cuccinelli, D., & De Groot, A.S. (1997). Put her in a cage: childhood sexual abuse, incarceration, and HIV infection. In Goldstein, N., & Manlowe, J.L. (Eds.), *The Gender Politics of HIV/AIDS in Women: Perspectives on the Pandemic in the United States* (pp.222–241). New York: New York University Press.

Cunningham, R.M., Stiffman, A.R., & Dore, P. (1994). The association of physical and sexual abuse with risk behaviors in adolescence and young adulthood: implications for public health. *Child Abuse and Neglect, 18*, 233–245.

Daley, S. (1998). Young, vulnerable and violated in the new South Africa. *The New York Times Magazine*, 12 July 1998, Section 6, pp.30–33.

Dansky, B.S., Brewerton, T.D., Kilpatrick, D.G., & O'Neil, P.M. (1997). The national women's study: relationship of victimization and post-traumatic stress disorder to bulimia nervosa. *International Journal of Eating Disorders, 21*, 213–228.

Educating Children for Parenting (1997). *Biennial Report*. Philadelphia, PA: Educating Children for Parenting.

Felitti, V.J. (1991). Long-term medical consequences of incest, rape, and molestation. *Southern Medical Journal, 84*, 328–331.

Felitti, V.J., Anda, R.F., Nordenberg, D., Williamson, D.F., Spitz, A.M., Edwards, V., Koss, M.P., & Marks, J.S. (1998). Relationship of childhood abuse and household dysfunction to many of the leading causes of death in adults. *American Journal of Preventive Medicine, 14*, 245–258.

Finkelhor, D. (1979). *Sexually Victimized Children*. New York: Free Press.

Finkelhor, D. (1994). Current information on the scope and nature of child sexual abuse. *The Future of Children, 4*, 31–53.

Finkelhor, D., & Berliner, L. (1995). Research on the treatment of sexually abused children: a review and recommendations. *Journal of the American Academy of Child & Adolescent Psychiatry, 34*, 1408–1423.

Finkelhor, D., & Browne, A. (1986). Initial and long-term effects: a conceptual framework. In Finkelhor, D., (Ed.), *A Sourcebook on Child Sexual Abuse* (pp. 180–198). Beverly Hills, CA: Sage.

Finkelhor, D., Hotaling, G., Lewis, I.A., & Smith, C. (1990). Sexual abuse in a national survey of adult men and women: prevalence, characteristics, and risk factors. *Child Abuse and Neglect, 14*, 19–28.

Finkelhor, D., Asdigian, N., & Dziuba-Leatherman, J. (1995). Victimization prevention programs for children: a follow-up. *American Journal of Public Health, 85*, 1684–1689.

Foa, E.B., Dancu, C.V., Hembree, E.A., Jaycox, L.H., Meadows, E.A., & Street, G.P. (1999). A comparison of exposure therapy, stress inoculation training and their combination for reducing PTSD in female assault victims. *Journal of Consulting and Clinical Psychology,* *67*, 194–200.

Frenken, J., & Van Stolk, B. (1990). Incest victims: inadequate help by professionals. *Child Abuse and Neglect, 14,* 253–263.

Friedman, L.S., Samet, J.H., Roberts, M.S., Hudlin, M., & Hans, P. (1992). Inquiry about victimization experiences. *Archives of Internal Medicine, 152,* 1186–1190.

Fromuth, M.E. (1986). The relationship of childhood sexual abuse with later psychological and sexual adjustment in a sample of college women. *Child Abuse and Neglect, 10,* 5–15.

Graziano, R. (1992) Treating women incest survivors: a bridge between "Cumulative Trauma" and "Post-Traumatic Stress". *Social Work in Health Care, 17,* 69–85.

Greenberg, J., Hennessy, M., Lifshay, J., Kahn-Krieger, S., Bartelli, D., Downer, A., & Bliss, M. (1999). Childhood sexual abuse and its relationship to high-risk behavior in women volunteering for an HIV and STD prevention intervention. *AIDS and Behavior 3,* 149–156.

Gutman, L., St Claire, K.K., Weedy, C., Herman-Giddens, M.E., Lane, B.A., Niemeyer, J.G., & McKinney, R.E. (1991). Human immunodeficiency virus transmission by child sexual abuse. *American Journal of Diseases of Children, 145,* 137–141.

Gutman, L.T., St Claire, K.K., Everett, V.D., Ingram, D.L., Soper, J., Johnston, W.W., Mulvaney, G.G., & Phelps, W.C. (1994). Cervical–vaginal and intra-anal human papillomavirus infection of young girls with external genital warts. *Journal of Infectious Diseases, 170,* 339–344.

Harber, K.D., & Pennebaker, J.W. (1992). Overcoming traumatic memories. In Christianson, S.A. (Ed.), *The Handbook of Emotion and Memory: Research and Theory* (pp.359–387). Hillsdale, NJ: Erlbaum.

Harvey, M.R., & Herman, J.L. (1994). Amnesia, partial amnesia, and delayed recall among survivors of childhood trauma. *Consciousness Cognition, 3,* 295–306.

Heise, L., Moore, K., & Toubia, N. (1995). *Sexual Coercion and Reproductive Health: A Focus on Research.* New York: Population Council.

Herman, J.L., & Schatzow, E. (1987). Recovery and verification of memories of childhood sexual trauma. *Psychoanalytic Psychology, 4,* 1–14.

Hewlett, S.A., & West, C. (1998) *The War Against Parents.* Boston: Houghton Mifflin Company.

Hyman, I., & Loftus, E. (1997). Some people recover memories that never really happened. In Appelbaum, P., & Uyehara, L. (Eds.), *Trauma and Memory: Clinical and Legal Controversies.* New York: Oxford University Press.

Jeffrey, T.B., & Jeffrey, L.K. (1991). Psychologic aspects of sexual abuse in adolescence. *Current Opinion in Obstetrics and Gynecology, 3,* 825–831.

Jones, W.P., & Emerson, S. (1994). Sexual abuse and binge eating in a nonclinical population. *Journal of Sex Education and Therapy, 20,* 47–55.

Kalichman, S.C. (1993). *Mandated Reporting of Suspected Child Abuse: Ethics, Law, & policy*. Washington, DC: American Psychological Association.

Kendall-Tackett, K.A., Williams, L.M., & Finkelhor, D. (1993). Impact of sexual abuse on children: a review and synthesis of recent empirical studies. *Psychological Bulletin, 113*, 164–180.

Kinsey, A.C., Pomeroy, W.B., Martin, C.E., & Gebhard, P.H. (1953). *Sexual Behavior in the Human Female*. Philadelphia: W.B. Saunders.

Korbin, J. (1987). Child sexual abuse: implications from the cross-cultural record. In Scheper-Hughes, N. (Ed.), *Child Survival: Anthropological Perspectives on the Treatment and Maltreatment of Children* (pp.247–265). Dordrecht: Kluwer.

Koss, M.P., & Dinero, T.E. (1989). Discriminant analysis of risk factors for sexual victimization among a national sample of college women. *Journal of Consulting and Clinical Psychology, 57*, 242–250.

Laumann, E., Gagnon, J., Michael, R., & Michaels, S. (1994). *The Social Organization of Sexuality: Sexual Practices in the United States*. Chicago: University of Chicago Press.

Lechner, M.E., Vogel M.E., Garcia-Shelton, L.M., Leichter, J.L., & Steibel, K.R. (1993). Self-reported medical problems of adult female survivors of childhood sexual abuse. *The Journal of Family Practice, 36*, 633–638.

Loftus, E.F. (1997). Repressed memory accusations: devastated families and devastated patients. *Applied Cognitive Psychology, 11*, 25–30.

Mullen, P.E., Martin, J.L., Anderson, J.C., Romans, S.E., & Herbison, G.P. (1994). The effect of child sexual abuse on social, interpersonal and sexual function in adult life. *British Journal of Psychiatry, 165*, 35–47.

National Center on Child Abuse and Neglect (1988). *Study of National Incidence and Prevalence of Child Abuse and Neglect: 1988 (NIS-2)* (chapter 5, p.26). Washington: US Department of Health and Human Services.

Neumann, D. (1994). Long-term correlates of childhood sexual abuse in adult survivors. *New Directions for Mental Health Services, 64*, 29–38.

Olds, D.L., Eckenrode, J., Henderson, C.R., Kitzman, H., Powers, J., Cole, R., Sidora, K., Morris, P., Pettitt, L.M., & Luckey, D. (1997). Long-term effects of home visitation on maternal life course and child abuse and neglect. *Journal of the American Medical Association, 278*, 637–643.

Plichta, S.B., & Abraham, C. (1996). Violence and gynecologic health in women < 50 years old. *American Journal of Obstetrics and Gynecology, 174*, 903–907.

"Raising Cain?" (1998). *The Philadelphia Inquirer*, 10 June 1998.

Rind, B., & Tromovitch, P. (1997). A meta-analytic review of findings from national samples on psychological correlates of child sexual abuse. *The Journal of Sex Research, 34*, 237–255.

Rosas, M. (1992). *Violencia Sexual y Politica Criminal*. Lima, Peru: Comite Latinoamericano para la Defensa del las Dereches de la Mujer (CLADEM), Informativo 6. [Cited in Heise et al., 1995.]

Rush, F. (1980). *The Best Kept Secret: Sexual Abuse of Children.* Englewood Cliffs: Prentice-Hall.

Russell, E.H. (1984). *Sexual Exploitation: Rape, Child Sexual Abuse, Sexual Harassment.* Beverly Hills, CA: Sage.

Simmons, K. (1998). 4 teens admit assaults on girls. *The Atlanta Journal – Constitution,* Local News, 13 October 1998, p.1.

Springs, F.E., & Friedrich, W.N. (1992). Health risk behaviors and medical sequelae of childhood sexual abuse. *Mayo Clinic Proceedings, 67,* 527–532.

Stock, J.L., Bell, M.A., Boyer, D.K., & Connell, F.A. (1997). Adolescent pregnancy and sexual risk-taking among sexually abused girls. *Family Planning Perspectives, 29,* 200–203, 227.

Thompson, N.J., Potter, J.S., Sanderson, C.A., & Maibach, E.W. (1997) The relationship of sexual abuse and HIV risk behaviors among heterosexual adult female STD patients. *Child Abuse and Neglect, 21,* 149–156.

Urquiza, A.J., & Goodlin-Jones, B.L. (1994). Child sexual abuse and adult revictimization with women of color. *Violence and Victims, 9,* 223–232.

Ussher, J.M., & Dewberry, C. (1995). The nature and long-term effects of childhood sexual abuse: a survey of adult women survivors in Britain. *British Journal of Clinical Psychology, 34,* 177–192.

Vermund, S.H., Alexander-Rodriquez, T., Macleod, S., & Kelley, K.F. (1990). History of sexual abuse in incarcerated adolescents with gonorrhea or syphilis. *Journal of Adolescent Health Care, 11,* 449–452.

Watts, W.D., & Ellis, A.M. (1993). Sexual abuse and drinking and drug use: implications for prevention. *Journal of Drug Education, 23,* 183–200.

Weiner, E.J., & Stephens, L. (1993). Sexual barrier weight: a new approach. Eating disorders. *The Journal of Treatment and Prevention, 1,* 241–249.

Weiss, M.J., & Wagner, S.H. (1998). What explains the negative consequences of adverse childhood experiences on adult health? Insights from cognitive and neuroscience research. *American Journal of Preventive Medicine, 14,* 356–360.

Widom, C.S., & Kuhns, J.B. (1996). Childhood victimization and subsequent risk for promiscuity, prostitution, and teenage pregnancy: a prospective study. *American Journal of Public Health, 86,* 1607–1612.

Wyatt, G.E. (1988). The relationship between child sexual abuse and adolescent sexual functioning in Afro-American and White American women. *Annals New York Academy of Sciences, 528,* 111–122.

Wyatt, G.E., Guthrie, D., & Notgrass, C.M. (1992). Differential effects of women's child sexual abuse and subsequent sexual revictimization. *Journal of Consulting and Clinical Psychology, 60,* 167–173.

Section 4

WOMEN AND PHYSICAL HEALTH

Chapter 16

Rheumatoid Arthritis: Pathophysiology, Epidemiology, and Treatment

Jennifer M. Grossman and Ernest Brahn

University of California at Los Angeles, School of Medicine, USA

Rheumatoid arthritis (RA) is the most common autoimmune inflammatory joint disease, affecting approximately 1–2% of the adult population. Although a principal feature of RA is an erosive and deforming arthritis, other organs that can be involved include the lungs, skin, nerves, eyes and blood vessels. Criteria for the diagnosis of RA have been developed by the American Rheumatism Association (Arnett et al., 1988) and are shown in Table 16.1.

EPIDEMIOLOGY OF RHEUMATOID ARTHRITIS

Rheumatoid arthritis is the most common inflammatory arthritis. Using five non-institutionalized populations, Lawrence and colleagues showed that the prevalence of RA in the United States is approximately 2.1 million persons, 1.5 million of which are women (Lawrence et al., 1998). A higher prevalence has been described in American Indian

Women, Health and the Mind
Edited by L. Sherr and J.S. St Lawrence. © 2000 John Wiley & Sons, Ltd

Table 16.1 Classification of rheumatoid arthritis[1]

Criterion	Definition
1. Morning stiffness	Morning stiffness in and around the joints lasting at least 1 hour before maximal improvement
2. Arthritis of three or more joint areas	At least three joint areas simultaneously having soft tissue swelling or fluid (not bony overgrowth alone) observed by a physician; the 14 possible joint areas are (right or left) PIP, MCP, wrist, elbow, knee, ankle, and MTP joints
3. Arthritis of hand joints	At least one joint area swollen as above in wrist, MCP, or PIP
4. Symmetrical arthritis	Simultaneous involvement of the same joint areas (as in criterion 2) on both sides of the body (bilateral involvement of PIP, MCP, or MTP joints is acceptable without absolute symmetry)
5. Rheumatoid nodules	Subcutaneous nodules over bony prominences or extensor surfaces, or in juxta-articular regions, observed by a physician
6. Serum rheumatoid factor	Demonstration of abnormal amounts of serum rheumatoid factor by any method that has been positive in < 5% of normal control subjects
7. Radiographic changes	Changes typical of RA on PA hand and wrist radiographs, which must include erosions or unequivocal bony decalcification localized to or most marked adjacent to the involved joints (osteoarthritis changes alone do not qualify)

Source: Arnett et al. (1988).
[1] For the purposes of classification, a patient is said to have RA if he or she has satisfied at least four of the seven criteria. Criteria 1–4 must be present for at least 6 weeks. Abbreviations: PIP, proximal interphalangeal; MCP, metacarpophalangeal; MTP, metatarsophalangeal; PA, posteroanterior

(Beasley et al., 1973) and in Finnish populations, while a lower prevalence has been reported in some African and Asian cohorts (Spector, 1990) even when adjustments for younger population samples in Third World countries are made (Abdel-Nasser et al., 1997). Two recent reviews have concluded that RA may be declining in prevalence and severity in the United States and Europe (Abdel-Nasser et al., 1997; Spector, 1990), but possibly increasing in severity in Africa (Abdel-Nasser et al., 1997).

Attempts have been made to identify risk factors for the development of RA. There is no relationship between the geographic latitude and prevalence, as has been implicated in multiple sclerosis (Lawrence, 1977); however, humidity has been related with increased symptoms (Rasker et al., 1986). Smoking has been associated with RA in one case–control study (Symmons et al., 1997), although it was protective against RA in another (Spector, 1990). Blood transfusions and obesity have also been identified as a risk factor for RA in one case–control study (Symmons et al., 1997), and gout and schizophrenia are negatively associated (Harris, 1997; Spector, 1990). Psychosocial stress may also play a role in the development of RA, but this has been difficult to evaluate given the insidious onset of disease (Spector, 1990).

HISTORY OF RHEUMATOID ARTHRITIS

Rheumatoid arthritis has been called a disease of modern society. Landre-Beauvais is credited with the first definitive description of RA in his thesis in 1800 in which he described nine women with a polyarticular onset of arthritis that led to disabling joint deformities over the course of a few years. At necropsy, cartilage ulcerations, bony destruction and osteopenia were evident (Short, 1974). The term "rheumatoid arthritis" was first applied to the disease by Sir Alfred Garrod in 1859 (Short, 1974). However, there are suggestions in archeology, as well as in paintings, that RA has existed for much longer. Skeletal remains of Indians in Alabama, dating back 3000 to 5000 years, have a symmetrical, erosive polyarthritis of the small and large joints (Rothschild et al., 1988). Similar changes were seen in 4050- to 4300-year-old skeletons unearthed in Kentucky whose sacroiliac joints were noted to be normal, further supporting the hypothesis that these bones manifest RA and not a seronegative spondyloarthropathy (Rothschild & Woods, 1990). Archeological findings are not uniform. A study of 800 skeletons from medieval England revealed only one skeleton with erosions suggestive of possible RA (Dieppe et al., 1987). Because this is not the expected prevalence for RA, it is less likely that this represents the disease as it is known today. Furthermore, skeletal remains of 443 subjects from sixteenth century Mexico did not reveal any evidence of RA (Aceves-Avila et al., 1998). This has led to a hypothesis that RA may be a disease that began in North America thousands of years ago and then spread.

Short (1974) suggests that there is no evidence of RA in paintings before 1800. Dequeker (1977), however, described subjects with swollen metacarpophalangeal (MCP) and proximal interphalangeal (PIP) joints in Flemish portraits from the 1400 to 1700 period. Rubens, a Flemish artist who lived from 1577 to 1640, suffered from an arthritis which some historians have called gout, although this diagnosis has been questioned since portraits of him reveal swollen MCP and PIP joints raising the possibility of RA (Appelboom et al., 1981). These examples cannot be used as conclusive evidence that RA existed during these time periods, however, because of the interpretative nature of painting. In summary, RA is a disease for which the first written description dates to 1800 but it may have existed in North America long before. These historical aspects may ultimately be helpful in understanding the etiopathogenesis of RA.

PATHOGENESIS OF RHEUMATOID ARTHRITIS

The pathogenesis of RA is unknown, but is most likely the result of an interaction of genetic and environmental factors. There are several lines of evidence that support the role of genetics in the development of RA. There is a reported 3- to 4-fold increased risk of RA in first-degree relatives (Spector, 1990) and a 30–50% concordance rate for monozygotic twins (Firestein, 1997). In addition, RA is associated with certain class II human leukocyte antigens (HLA), especially HLA-DR4. Gran et al. (1983) have found a gene frequency of the HLA-DR4 allele of 60–70% in Caucasian RA patients compared with 27–35% in controls. The HLA-DR allele contains a locus, DRB1, that encodes the HLA-DRB1 chain. In a study by Weyand et al. (1992) of 102 RA patients who were rheumatoid factor positive, the HLA-DRB1 alleles known as 0401, 0404, 0101 and 1402 were associated with increased disease severity as measured by the presence of extra-articular disease and the need for joint surgery. The third hypervariable region of these alleles contains the same amino acid sequence, glutamine-lysine-arginine-alanine-alanine, which plays an important role in T-cell recognition. This amino acid sequence is also found in the gp110 protein of the Epstein–Barr virus (Roudier et al., 1989) and a heat shock protein produced by *E. coli* (Auger & Roudier, 1997). This observation has led to the hypothesis that RA may be caused by molecular mimicry in which T cells first respond to a foreign antigen and then cross-react with an autoantigen.

A T cell paradigm becomes less straightforward as the nature of the complex cell–cell interactions in the RA synovium unfolds. Numerous studies have searched for an infectious trigger including *Chlamydia*, *Mycoplasma*, *Mycobacteria*, and various viruses such as Epstein–Barr, parvovirus, and retroviruses (Harris, 1990). There have been no consistent data to implicate any of these agents as an etiology for RA. Whatever the initiating event, it is clear that there are a variety of cells and compounds that are responsible for the propagation of inflammation and joint damage. This is depicted in Figure 16.1. The cells involved include monocytes, macrophages, fibroblasts, lymphocytes (both T and B cells), neutrophils, and endothelial cells. These cells produce and are subsequently regulated by proteins called cytokines. Interleukin 1 (IL-1), interleukin 2 (IL-2), interleukin 4 (IL-4), interleukin 6 (IL-6), interleukin 8 (IL-8), interleukin 10 (IL-10), and tumor necrosis factor α (TNF-α) are some of the cytokines that have been shown to play a role in the inflammation. Metalloproteinases are enzymes that are responsible for the degradation of proteoglycans, cartilage and bone. Angiogenesis, the formation of new blood vessels, is another important component in the development of the RA pannus (Koch, 1998). These molecules and cells are all becoming targets for therapeutic interventions with biologic agents.

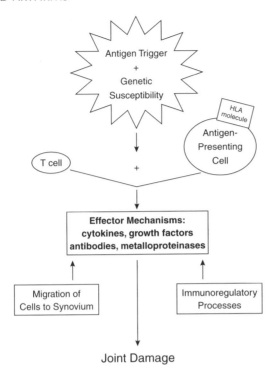

Figure 16.1 Theoretical pathophysiologic processes in rheumatoid arthritis

HORMONES AND RHEUMATOID ARTHRITIS

There are several lines of evidence that support the theory that sex hormones can influence RA. It is a disease of female predominance, with a peak incidence in women that occurs around the time of menopause, although it can affect all ages (Goemaere et al., 1990). Women with RA also have a statistically significant decrease in pain and morning stiffness during the postovulatory phase of the menstrual cycle when plasma levels of estrogen and progesterone are increased (Latman, 1983). In males, the incidence of RA rises with increased age. Since androgen levels decline with aging, one could postulate that androgens function as a suppressive force in the development of RA. While levels of female sex hormones in patients with active RA have not been shown to be significantly different from healthy controls, most studies demonstrate suppressed androgen levels in RA patients. In one study of pre- and postmenopausal women, androgen levels correlated inversely with disease activity (Feher et al., 1986).

Sex steroids may have direct effects on the immune system, although, the precise biologic mechanisms are unknown. In general, androgens tend to suppress the immune system (Wilder, 1996) while prolactin can stimulate it. Estrogen can both stimulate the immune system, as illustrated by increased immunoglobulin synthesis in females compared with males, and inhibit the immune system, by suppressing T cell dependent functions (Grossman, 1985). In collagen-induced arthritis and adjuvant arthritis, experimental models of RA in rats, castration of female rats can enhance susceptibility of disease, whereas estrogen treatment of castrated animals suppresses disease development (Holmdahl et al. 1989).

There has been a great deal of interest in the relationship between disease activity in RA and the use of supplemental estrogen preparations, both hormone replacement therapy and oral contraceptives. In a population-based study in Olmstead County, Minnesota, from 1950 to 1974, Linos et al. (1980) found a decrease in the RA incidence rates in females during the last 10 years, whereas the rates for males were relatively constant. This change coincided with the increased use of exogenous hormones, leading the authors to postulate that hormone therapy may have a protective role in the development of RA. However, Jacobsson et al. (1994) found a decreasing prevalence and incidence in RA in Pima Indians even when exogenous estrogen use was controlled for, suggesting that another factor, such as an environmental exposure, may be responsible for this decline. Numerous studies have attempted to decipher this relationship. The results of these studies are shown in Tables 16.2 and 16.3 and, as is evident, there are discrepant results. Problems with the studies include a lack of definitive criteria for the diagnosis of RA, a recall bias in regards to oral contraceptive and hormone replacement therapy use, a variety of different controls, and the reliance on medical records alone as the source of the medication history. Two meta-analyses have examined oral contraceptive use and risk of RA. Romieu et al. (1989) found that case-controlled studies demonstrated a small but not statistically significant protective effect. Spector and Hochberg (1990) noted a statistically significant protective effect of oral contraceptives in which the benefit was seen in hospital-based clinics, but not in population-based clinics. This suggests that the benefits seen in some RA patients may result from a modulating effect only in those with more severe disease (Spector & Hochberg, 1990).

The relationship of disease activity and pregnancy provides another aspect of potential disease modification by sex hormones. Nulliparity is a risk factor for rheumatoid arthritis (Hazes et al., 1990a; Spector et al., 1990). One study, however, found that more than three pregnancies was associated with more severe disease (Jorgensen et al., 1996). In RA patients who become pregnant, there is an amelioration of disease about 80% of the time, with approximately 25% flaring post-partum. Several potential explanations have included increased cortisol levels during pregnancy, alterations in sex hormones, and increased pregnancy-specific α-glycoprotein (Spector & Da Silva, 1992). Brennan &

Table 16.2   Post-menopausal hormone use and the risk of rheumatoid arthritis[1]

Reference	Study design	Sample size	Outcome
Linos et al., 1983	Case–control	Cases = 229 Controls = 458	If used HRT during menopause transition, RR = 2.2–2.9 depending on duration of use If used after menopause transition, RR = 0.8–1.2 depending on duration of use; all the 95% CI encompass 1.0
Vanden-broucke et al., 1986	Case–control	Cases = 310 Controls (OA or STR) = 353	If used HRT before onset of disease, odds ratio = 0.32 (0.16–0.64)
Carette et al., 1989	Case–control	Cases = 111 Controls (OA or STR) = 305	If past use of HRT before symptoms, RR = 0.95 (0.56–1.60) If current use at symptom onset, RR = 0.89 (0.49–1.63)
Hernandez-Avila et al., 1990	Prospective population study	Cases = 123 (RA and undifferentiated polyarthritis) Total sample = 906 851 person-years	If current use of HRT at symptom onset, RR = 1.3 (0.9–2.0) If ever used before symptoms, RR = 1.0 (0.7–1.4) If past use before symptoms, RR = 0.7 (0.5–1.2)
Spector et al., 1991	Retrospective cohort	New diagnosis of RA = 6 in an HRT cohort of 1075 New diagnosis of RA = 8 in a control cohort of 1542	If ever used HRT before symptoms, RR = 1.62 (0.56–4.74)
Koepsell et al., 1994	Population-based, case–control	Cases = 135 Controls = 592	If ever used HRT before symptoms, RR = 1.04 (0.7–1.55) If current use at symptom onset, RR = 0.81 for estrogen and progesterone, RR = 0.97 for estrogen only use, with both 95% CI encompassing 1.0
Van den Brink et al., 1993	Double-blind, randomized, placebo controlled trial of 12 months	n = 15 in treatment arm, n = 18 in placebo arm that completed the study	No beneficial effect of HRT on disease activity

(*continued overleaf*)

Table 16.2 *(continued)*

Reference	Study design	Sample size	Outcome
Hall et al., 1994	Single-blind, randomized, placebo controlled trial of 6 months' duration	*n* = 91 in treatment arm, *n* = 77 in placebo arm	No overall effect of HRT on disease activity, but when analyzed for compliant participants, improvement in articular index, pain, and morning stiffness in the treatment group (*P* < 0.05)
MacDonald et al., 1994	Double-blind placebo-controlled trial of 48 weeks	*n* = 31 in treatment arm *n* = 13 in placebo arm that completed the study	Treatment group had increased sense of well-being (*P* < 0.01) and an improvement in articular index (*P* < 0.05)

[1] Abbreviations: RR ( ), relative risk of developing RA (95% confidence intervals); OA, osteoarthritis; STR, soft tissue rheumatism; CI, confidence interval; HRT, hormone replacement therapy

Silman (1994a) found an increased prevalence of breastfeeding among women who developed RA within 12 months after a first pregnancy. They suggested that in susceptible women, hormonal influences, in particular the proinflammatory prolactin, may increase the risk of RA. Nelson et al. (1993) demonstrated that an improvement in RA during pregnancy occurs most frequently when the maternal and fetal HLA class II antigens differ. The mechanism by which this occurs is unknown. In a case–control study, Silman et al. (1992) found that there was a decreased relative risk of disease onset during pregnancy and a subsequent increased risk during the first 3 months post-partum that persists, although is slightly less, for the next 9 months. In summary, the relationship of sex hormones to RA is complex, with numerous studies yielding conflicting results. Further work is needed.

CLINICAL MANIFESTATIONS OF RHEUMATOID ARTHRITIS

The diagnosis of RA is based on the history, physical examination, laboratory tests, and radiographic findings. A patient is classified as having RA when at least four of seven criteria are fulfilled (Table 16.1). These criteria have a sensitivity of 92% and a specificity of 89% (Arnett et al., 1988). Some diseases that can mimic RA include gout, pseudo-gout, systemic lupus erythematosus, spondyloarthropathies (such as Reiter's and psoriatic arthritis), adult onset Still's disease, amyloid arthropathy, palindromic rheumatism, hemachromatosis, Lyme disease, and viral infections such as hepatitis B, hepatitis C, and parvovirus.

The predominant feature evident from the history and physical examination is a symmetric polyarthritis. The majority of patients experience

Table 16.3 Oral contraceptives and the risk of rheumatoid arthritis[1]

Reference	Study design	Sample size	Outcome
Wingrave & Kay, 1978	Prospective survey of oral contraceptive use	23 000 OCP users with 37 cases of RA 23 000 controls with 57 cases of RA	Rate of reporting RA per 1000 women-years If current users at symptom onset = 0.31 If ex-users at symptom onset = 0.53 If never user = 0.63
Vanden- broucke et al., 1982	Case–control	Cases = 228 Controls (OA and STR) = 302	OR for developing RA If ever users before symptoms = 0.42 (0.27–0.65) If ex-users before symptoms = 0.40 (0.22–0.72) If current users at symptom onset = 0.45 (0.28–0.75)
Linos et al., 1983	Case–control	Cases = 229 Controls = 458	RR = 0.7–1.3 depending on duration of usage with all 95% CI overlapping 1.0
Allebeck et al., 1984	Case–control	Cases = 76 Controls = 152	RR if prior OCP use > 1 year = 0.7 (0.40–1.24)
Del Junco et al., 1985	Population- based Case–control	Cases = 182 Controls = 182	If prior OCP before symptoms, RR = 1.1 (0.7–1.7) If current use at symptom onset, RR = 1.3 (0.7–2.4)
Vanden- broucke et al., 1986	Case–control	Cases = 246 Controls (OA and STR) = 323	If prior oral contraceptive use before symptoms, RR = 0.52 (0.3–0.9)
Darwish & Armenian, 1987	Case–control	Cases = 100 Controls = 100	If oral contraceptive use, RR = 1.29 (0.64–2.58)
Vessey et al., 1987	Prospective cohort	Cases = 78 Sample size = 17 032	Rate per 1000 woman-years: If current use of OCP at symptom onset = 0.44 If ex-use of OCP before symptoms = 0.33 If never use of OCP = 0.33
Hazes et al., 1990c	Case–control	Cases = 86 Controls (sisters) = 118	Adjusted OR for premorbid OCP use = 0.60 (0.21–1.71)
Moskowitz et al., 1990	Case–control	Cases = 71 Controls = 280	If current use at symptom onset, RR = 2.0 (0.97–4.21) If past use before symptoms, RR = 1.0 (0.4–2.2)

(continued overleaf)

Table 16.3 (*continued*)

Reference	Study design	Sample size	Outcome
Hazes et al., 1990b	Case–control	Cases = 135 Controls (OA and STR) = 378	If ever use of OCP before symptoms, RR = 0.39 (0.24–0.63) If current use of OCP at symptom onset, RR = 0.58 (0.32–1.04)
Spector et al., 1990	Case–control	RA cases = 270 OA controls = 292 Population controls = 245	For RA versus OA, if OCP use before age 35, RR = 0.56 (0.29–1.12) For RA versus population controls if OCP use before age 35, RR = 0.60 (0.30–1.17)
Hannaford et al., 1990	Prospective study, a follow up of Wingrave & Kay (1978)	Initial cohort of 23 000 pill users, and 23 000 con- trols. (nearly 65% original of partici- pants lost to follow- up)	Standardized risk ratio for RA Between current and never users = 0.82 (0.59–1.15) Between former and never users = 0.94 (0.72–1.22)
Hernandez- Avila et al., 1990	Prospective population study	115 cases of RA in 121 700 female nurses in the population cohort	Age-adjusted RR If OCP use for 1–23 months, RR = 0.9 (0.5–1.6) If OCP use for 24–59 months, RR = 0.7 (0.4–1.6) If OCP use for > 60 months, RR = 1.2 (0.7–2.0)
van Zeben et al., 1990	Case–control	Definite RA = 121 Probable RA = 52 Controls (OA or STR) = 378	RR if OCP use before onset of symptoms For probable RA, RR = 0.72 (0.27–1.89) For mild RA, RR = 0.79 (0.21–2.79) For severe RA, RR = 0.33 (0.19–0.57)
Brennan and Silman, 1994b	Matched case–control from a study population of twins	35 monozygotic twin pairs discor- dant for disease, 31 dizygotic twin pairs discordant for disease, and 60 mixed cases and 160 population controls	OR for ever use of OCP before disease For monozygotic cases, OR = 0.25 (0.03–2.24) For dizygotic cases, OR = 0.75 (0.17–3.35) For mixed cases versus population controls, OR = 0.43 (0.17–1.09)

Table 16.3 (*continued*)

Reference	Study design	Sample size	Outcome

Jorgensen et al., 1996	Case–control	Cases of mild RA = 89
		Cases of severe RA = 82
		Controls = 145
			Adjusted odds ratio for developing RA
			  If < 5 years OCP use, RR = 0.713 (0.41–1.23)
			  If > 5 years OCP use, RR = 0.76 (0.5–1.14)
			  If severe disease with > 5 years OCP use, RR = 0.1 (0.01–0.6)

Brennan et al., 1997	Population-based case–control	Cases = 115
		Controls = 115
			Adjusted OR
			  If ever use of OCP before symptoms, OR = 0.88 (0.47–1.64)
			  If current use at disease onset, OR = 0.22 (0.06–0.85)

[1] Abbreviations: OCP, oral contraceptive pill; RR ( ), relative risk of developing RA (95% confidence intervals); OR, odds ratio; OA, osteoarthritis; STR, soft tissue rheumatism.

an insidious onset of disease with symptoms developing over several months; however, 8–15% can present with an acute onset and 15–20% with an intermediate onset of a few days to weeks (Harris, 1997). On examination, joint inflammation presents as tenderness along the joint line or pain with passive range of motion and/or swelling. The most frequently affected joints in early RA are the MCP, PIP, and wrist joints (Harris, 1997). Morning stiffness lasting more than 1 hour is a common complaint in patients with active RA. Rheumatoid nodules are another feature of RA that are seen in 20–35% of seropositive patients. They typically occur along extensor surfaces and histologically demonstrate an area of central necrosis surrounded by palisading fibroblasts, collagenous material, and perivascular inflammation. Rheumatoid nodules should be differentiated from other types of nodules, including xanthomas, granuloma annulare, and tophi. Some patients may also have low-grade fever and lymphadenopathy.

Rheumatoid factors, typically autoantibodies against the Fc fragments of IgG immunoglobulin, are a component of the laboratory evaluation of RA. They are seen in approximately 75% of patients with RA but are also seen in chronic bacterial infections such as subacute bacterial endocarditis, osteomyelitis, tuberculosis, leprosy, viral infections (e.g. hepatitis B and C and mononucleosis), cancers after radiation or chemotherapy, chronic liver disease, and other rheumatic diseases such as systemic lupus erythematosus and Sjögren's syndrome. Thus, a positive rheumatoid factor is neither sensitive or specific for rheumatoid arthritis (Shmerling & Delbanco, 1992). Whether rheumatoid factors are a cause or a consequence of inflammation in RA remains to be determined.

Other laboratory abnormalities seen in RA include an anemia of chronic disease, elevated sedimentation rate, increased C-reactive protein, and thrombocytosis all of which occur as a consequence of inflammation. The joint fluid of these patients is inflammatory with a white blood cell count ranging in general from 2000 to 75 000 with a polymorphonuclear cell predominance. Glucose levels in the synovial fluid of RA are frequently low (Harris, 1997).

The radiographic findings in RA include soft tissue swelling, peri-articular osteopenia, joint space narrowing, and marginal erosions (Resnick et al., 1997). Classically, these changes are symmetric. They are not specific for RA, but they are helpful in confirming a diagnosis and in following disease progression.

Because RA is a systemic autoimmune disease, some patients have extra-articular features that can be life-threatening (Anderson, 1997). One of the most dangerous is vasculitis. Vasculitis causes digital gangrene, periungual infarcts, cutaneous ulceration, palpable purpura, and peripheral neuropathy. It can also affect the arteries of major organs, including the bowel, heart, lungs, liver, spleen, and pancreas. Pulmonary complications of RA include pleural effusions, pulmonary nodules, and interstitial lung disease. Ocular involvement is manifested by scleritis, episcleritis, uveitis, and keratoconjunctivitis sicca. Cardiac complications include pericarditis with pericardial effusions and/or constrictive pericarditis, myocarditis, and, rarely, valvular disease and conduction disturbances. Patients with Felty's syndrome, a complication of long-standing, usually severe seropositive disease, have splenomegaly, leukopenia, and frequently thrombocytopenia. They sometimes respond to increased treatment of the underlying RA.

The disease course in RA is typically progressive, although 15–20% can have intermittent episodes, and about 10% can have long-term clinical remissions (Harris, 1997). There has been interest in early identification of patients who will have more aggressive disease so that treatment can be intensified. The parameters that have been associated with a poor prognosis include rheumatoid factor positivity, subcutaneous nodules, early age of disease onset, extra-articular disease, certain HLA class II markers, and a lower socio-economic status (Alarcón, 1997).

TREATMENT OF RHEUMATOID ARTHRITIS

The treatment of RA requires a multidisciplinary approach. Patient education about RA is important, especially since poorer outcomes have been associated with patients who have less formal education. Arthritis self-help courses can improve knowledge, recommend adaptive behaviors, and improve pain (Lorig et al., 1993). Physical therapy is an important component of the treatment of RA. During periods of increased disease activity, patients should be encouraged to rest but also to continue passive range of motion exercises. When the disease is less active, physical therapy with strengthening exercises can improve function, stabilize gait, and protect joints. Occupational therapy (OT) helps patients cope with the tasks of daily living. It offers a wide range of services, including splints to correct subluxation and decrease pain, adaptive aids such as built-up pens and cutlery, and assistive devices to help with dressing and ambulation.

The mainstays of medical therapy for RA have been non-steroidal anti-inflammatory drugs (NSAIDs) and immunosuppressive agents. Traditionally, a pyramid approach has been used in the treatment of RA. This strategy began at the base of the pyramid with education, rest, physical therapy, and the use of NSAIDs. For patients who had an incomplete response, a disease modifying anti-rheumatic drug (DMARD) was added. At the top of the pyramid, patients who failed with these agents were begun on cytotoxic and experimental therapies. Corticosteroids – either intra-articular and/or oral – as well as surgical interventions were used as needed during the course of therapy. Over the past two decades there has been a trend to begin therapy with a DMARD early in the course of the disease. There are several lines of evidence to support this approach. Sherrer et al. (1986) evaluated 681 consecutive patients for factors that predicted the development of disability. They found that disability developed most rapidly within the first few years of disease. Other studies have demonstrated that erosions also develop within the first 2 years of onset (Brooks & Corbett, 1977; Fuchs et al., 1989). A randomized trial found that using a DMARD early on modified the course of disease (Borg et al., 1988). This suggests that there may be a window of opportunity in which to begin DMARD therapy to achieve maximal benefit.

The DMARDs that are currently used include glucocorticoids, auranofin, parenteral gold, methotrexate, sulfasalazine, hydroxychloroquine, minocycline, D-penicillamine, azathioprine, cyclophosphamide, and cyclosporin. The effectiveness, advantages and disadvantages are briefly reviewed below.

Glucocorticoids function as anti-inflammatory agents and as immunosuppressives. Typically, daily prednisone/prednisolone in a dose of 5–10mg is used for the treatment of joint disease. In a randomized trial, 7.5mg of prednisolone was associated with a decreased rate of joint erosion as compared with placebo (Kirwan, 1995). Other trials have not been able to demonstrate a statistically significant benefit of glucocorticoids in terms of radiographic progression (Empire Rheumatism Council, 1957; van Schaardenburg et al., 1995). Doses greater than 10mg should be avoided if possible because of increased side-effects. Complications of glucocorticoid therapy include osteoporosis, weight gain, hypertension, acceleration of cataract formation, glaucoma, steroid myopathy, psychosis, osteonecrosis, acne, alopecia, skin atrophy, and predisposition to infection.

Gold salts include auranofin, which is an oral preparation, gold sodium thiomalate and gold sodium thioglucose. In a double-blind controlled trial in 1960, the use of a total cumulative dose of 1g sodium aurothiomalate resulted in a better outcome in functional capacity, joint involvement, grip strength, and pain control than was seen in controls (Research Sub-committee of the Empire Rheumatism Council, 1961). Several studies have suggested that gold can decrease the rate of erosion progression (Borg et al., 1988; Luukkainen et al., 1977). In a meta-analysis, parenteral gold, but not oral gold, was found to be as effective as methotrexate, sulfasalazine, and D-penicillamine (Felson et al., 1990). However, in a large study of 822 patients with RA, the use of parenteral gold for at least 2 consecutive years was not associated with an improved outcome in function or number of painful joints, compared with those who had not received any gold therapy (Epstein et al., 1991). Thus, the degree of benefit derived from gold therapy may be modest. Parenteral gold has a relatively high toxicity profile, with proteinuria, rash, and cytopenias as notable complications.

Methotrexate is one of the most effective and most popular agents in the treatment of RA. Four randomized, placebo-controlled trials, two with oral and two with intra-muscular preparations, demonstrated improvement in joint swelling (Andersen et al., 1985; Thompson et al., 1984; Weinblatt et al., 1985; Williams et al., 1985). It has also been shown to retard radiographic progression (Weinblatt, 1995). Patients may be more likely to stay on methotrexate for prolonged periods than other DMARDs (Pincus et al., 1992). The side-effects of methotrexate include stomatitis, diarrhea, hepatotoxicity, bone marrow suppression, increased susceptibility to infections, and pneumonitis.

Sulfasalazine is a compound comprised of anti-inflammatory, salicylic acid, and anti-bacterial, sulfapyridine, components. In a randomized, placebo-controlled trial, sulfasalazine treatment produced a significant improvement in swollen joint count and a trend towards improvement in radiographic scores (Hannonen et al., 1993). The side-effects of sulfasalazine are stomach upset, rash, cytopenias and, rarely, aplastic anemia and hepatic injury.

Hydroxychloroquine is an anti-malarial agent that is one of the most well tolerated DMARDs used in the treatment of RA. Maximal improvement may take six months or longer to achieve (Rynes, 1997). Several double-blind placebo-controlled trials have demonstrated improvement in disease activity; however, a definitive benefit on radiographic progression has not been established (Rynes, 1997). Toxicities include diarrhea, nausea and, rarely, retinal damage.

Minocycline, an antibiotic, was initially used in the treatment of RA with the goal of treating a potential infectious agent but is currently used for its capacity to inhibit matrix metalloproteinases that are involved in cartilage degradation. Two investigations have demonstrated efficacy, one in early RA (O'Dell et al., 1997), the other in mild to moderate disease (Tilley et al., 1995). The most common side-effect is dizziness.

The Multi-Center Trial Group was one of the first studies demonstrating D-penicillamine's effectiveness in RA. Improvement was seen in all parameters except joint erosions (Multicentre Trial Group, 1973). A meta-analysis suggested similar efficacy compared to other DMARDs (Felson et al., 1990). Toxicities including proteinuria, leukopenia, thrombocytopenia, rashes, altered taste, and autoimmune syndromes such as myasthenia gravis, however, have limited its current use in clinical practice.

Azathioprine is a purine analog that is used as an immunosuppressive agent in the treatment of RA. It has been shown in some studies to decrease the rate of joint progression as well as improve symptoms (McKendry, 1992). A double-blind randomized study comparing methotrexate with azathioprine found methotrexate to be superior (Jeurissen et al., 1991). Toxicities of azathioprine include bone marrow suppression, gastrointestinal intolerance and increased susceptibility to infection.

Cyclophosphamide is an alkylating agent that has been used in RA. Because of its significant toxicities that include bone marrow suppression, increased risk of hematologic malignancies, hemorrhagic cystitis, susceptibility to infection, and infertility, it has obvious limitations. It is typically used in the treatment of refractory disease or severe extra-articular manifestations.

Cyclosporin is another immunosuppressive agent that has been shown in randomized controlled trials to improve RA (Dougados et al., 1988; Tugwell et al., 1990). It has limited benefit as a single agent in RA because of the side-effects of hypertension, decreased renal function and excessive hair growth seen at higher doses.

Because of side-effects or loss of efficacy, the duration of therapy for an individual DMARD may be limited to 2–3 years (Wolfe et al., 1990). For this reason, alternative approaches have been proposed. These include a step-down approach and combination therapy. In step-down protocols, multiple DMARDS are instituted simultaneously and withdrawn gradually as control of inflammation is achieved (Wilske, 1993). Combination therapy employs several simultaneous DMARDs, whose mechanisms of action differ, in an attempt to attack the inflammation at multiple steps. Some combinations that have been evaluated include hydroxychloroquine, sulfasalazine, and methotrexate (O'Dell et al., 1996), and methotrexate with cyclosporin (Tugwell et al., 1995). A meta-analysis suggested that combination therapy reduces tender joint counts more effectively but is accompanied by higher toxicity rates (Felson et al., 1994).

As an understanding of events at the cellular and molecular level in RA advances, new therapies for RA develop. An inducible form of cyclo-oxygenase, COX-2, an enzyme involved in the prostaglandin pathway of inflammation, has recently been identified. Specific inhibition of this enzyme can decrease swelling and improve pain without the toxic side-effects of gastric erosions and platelet inhibition that are

Table 16.4 Biologic agents used in rheumatoid arthritis

Agent	Target
Interferon γ	Suppression of inflammatory response via effects on multiple cells
Anti-CD5 antibody	CD5 antigen on T cells + B cell subset
Anti-CD4 antibody	CD4 antigen on T cells
Campath 1H antibody	Monocytes and lymphocytes
Anti-IL 2 antibody	IL-2 receptor on activated lymphocytes
Anti-IL 6 antibody	IL-6
Anti-TNF α antibody	TNF
TNF α receptor antagonist	TNF
IL-1 receptor antagonist	IL-1
IL-10	Downregulation of monocytes, macrophages and T cells
Anti-ICAM-1 antibody	ICAM-1, an adhesion molecule used for transmigration by inflammatory cells
T cell receptor peptide vaccine	Downregulate T cells
Oral collagen type II	Downregulate T cells?

seen with NSAIDs (Simon et al., 1998). Biologic agents are a new component of the armamentarium in the treatment of RA. This topic has recently been reviewed (Moreland et al., 1997b). Table 16.4 provides a list of some of the biologic agents that have been used or are currently being studied. These drugs inhibit T cell function, block inflammatory mediators, or interfere with cell migration. Dramatic responses have been noted with the TNF-α receptor inhibitor that is now approved by the Food and Drug administration in the United States (Moreland et al., 1997a). Oral collagen is a different type of biologic agent that may downregulate arthritogenic T cells. A modest, but not statistically significant benefit has been seen in one study (Sieper et al., 1996). It is anticipated that most of these compounds will be used in combination, either with DMARDs or with other biologic agents (Strand, 1996).

DIET AND SUPPLEMENTS IN RHEUMATOID ARTHRITIS

Numerous self-help books have been written about how dietary manipulations can improve RA. There is little scientific evidence to support this. A well-balanced diet is recommended, with care taken to prevent the development of obesity, which can accelerate damage in weight-bearing joints. The use of fish or plant oils, which have an in vitro ability to reduce certain inflammatory mediators combined with avoidance of animal fats, may be beneficial for patients. Studies using omega-3 fatty acid (Kremer et al., 1995) and gamma-linolenic acid (an extract of borage seed or evening primrose) (Leventhal et al., 1993) have shown modest clinical benefit. However, the amount of these oils needed to achieve this benefit may be more than most patients are willing to take. A recent book for the lay person (Theodosakis et al., 1997) states that the nutritional supplements glucosamine and chondroitin sulfate can halt or reverse osteoarthritis, but there are few data to support this. Several small studies have suggested a small improvement in symptoms but no resolution of the underlying disease. There are no published investigations of combination glucosamine and chondroitin sulfate in rheumatoid arthritis, although a study is planned.

ECONOMICS OF RHEUMATOID ARTHRITIS

The costs of RA result from both direct and indirect costs. Direct costs include physician fees, medications, surgeries, laboratory studies, and therapy. Indirect costs are a consequence of lost wages, increased disability, increased mortality, and interference with social function. In 1994, the total cost of RA in the United States was estimated to be $8.74 billion, 0.3% of the gross domestic product, with direct annual medical costs per patient between $1686 and $5741 and indirect costs between $9700 and $16 831 (Yelin, 1996). A Canadian study found that annual direct costs of RA in the early 1990s were $4656 with indirect costs $1597 (in 1994 Canadian dollars). The lower indirect costs reflects an older population that was retired and had less loss of wages (Clarke et al., 1997). In England, RA cost £1.256 billion in 1992, over half of which was attributable to indirect costs (McIntosh, 1996).

MORBIDITY IN RHEUMATOID ARTHRITIS

Rheumatoid arthritis is associated with significant disability. As noted earlier by Sherrer et al. (1986), disability tends to develop within the first few years of disease onset. In this study, with an average follow-up of 11.9 years, only 17% of participants were without any functional disability. Factors associated with the development of disability were older age, radiographic damage, female sex, and initial functional class. The use of DMARDs was not related to decreased disability; however, patients used DMARDs for only 30% of the study period, perhaps not long enough to have achieved benefit. Other studies have also shown female sex to be a predictor of the development of disability (Allaire, 1996; Smedstad et al., 1995). Leigh & Fries (1992) found that the initial level of disability was the most important factor in the prediction of subsequent decline and permanent disability. A lower educational level has been associated with increased morbidity in several studies (Callahan & Pincus, 1988; Leigh & Fries, 1991). Others have found that social and work factors such as job characteristics and autonomy over work pace were the more important determinants of inability to work than disease severity or medical therapy (Yelin et al., 1980). Reisine et al. (1989) found that in addition to factors related to physical demands of the job and social support at home, disease severity was an important contributor to the female RA patient's inability to work outside the home.

The influence of gender on the development of disability has been recently reviewed by Allaire (1996). Briefly, women with RA, in general, have increased functional limitations and poorer perceptions of health status. Possible explanations include more severe disease, increased reporting of health problems by women, and different social roles and tasks. Because women as a whole are statistically less educated than men and hold jobs that are more likely to require manual dexterity, they are more likely to suffer work-related losses. Women with RA apply less often and are accepted less frequently than men with RA for Social Security Disability Income (SSDI). When accepted, their benefits are lower because previous wages were lower. Methods of accounting for disability in the home-making role need to be integrated into the assessment of limitations and financial compensation.

Depression, another aspect of morbidity, is present at some point in 17–21% of patients with RA (Wright et al., 1996) and is associated with pain and disability (Parker & Wright, 1995). Risk factors for depression are the number of average daily stressors, confidence in one's ability to cope, and physical disability. Some of these risk factors may be preventable (Wright et al., 1996). Greater depression is associated with the inability to work (Allaire, 1996). Future research efforts need to examine the impact of job retraining on disability and depression. Because depression is a treatable condition by both behavioral and pharmacological therapy, there should be a significant effort to make an early diagnosis.

MORTALITY IN RHEUMATOID ARTHRITIS

Overall, patients with RA have a shorter life expectancy. One study found that women with RA died 10 years younger and men died 4 years younger than a sex-matched general population (Mitchell et al., 1986). The 5-year survival rate for patients with functional class IV status is 40–60%, the same as for patients with stage IV Hodgkin's disease or triple-vessel coronary artery disease (Pincus et al., 1994). The most common cause of death in RA patients is cardiovascular disease (42%), followed by cancer (14%), infection (9%), renal disease (7.8%), respiratory disease (7.2%), and RA (5.3%) (Pincus & Callahan, 1986). The increasing use of immunosuppressant agents to treat RA has led investigators to question whether the incidence of malignancies in RA will be greater than the general population. In a study of 862 RA patients, fewer cancers were seen than expected (Cibere et al., 1997). The decrease occurred mostly in colorectal cancers. There was an increased incidence of leukemia but not Hodgkin's disease or non-Hodgkin's lymphoma. Future studies will need to re-address this issue as pharmacologic and biologic therapy for RA changes or its use is expanded.

SUMMARY

Rheumatoid arthritis is an autoimmune inflammatory disease, of which the predominant feature is a destructive arthritis. It is associated with significant morbidity and mortality. Advances are occurring rapidly both in understanding the pathogenesis of RA and in its treatment. The goal of these advances is a reduction in disability with more effective, less toxic drugs.

REFERENCES

Abdel-Nasser, A.M., Rasker, J.J., & Valkenburg, H.A. (1997). Epidemiological and clinical aspects relating to the variability of rheumatoid arthritis. *Seminars in Arthritis and Rheumatism, 27*, 123–140.

Aceves-Avila, F.J., Baez-Molgado, S., Medina, F., & Fraga, A. (1998). Paleopathology in osseous remains from the 16th century. A survey of rheumatic diseases. *Journal of Rheumatology, 25*, 776–782.

Alarcón, G.S. (1997). Predictive factors in rheumatoid arthritis. *American Journal of Medicine, 103(6A)*, 19S–24S.

Allaire, S.H. (1996). Gender and disability associated with arthritis: differences and issues. *Arthritis Care and Research, 9*, 435–440.

Allebeck, P., Ahlbom, A., Ljungström, K., & Allander, E. (1984). Do oral contraceptives reduce the incidence of rheumatoid arthritis? *Scandinavian Journal of Rheumatology, 13*, 140–146.

Andersen, P.A., West, S.G., O'Dell, J.R., Via, C.S., Claypool, R.G., & Kotzin, B.L. (1985). Weekly pulse methotrexate in rheumatoid arthritis. Clinical and immunologic effects in a randomized, double-blind study. *Annals of Internal Medicine, 103*, 489–496.

Anderson, R.J. (1997). Rheumatoid arthritis: clinical and laboratory feature. In Klippel, J.H. (Ed.), *Primer on the Rheumatic Diseases*, 11th Edition (pp.161–167). Atlanta, Georgia: The Arthritis Foundation.

Appelboom, T., de Boelpaepe, C., Ehrlich, G.E., & Famaey, J.P. (1981). Rubens and the question of antiquity of RA. *Journal of the American Medical Association, 245*, 483–486.

Arnett, F.C., Edworthy, S.M., Bloch, D.A., McShane, D.J., Fries, J.F., Cooper, N.S., Healy, L.A., Kaplan, S.R., Liang, M.H., & Luthra, H.S. (1988). The American Rheumatism Association revised 1987 criteria for the classification of rheumatoid arthritis. *Arthritis and Rheumatism*, *31*, 315–324.

Auger, I., & Roudier, J. (1997). A function for the QKRAA amino acid motif mediating binding of DnaJ to DnaK. Implications for the association of rheumatoid arthritis with HLA-DR4. *Journal of Clinical Investigation*, *99*, 1818–1822.

Beasley, R.P., Willkens, R.F., & Bennett, P.H. (1973). High prevalence of rheumatoid arthritis in Yakima Indians. *Arthritis and Rheumatism*, *16*, 743–748.

Borg, G., Allender, E., Lund, B., Berg, E., Brodin, U., Pettersson, H., & Trang, L. (1988). Auranofin improves outcome in early rheumatoid arthritis. Results from a 2-year, double blind, placebo controlled study. *Journal of Rheumatology*, *15*, 1747–1754.

Brennan, P., & Silman, A. (1994a). Breast-feeding and the onset of rheumatoid arthritis. *Arthritis and Rheumatism*, *37*, 808–813.

Brennan, P., & Silman, A.J. (1994b). An investigation of gene-environment interaction in the etiology of rheumatoid arthritis. *American Journal of Epidemiology*, *140*, 453–460.

Brennan, P., Bankhead, C., Silman, A., & Symmons, D. (1997). Oral contraceptives and rheumatoid arthritis: results from a primary care-based incident case-control study. *Seminars in Arthritis and Rheumatism*, *26*, 817–823.

Brooks, A., & Corbett, M. (1977). Radiographic changes in early rheumatoid disease. *Annals of Rheumatic Diseases*, *36*, 71–73.

Callahan, L.F., & Pincus, T. (1988). Formal education level as a significant marker of clinical status in rheumatoid arthritis. *Arthritis and Rheumatism*, 31, 1346–1357.

Carette, S., Marcoux, S., & Gingras, S. (1989). Postmenopausal hormones and the incidence of rheumatoid arthritis. *Journal of Rheumatology, 16*, 911–913.

Cibere, J., Sibley, J., & Haga, M. (1997). Rheumatoid arthritis and the risk of malignancy. *Arthritis and Rheumatism, 40*, 1580–1586.

Clarke, A.E., Zowall, H., Levinton, C., Assimakopoulos, H., Sibley, J.T., Haga, M., Shiroky, J., Neville, C., Lubeck, D.P., Grover, S.A., & Esdaile, J.M. (1997). Direct and indirect medical costs incurred by Canadian patients with rheumatoid arthritis: a 12 year study. *Journal of Rheumatology, 24*, 1051–1060.

Darwish, M.J., & Armenian, H.K. (1987). A case–control study of rheumatoid arthritis in Lebanon. *International Journal of Epidemiology, 16*, 420–424.

del Junco, D.J., Annegers, J.F., Luthra, H.S., Coulam, C.B., & Kurland, L.T. (1985). Do oral contraceptives prevent rheumatoid arthritis? *Journal of the American Medical Association, 254*, 1938–1941.

Dequeker, J. (1977). Arthritis in Flemish paintings (1400–1700). *British Medical Journal*, *1*, 1203–1205.

Dieppe, P., Heywood, A., Rogers, J., Waldron, T., & Watt, I. (1987). The paleopathology of rheumatic diseases. In Appelboom, T. (ed.), *Art, History and Antiquity of Rheumatic Disease* (pp.109–112). Brussels: Elsevier.

Dougados, M., Awada, H., & Amor, B. (1988). Cyclosporin in rheumatoid arthritis: a double blind, placebo controlled study in 52 patients. *Annals of Rheumatic Diseases*, *47*, 127–133.

Empire Rheumatism Council (1957). Multi-centre controlled trial comparing cortisone acetate and acetyl salicylic acid in the long-term treatment of rheumatoid arthritis. *Annals of Rheumatic Diseases*, *16*, 277–288.

Epstein, W.V., Henke, C.J., Yelin, E.H., & Katz, P.P. (1991). Effect of parenterally administered gold therapy on the course of adult rheumatoid arthritis. *Annals of Internal Medicine*, *114*, 437–444.

Feher, K.G., Feher, T., & Meretey, K. (1986). Interrelationship between immunological and steroid hormone parameters in rheumatoid arthritis. *Annals of Internal Medicine*, *87*, 38–42.

Felson, D.T., Anderson, J.J., & Meenan, R.F. (1990). The comparative efficacy and toxicity of second-line drugs in rheumatoid arthritis. *Arthritis and Rheumatism*, *33*, 1449–1461.

Felson, D.T., Anderson, J.J., & Meenan, R.F. (1994). The efficacy and toxicity of combination therapy in rheumatoid arthritis: a meta-analysis. *Arthritis and Rheumatism*, *37*, 1487–1491.

Firestein, G.S. (1997). Etiology and pathogenesis of rheumatoid arthritis. In Kelley, W.N., Harris, E.D. Jr, Sledge, C.B., & Ruddy, S. (Eds.), *Textbook of Rheumatology*, 5th Edition (pp.851–897). Philadelphia: W.B. Saunders.

Fuchs, H.A., Kaye, J.J., Callahan, L.F., Nance, E.P., & Pincus, T. (1989). Evidence of significant radiographic damage in rheumatoid arthritis within the first 2 years of disease. *Journal of Rheumatology*, *16*, 585–591.

Goemaere, S., Ackerman, C., Goethals, K., De Keyser, F., Van der Straeten, C., Verbruggen, G., Mielants, H., & Veys, E.M. (1990). Onset of symptoms of rheumatoid arthritis in relation to age, sex and menopausal transition. *Journal of Rheumatology*, *17*, 1620–1622.

Gran, J.T., Husby, G., & Thorsby, E. (1983). The association between rheumatoid arthritis and HLA antigen DR4. *Annals of Rheumatic Diseases*, *42*, 292–296.

Grossman, C.J. (1985). Interactions between the gonadal steroids and the immune system. *Science*, *227*, 257–261.

Hall, G.M., Daniels, M., Huskisson, E.C., & Spector, T.D. (1994). A randomised controlled trial of the effect of hormone replacement therapy on disease activity in postmenopausal rheumatoid arthritis. *Annals of Rheumatic Diseases*, *53*, 112–116.

Hannaford, P.C., Kay, C.R., & Hirsch, S. (1990). Oral contraception and rheumatoid arthritis: new data from the Royal College of General

Practitioners' oral contraception study. *Annals of Rheumatic Diseases*, 49, 744–746.

Hannonen, P., Mottonen, T., Hakola, M., & Oka, M. (1993). Sulfasalazine in early rheumatoid arthritis. A 48-week double-blind, prospective, placebo-controlled study. *Arthritis and Rheumatism*, 36, 1501–1509.

Harris, E.D. Jr. (1990). Rheumatoid arthritis: pathophysiology and implications for therapy. *New England Journal of Medicine*, 322, 1277–1289.

Harris, E.D. Jr. (1997). Clinical features of rheumatoid arthritis. In Kelley, W.N., Harris, E.D. Jr., Sledge, C.B., & Ruddy, S. (Eds.), *Textbook of Rheumatology*, 5th Edition (pp.898–932). Philadelphia: W.B. Saunders.

Hazes, J.M.W., Dijkmans, B.A.C., Vandenbroucke, J.P., de Vries, R.R.P., & Cats, A. (1990a). Pregnancy and the risk of developing rheumatoid arthritis. *Arthritis and Rheumatism*, 33, 1770–1775.

Hazes, J.M.W., Dijkmans, B.A.C., Vandenbroucke, J.P., de Vries, R.R.P., & Cats, A. (1990b). Reduction of the risk of rheumatoid arthritis among women who take oral contraceptives. *Arthritis and Rheumatism*, 33, 173–179.

Hazes, J.M.W., Silman, A.J., Brand, R., Spector, T.D., Walker, D.J., & Vandenbrouke, J.P. (1990c). Influence of oral contraception on the occurrence of rheumatoid arthritis in female sibs. *Scandinavian Journal of Rheumatology*, 19, 306–310.

Hernandez-Avila, M., Liang, M.H., Willett, W.C., Stampfer, M.J., Colditz, G.A., Rosner, R., Chang, R.W., Henne Keng, C.H., & Speizer, F.E. (1990). Exogenous sex hormones and the risk of rheumatoid arthritis. *Arthritis and Rheumatism*, 33, 947–953.

Holmdahl, R., Carlsten, H., Jansson, L., & Larsson, P. (1989). Oestrogen is a potent immunmodulator of murine experimental rheumatoid disease. *British Journal of Rheumatology*, 28(Suppl I), 54–58.

Jacobsson, L.T.H., Hanson, R.L., Knowler, W.C., Pillemer, S., Pettit, D.J., McCance, D.R., & Bennett, P.H. (1994). Decreasing incidence and prevalence of rheumatoid arthritis in Pima Indians over a twenty-five-year period. *Arthritis and Rheumatism*, 37, 1158–1165.

Jeurissen, M.E.C., Boerbooms, A.M.R., van de Putte, L.B.A., Doesburg, W.H., Mulder, J., Rasker, J.J., Kruijsen, M.W.M., Haverman, J.F., van Beusekom, H.J., Muller, W.H., Franssen, M.J.A.M., & de Rooy, D.-J.R.A.M. (1991). Methotrexate versus azathioprine in the treatment of rheumatoid arthritis. A forty-eight-week randomized, double-blind trial. *Arthritis and Rheumatism*, 34, 961–972.

Jorgensen, C., Picot, M.C., Bologna, C., & Sany, J. (1996). Oral contraception, parity, breast feeding, and severity of rheumatoid arthritis. *Annals of Rheumatic Diseases*, 55, 94–98.

Kirwan, J.R. (1995). The effect of glucocorticoids on joint destruction in rheumatoid arthritis. *New England Journal of Medicine*, 333, 142–146.

Koch, A.E. (1998). Angiogenesis. Implications for rheumatoid arthritis. *Arthritis and Rheumatism*, 41, 951–962.

Koepsell, T.D., Dugowson, C., Nelson, J.L., Voight, L.F., & Daling, J.R.

(1994). Non-contraceptive hormones and the risk of rheumatoid arthritis in menopausal women. *International Journal of Epidemiology*, 23, 1248–1255.

Kremer, J.M., Lawrence, D.A., Petrillo, G.F., Litts, L.L., Mullaly, P.M., Rynes, R.I., Stocker, R.P., Parhami, N., Greenstein, N.S., Fuchs, B.R., Mathur, A., Robinson, D.R., Sperling, R.I., & Bigaouette, J. (1995). Effects of high-dose fish-oil on rheumatoid arthritis after stopping nonsteroidal antiinflammatory drugs: clinical and immune correlates. *Arthritis and Rheumatism*, 38, 1107–1114.

Latman, N.S. (1983). Relation of menstrual cycle phase to symptoms of rheumatoid arthritis. *American Journal of Medicine*, 74, 957–960.

Lawrence, J.S. (1977). *Rheumatism in Populations*. London: William Heinneman Medical.

Lawrence, R.C., Helmick, C.G., Arnett, F.C., Deyo, R.A., Felson, D.T., Giannini, E.H., Heyse, S.P., Hirsch, R., Hochberg, M.C., Hunder, G.G., Liang, M.H., Pillemer, S.R., Steen, V.D., & Wolfe, F. (1998). Estimates of the prevalence of arthritis and selected musculoskeletal disorders in the United States. *Arthritis and Rheumatism*, 41, 778–799.

Leigh, J.P., & Fries, J.F. (1991). Education level and rheumatoid arthritis: evidence from five data centers. *Journal of Rheumatology*, 18, 24–34.

Leigh, J.P., & Fries, J.F. (1992). Predictors of disability in a longitudinal sample of patients with rheumatoid arthritis. *Annals of Rheumatic Diseases*, 51, 581–587.

Leventhal, L.J., Boyce, E.G., & Zurier, R.B. (1993). Treatment of rheumatoid arthritis with gammalinolenic acid. *Annals of Internal Medicine*, 119, 867–973.

Linos, A., Worthington, J.W., O'Fallon, W.M., & Kurland, L.T. (1980). The epidemiology of rheumatoid arthritis in Rochester, Minnesota: a study of incidence, prevalence, and mortality. *American Journal of Epidemiology*, 111, 87–98.

Linos, A., Worthington, J.W., O'Fallon, W.M., & Kurland, L.T. (1983). Case–control study of rheumatoid arthritis and prior use of oral contraceptives. *Lancet*, i, 1299–1300.

Lorig, K.R., Mazonson, P.D., & Holman, H.R. (1993). Evidence suggesting that health education for self-management in patients with chronic arthritis has sustained health benefits while reducing health care costs. *Arthritis and Rheumatism*, 36, 439–446.

Luukkainen, R., Kajander, A., & Isomaki, H. (1977). Effect of gold treatment on the progression of erosions in rheumatoid arthritis patients. *Scandinavian Journal of Rheumatology*, 6, 189–192.

MacDonald, A.G., Murphy, E.A., Capell, H.A., Bankowska, U.Z., & Ralston, S.H. (1994). Effects of hormone replacement therapy in rheumatoid arthritis: a double blind placebo-controlled study. *Annals of Rheumatic Diseases*, 53, 54–57.

McIntosh, E. (1996). The cost of rheumatoid arthritis. *British Journal of Rheumatology*, 35, 781–790.

McKendry, R.J.R. (1992). Purine Analogs. In Dixon, J.S., & Furst, D.E. (Eds.), *Second-Line Agents in the Treatment of Rheumatic Diseases* (pp.223–243). New York: Marcel Dekker.

Mitchell, D.M., Spitz, P.W., Young, D.Y., Bloch, D.A., McShane, D.J., & Fries, J.F. (1986). Survival, prognosis and causes of death in rheumatoid arthritis. *Arthritis and Rheumatism, 29,* 706–714.

Moreland, L.W., Baumgartner, S.W., Schiff, M.H., Tindall, E.A., Fleischmann, R.M., Weaver, A.L., Ettlinger, R.E., Cohen, S., Koopman, W.J., Mohler, K., Widmer, M.B., & Blosch, C.M. (1997a). Treatment of rheumatoid arthritis with a recombinant human tumor necrosis factor receptor (p75) – Fc fusion protein. *New England Journal of Medicine, 337,* 141–147.

Moreland, L.W., Heck, L.W. Jr, & Koopman, W.J. (1997b). Biologic agents for treating rheumatoid arthritis: concepts and progress. *Arthritis and Rheumatism, 40,* 397–409.

Moskowitz, M.A., Jick, S.S., Burnside, S., Wallis, W.J., Dickson, J.F., Hunter, J.R., & Jick, H. (1990). The relationship of oral contraceptive use to rheumatoid arthritis. *Epidemiology, 1,* 153–156.

Multicentre Trial Group (1973). Controlled trial of D(-)penicillamine in severe rheumatoid arthritis. *Lancet, i,* 275–280.

Nelson, J.L., Hughes, K.A., Smith, A.G., Nisperos, B.B., Branchaud, A.M., & Hansen, J.A. (1993). Maternal–fetal disparity in HLA class II alloantigens and the pregnancy-induced amelioration of rheumatoid arthritis. *New England Journal of Medicine, 329,* 466–471.

O'Dell, J.R., Haire, C.E., Erikson, N., Drymalski, W., Palmer, W., Eckhoff, P.J., Garwood, V., Maloley, P., Klassen, L.W., Wees, S., Slein, H., & Moore, G.F. (1996). Treatment of rheumatoid arthritis with methotrexate alone, sulfasalazine and hydroxychloroquine or a combination of all three medications. *New England Journal of Medicine, 334,* 1287–1291.

O'Dell, J.R., Haire, C.E., Palmer, W., Drymalski, W., Wees, S., Blakely, K., Churchill, M., Eckhoff, P.J., Weaver, A., Doud, D., Erickson, N., Dietz, F., Olson, R., Maloley, P., Klassen, L.W., & Moore, G.F. (1997). Treatment of early rheumatoid arthritis with minocycline or placebo. *Arthritis and Rheumatism, 40,* 842–848.

Parker, J.C., & Wright, G.E. (1995). The implications of depression for pain and disability in rheumatoid arthritis. *Arthritis Care and Research, 8,* 279–283.

Pincus, T., & Callahan, L.F. (1986). Taking mortality in rheumatoid arthritis seriously. Predictive markers, socioeconomic status and comorbidity. *Journal of Rheumatology, 13,* 841–845.

Pincus, T., Marcum, S.B., & Callahan, L.F. (1992). Longterm drug therapy for rheumatoid arthritis in seven rheumatology private practices: II. Second line drugs and prednisone. *Journal of Rheumatology, 19,* 1885–1894.

Pincus, T., Brooks, R.H., & Callahan, L.F. (1994). Prediction of long-term mortality in patients with rheumatoid arthritis according to simple questionnaire and joint count measures. *Annals of Internal Medicine*, 120, 26–34.

Rasker, J., Peters, H., & Boon, K. (1986). Influence of weather on stiffness and force in patients with rheumatoid arthritis. *Scandinavian Journal of Rheumatology*, 15, 27–36.

Reisine, S.T., Grady, K.E., Goodenow, C., & Fifield, J. (1989). Work disability among women with rheumatoid arthritis: the relative importance of disease, social work, and family factors. *Arthritis and Rheumatism*, 32, 538–543.

Research Sub-committee of the Empire Rheumatism Council (1961). Gold therapy in rheumatoid arthritis. Final report of a multicentre controlled trial. *Annals of Rheumatic Diseases*, 20, 315–333.

Resnick, D., Yu, J.S., & Sartoris, D. (1997). Imaging. In Kelley, W.N., Harris, E.D. Jr., Ruddy, S., & Sledge, C.B. (Eds.), *Textbook of Rheumatology*, 5th Edition (pp.626–686). Philadelphia: W.B. Saunders.

Romieu, I., Hernandez-Avila, M., & Liang, M.H. (1989). Oral contraceptives and the risk of rheumatoid arthritis: a meta-analysis of a conflicting literature. *British Journal of Rheumatology*, 28(Suppl 1), 13–17.

Rothschild, B.M., & Woods, R.J. (1990). Symmetrical erosive disease in archaic indians: the origin of rheumatoid arthritis in the New World. *Seminars in Arthritis and Rheumatism*, 19, 278–284.

Rothschild, B.M., Turner, K.R., & Deluca, M.A. (1988). Symmetrical erosive peripheral polyarthritis in the late archaic period of Alabama. *Science*, 241, 1498–1501.

Roudier, J., Petersen, J., Rhodes, G.H., Luka, J., & Carson, D.A. (1989). Susceptibility to rheumatoid arthritis maps to a T-cell epitope shared by the HLA Dw4 DR beta-1 chain and the Epstein–Barr virus glycoprotein gp110. *Proceedings of the National Academy of Science USA*, 86, 5104–5108.

Rynes, R.I. (1997). Antimalarial drugs. In Kelley, W.N., Harris, E.D. Jr., Ruddy, S., & Sledge, C.B. (Eds.), *Textbook of Rheumatology*, 5th Edition (pp.747–758). Philadelphia: W.B. Saunders.

Sherrer, Y.S., Bloch, D.A., Mitchell, D.M., Young, D.Y., & Fries, J.F. (1986). The development of disability in rheumatoid arthritis. *Arthritis and Rheumatism*, 29, 494–500.

Shmerling, R.H., & Delbanco, T.L. (1992). How useful is the rheumatoid factor? An analysis of sensitivity, specificity and predictive value. *Archives of Internal Medicine*, 152, 2417–2420.

Short, C.L. (1974). The antiquity of rheumatoid arthritis. *Arthritis and Rheumatism*, 17, 193–205.

Sieper, J., Kary, S., Sörensen, H., Alten, R., Eggens, U., Hüge, W., Hiepe, F., Kühne, A., Listing, J., Ulbrich, N., Braun, J., Zink, A., & Mitchinson, N.A. (1996). Oral type II collagen treatment in early rheumatoid arthritis: a double-blind, placebo-controlled, randomized trial. *Arthritis and Rheumatism*, 39, 41–51.

Silman, A., Kay, A., & Brennan, P. (1992). Timing of pregnancy in relation to the onset of rheumatoid arthritis. *Arthritis and Rheumatism*, 35, 152–155.

Simon, L.S., Lanza, F.L., Lipsky, P.E., Hubbard, R.C., Talwalker, S., Schwartz, B.D., Isakson, P.C., & Geis, G.S. (1998). Preliminary study of the safety and efficacy of SC-58635, a novel cyclo-oxygenase 2 inhibitor. *Arthritis and Rheumatism*, 41, 1591–1602.

Smedstad, L.M., Kvien, T.K., Moum, T., & Vaglum, P. (1995). Life events, psychosocial factors, and demographic variables in early rheumatoid arthritis: relations to one-year changes in functional disability. *Journal of Rheumatology*, 22, 2218–2225.

Spector, T.D. (1990). Epidemiology of rheumatoid arthritis. *Rheumatic Disease Clinics of North America*, 16, 513–538.

Spector, T.D., & Da Silva, J.A.P. (1992). Pregnancy and rheumatoid arthritis: an overview. *American Journal of Reproductive Immunology*, 28, 222–225.

Spector, T.D., & Hochberg, M.C. (1990). The protective effect of the oral contraceptive pill on rheumatoid arthritis: an overview of the analytic epidemiological studies using meta-analysis. *Journal of Clinical Epidemiology*, 43, 1221–1230.

Spector, T.D., Roman, E., & Silman, A.J. (1990). The pill, parity, and rheumatoid arthritis. *Arthritis and Rheumatism*, 33, 782–789.

Spector, T.D., Brennan, P., Harris, P., Studd, J.W.W., & Silman, A.J. (1991). Does estrogen replacement therapy protect against rheumatoid arthritis. *Journal of Rheumatology*, 18, 1473–1476.

Strand, V. (1996). The future use of biologic therapies in combination for the treatment of rheumatoid arthritis. *Journal of Rheumatology*, 23(Suppl 44), 91–96.

Symmons, D.P., Bankhead, C.R., Harrison, B.J., Brennan, P., Barrett, E.M., Scott, D.G., & Silman, A.J. (1997). Blood transfusion, smoking, and obesity as risk factors for the development of rheumatoid arthritis. *Arthritis and Rheumatism*, 40, 1955–1961.

Theodosakis, J., Adderly, B., & Fox, B. (1997). *The Arthritis Cure*. New York: St Martin's Press.

Thompson, R.N., Watts, C., Edelman, J., Esdaile, J., & Russell, A.S. (1984). A controlled two-centre trial of parenteral methotrexate therapy for refractory rheumatoid arthritis. *Journal of Rheumatology*, 11, 760–763.

Tilley, B.C., Alarcón, G.S., Heyse, S.P., Trentham, D.E., Neuner, R., Kaplan, D.A., Clegg, D.O., Leisen, J.C.C., Buckley, L., Cooper, S.M., Duncan, H., Pillemer, S.R., Tuttleman, M., & Fowler, S.E. (1995). Minocycline in rheumatoid arthritis: a 48-week, double-blind placebo-controlled trial. *Annals of Internal Medicine*, 122, 81–89.

Tugwell, P., Bombardier, C., Gent, M., Bennett, K.J., Bensen, W.G., Carette, S., Chalmers, A., Esdaile, J., Klinkhoff, A.V., Kraag, G.R., Ludwin, D., & Roberts, R.S. (1990). Low-dose cyclosporin versus placebo in patients with rheumatoid arthritis. *Lancet*, 335, 1051–1055.

Tugwell, P., Pincus, T., Yocum, D., Stein, M., Gluck, O., Kraag, G., McKendry, R., Tesser, J., Baker, P., & Wells, G. (1995). Combination therapy with cyclosporine and methotrexate in severe rheumatoid arthritis. *New England Journal of Medicine, 333*, 137–141.

van den Brink, H.R., van Everdingen, A.A., van Wijk, M.J.G., Jacobs, J.W.G., & Bijlsma, J.W.J. (1993). Adjuvant oestrogen therapy does not improve disease activity in postmenopausal patients with rheumatoid arthritis. *Annals of Rheumatic Diseases, 52*, 862–865.

van Schaardenburg, D., Valkema, R., Dijkmans, B.A.C., Papapoulos, S., Zwinderman, A.H., Han, K.H., Pauwels, E.K.J., & Breedveld, F.C. (1995). Prednisone treatment of elderly-onset rheumatoid arthritis. Disease activity and bone mass in comparison with chloroquine treatment. *Arthritis and Rheumatism, 38*, 334–342.

van Zeben, D., Hazes, J.M.W., Vandenbroucke, J.P., Dijkmans, B.A.C., & Cats, A. (1990). Diminished incidence of severe rheumatoid arthritis associated with oral contraceptive use. *Arthritis and Rheumatism, 33*, 1462–1465.

Vandenbroucke, J.P., Valkenburg, H.A., Boersma, J.W., Cats, A., Festen, J.J.M., Huber-Bruning, O., & Rasker, J.J. (1982). Oral contraceptives and rheumatoid arthritis: further evidence for a preventive effect. *Lancet, ii*, 839–842.

Vandenbroucke, J.P., Witteman, J.C.M., Valkenburg, H.A., Boersma, J.W., Cats, A., Festen, J.J.M., Hartman, A.P., Huber-Bruning, O., Rasker, J.J., & Weber, J. (1986). Noncontraceptive hormones and rheumatoid arthritis in perimenopausal and postmenopausal women. *Journal of the American Medical Association, 255*, 1299–1303.

Vessey, M.P., Villard-Mackintosh, L., & Yeates, D. (1987). Oral contraceptives, cigarette smoking and other factors in relation to arthritis. *Contraception, 35*, 457–464.

Weinblatt, M.E. (1995). Efficacy of methotrexate in rheumatoid arthritis. *British Journal of Rheumatology, 34(Suppl 2)*, 43–48.

Weinblatt, M.E., Coblyn, J.S., Fox, D.A., Fraser, P.A., Holdsworth, D.E., Glas, D.N., & Trentham, D.E. (1985). Efficacy of low-dose methotrexate in rheumatoid arthritis. *New England Journal of Medicine, 312*, 818–822.

Weyand, C.M., Hicok, K.C., Conn, D.L., & Goronzy, J.J. (1992). The influence of HLA-DRB-1 genes on disease severity in rheumatoid arthritis. *Annals of Internal Medicine, 117*, 801–806.

Wilder, R.L. (1996). Adrenal and gonadal steroid hormone deficiency in the etiopathogenesis of rheumatoid arthritis. *Journal of Rheumatology, 23(Suppl 44)*, 10–12.

Williams, H.J., Willkens, R.F., Samuelson, C.O.J., Alarcón, G.S., Guttadauria, M., Yarboro, C., Polisson, R.P., Weiner, S.R., Luggen, M.E., & Billingsley, L.M. (1985). Comparison of low-dose oral pulse methotrexate and placebo in the treatment of rheumatoid arthritis. A controlled clinical trial. *Arthritis and Rheumatism, 28*, 721–730.

Wilske, K.R. (1993). Approach to the management of rheumatoid arthritis: rationale for early combination therapy. *Journal of Rheumatology, 32(Suppl 1)*, 24–25.

Wingrave, S.J., & Kay, C.R. (1978). Reduction in incidence of rheumatoid arthritis associated with oral contraceptives. *Lancet, i,* 569–571.

Wolfe, F., Hawley, D.J., & Cathey, M.A. (1990). Termination of slow acting antirheumatic therapy in rheumatoid arthritis: a 14-year prospective evaluation of 1017 consecutive starts. *Journal of Rheumatology, 17,* 994–1002.

Wright, G.E., Parker, J.C., Smarr, K.L., Schoenfeld-Smith, K., Buckelew, S.P., Slaughter, J.R., Johnson, J.C., & Hewett, J.E. (1996). Risk factors for depression in rheumatoid arthritis. *Arthritis Care and Research, 9,* 264–272.

Yelin, E. (1996). The costs of rheumatoid arthritis: absolute, incremental, and marginal estimates. *Journal of Rheumatology, 23(Suppl 44),* 47–51.

Yelin, E., Meenan, R., Nevitt, M., & Epstein, W. (1980). Work disability in rheumatoid arthritis: effects of disease, social, and work factors. *Annals of Internal Medicine, 93,* 551–556.

Chapter 17

Women and HIV

Lisa Belcher and Janet St Lawrence

Centers for Disease Control and Prevention, United States

NATIONAL AND INTERNATIONAL HIV EPIDEMIOLOGY AND SURVEILLANCE

Since its initial discovery in the early 1980s, more than 30 million people worldwide have contracted the human immunodeficiency virus (HIV) infection (UNAIDS, 1997). From this number, six million people have died of complications caused by acquired immune deficiency syndrome (AIDS) (UNAIDS, 1997). The vast majority of HIV infections, about 90%, occurred in developing countries and almost half were among women (AIDSCAP/Family Health International/Harvard School of Public Health, & UNAIDS, 1996). In some Sub-Saharan countries, such as Zambia and Malawi, more than one out of every four pregnant women are infected with HIV (World Bank, 1997a,b). Among women attending antenatal clinics in cities in Botswana and Zimbabwe, 40% are infected (World Bank, 1997a,b). In Southeast Asia, where the most common mode of transmission is heterosexual intercourse, HIV is also spreading rapidly (World Bank, 1997a,b). The World Health Organisation estimated that by the year 2000, it would be quite possible that the number of HIV infected women in Asia exceeded the number of infected women in Africa (Mann, 1992). In Latin America and the Caribbean a steady increase of new HIV infections of about 200 000 per year has been recorded for the past several years (UNAIDS, 1997).

Women, Health and the Mind
Edited by L. Sherr and J.S. St Lawrence. © 2000 John Wiley & Sons, Ltd

The early HIV epidemic in the United States was concentrated among gay men in urban areas, such as San Francisco and New York City. However, heterosexual women and women who used intravenous drugs were among the first to be diagnosed with the immune-suppressed condition that would eventually come to be know as AIDS (Shilts, 1987). In 1998, almost two decades into the AIDS epidemic, it is estimated that approximately 250 000 people in the United States are living with AIDS and between 650 000 and 900 000 people are living with HIV, and that 40 000 new HIV infections occur each year. Women represent more than 17% of all current AIDS case in the United States and roughly 28% of HIV cases in the 25 states that currently report HIV cases (Centers for Disease Control and Prevention, 1998a). Since 1981, more than 90 000 American women have been diagnosed with AIDS (Centers for Disease Control and Prevention, 1998a).

In the United States, women are most often infected with HIV through the sharing of needles while using intravenous drugs or through sexual intercourse with an infected intravenous drug-using partner. National surveillance data compiled by the Centers for Disease Control and Prevention (1997) estimates that 45% of national AIDS cases among women can be attributed to intravenous drug use, whereas 38% are attributable to heterosexual transmission. African-American and Hispanic women have been disproportionately affected by AIDS in the United States, representing 79% of all AIDS cases among women in 1996 (Centers for Disease Control and Prevention, 1998a), while accounting for only 24% of the population (US Census Bureau, 1998).

Recent developments in treatment regimens have improved the prognosis for those already infected with HIV or living with AIDS. Antiretroviral therapies delay the progression of HIV infection to AIDS and from AIDS to death. In 1996, largely due to treatment advances, the United States observed its first reduction in the annual incidence of AIDS and the number of deaths caused by AIDS since the beginning of the epidemic. This trend was replicated in the first half of 1997, with national AIDS cases declining 15% and AIDS deaths declining an amazing 45% compared with the first half of 1996. Among women, decreases were somewhat less dramatic but none the less hopeful, with an 8% decrease in AIDS cases and 32% decrease in AIDS deaths (Centers for Disease Control and Prevention, 1998b).

Although reductions in AIDS diagnoses and deaths provide hope for those who are, and those who will become, infected with HIV, the dynamics of disease transmission have also changed. With each coming year, more people with HIV will be living, working, and enjoying life without the constant threat of opportunistic infection and illness. In the absence of an HIV vaccine, it is now more important than ever to complement ground-breaking medical treatment advances with effective behavioural prevention strategies.

HIV TRANSMISSION

Sexual transmission of HIV is by far the most common route of infection, with the majority of these transmissions occurring between male and female sex partners. In fact, heterosexual transmission of HIV accounts for over 70% of all infections worldwide (Centers for Disease Control and Prevention, 1997). In particular, vaginal intercourse without any form of barrier protection, such as a latex condom, presents the greatest risk of infection for women. It is estimated that male-to-female transmission of HIV is eight times more efficient than female-male-transmission (Padian et al., 1997). The other major mode of HIV transmission among women is from sharing of unsterilised needles with drug users. Intravenous drug use accounts for almost half of all HIV infections among women in the United States (Centers for Disease Control and Prevention, 1998 a,b), and is the primary mode of transmission in China, India, and Pakistan (World Bank, 1997a,b).

Many social, economic, and behavioural factors influence women's risk of HIV infection and it is important to consider and understand each in making steps towards prevention. Although it is important to have thorough and accurate estimates of the prevalence, incidence, and transmission dynamics of HIV and AIDS across the world, these data represent only the beginning of the process by which individual, community, national, and global responses to the AIDS epidemic are formed. Additional pieces to the complex puzzle of this disease need to be better understood, including cultural, biological developmental, gender-related, and psychological issues. This chapter will focus on our current empirical understanding of women's HIV risks and the strategies that have been effective in reducing those risks.

SOCIO-ECONOMIC AND SOCIOCULTURAL CORRELATES OF SEXUAL RISK

Socio-economic Influence

Many studies document correlations between socio-economic status and health. Indicators of lower socio-economic status, such as lower levels of education or income, are consistently correlated with behaviours that negatively affect health, reduced access to health services, increased disease risk, increased risk of an adverse health outcome, and increased rates of mortality (Adler et al., 1993; Pappas et al., 1993). In fact, history tells us that most epidemics have disproportionately affected the poor, and within the context of HIV and AIDS there is growing evidence to suggest that this epidemic is no different. This phenomenon is perhaps most evident when considering the socio-economic status of women as it relates to HIV infection. In a recent article, Fournier & Carmichael

(1998) eloquently stated that around the world, women's cultural and economic status is inversely correlated with their risk of acquiring HIV infection. Where women lack self-sufficiency, where they are denied choices about their economic livelihood and their sexuality, and where they are confined to a narrow social sphere, HIV transmission will be facilitated. Poverty is also highly correlated with prostitution and the trade of sex for survival among men and women. The sex trade industry is, in turn, characterised by high rates of drug use, inner-city habitation, incarceration, and homelessness. The tremendous overlap of these contextual risk factors underscores the importance of considering the social and economic backdrop of the AIDS epidemic in the development of prevention strategies.

One example of the intersection of these multiple socio-economic influences is illustrated in a study by Edlin et al. (1994) that examines the interrelationships of crack cocaine and HIV infection in urban areas within the context of other social issues such as sex trading and homelessness. The sale of crack, a highly addictive synthetic form of cocaine correlated with hypersexuality (Weiner et al., 1992) has become an enormous industry in urban areas in the United States because it is extremely affordable and can be bartered directly for sex. Increased high-risk sexual behaviours parallel the introduction of crack cocaine and are also related to the spread of other sexually transmitted diseases (STDs). In a review of epidemiological evidence examining the relationship of drug use, sexual behaviour, and STDs, Marx et al. (1991) found that crack use in the United States paralleled both the temporal and population trends for syphilis, gonorrhoea, chancroid, and HIV infection. Another study found that crack use among women was related to an increased risk for syphilis (Finelli et al., 1993).

Socio-economic status and HIV was examined in another large survey of patients attending state and city health departments in the United States. In this study, Diaz et al. (1994) found that among women living with AIDS, 29% of white women and 63% of black women had not completed 12 years of school; 90% were unemployed; and 84% of female intravenous drug users (IDUs) with AIDS reported an annual household income of $10 000 or less. Research has shown that in the United States, African-American women, in particular, are more likely to be poor and live within inner-city areas with higher prevalence of injection drug use and HIV infection (Sobo, 1993). Evidence of a socio-economic influence on the AIDS epidemic has also emerged internationally. For example, among 600 female sex workers in Sao Paulo State, Brazil, Lurie et al. (1995) found that women with lower socioeconomic status were significantly more likely to be infected with HIV-1 (17 versus 4%), syphilis (66 versus 24%), and hepatitis B (52 versus 26%) than were women with higher socio-economic status.

In a recent study, Wingood & DiClemente (1998) observed similar trends in socio-economic factors as they relate to HIV risk behaviour. They found that women who received government financial support for dependent children (AFDC) were three times as likely to report not using condoms in the previous 3-month period than women who were working outside of the home. The authors of this study provided two explanations for this finding. First, they proposed that when compared with other competing expenses, such as food, housing, and care for children, the priority placed on the purchase of condoms by women receiving limited government benefits may be lower than that of women who work for pay. Second, the authors suggested that some economically disadvantaged women, or women who are financially dependent on a male partner may feel uncomfortable being sexually assertive given the potential power differential and traditional gender roles within these relationships (Wingood & DiClemente, 1998).

Partner Influences

Because the vast majority of HIV-infected women worldwide are infected through heterosexual contact, and sexual risk behaviour involves two partners, a more thorough understanding of male partners' roles in heterosexual relationships may lead to the development of more effective prevention strategies. Although the value of understanding the male partner's influence within the context of heterosexual HIV risk is widely agreed upon, partner dynamics such as power and gender roles have not received a great deal of attention in the field of HIV prevention (Amaro, 1995). Although this has recently begun to change with the initiation of several couples-based HIV intervention studies, most HIV prevention efforts thus far have been directed at individual women and men outside of the relationship context (Belcher et al., 1998; Carey et al., 1997; DiClemente & Wingood, 1995; Hobfoll et al., 1994; Kamb et al., 1998; Kelly et al., 1994; NIMH Multisite Trial, 1997). Therefore, the extent to which the male partner influences decision-making on issues such as condom use and sexual risk behaviour is, as yet, not well understood.

The issue of relationship power among heterosexual couples is important in understanding a woman's ability to successfully negotiate HIV protective behaviours, such as condom use, and is likely to be an important predictor of her future sexual health. Relationship power is defined not only by emotional dependence and trust, but also by economic issues and concerns about physical safety. A woman who is financially dependent on her sex partner to provide basic resources such as food and housing can perceive herself to be vulnerable to her partner's decisions about sexual risk practices.

In addition to emotional and financial dependence, women can be significantly impacted by fear of physical and sexual abuse in intimate relationships. In one study, women attending emergency departments in the United States were interviewed about their personal experience with partner violence (Abbott et al., 1995). Over half of the women in the study had been the victim of intimate partner violence at some time in their lives and 11% of women with current male partners reported partner abuse as the reason for the hospital visit (Abbott et al., 1995). Fear of physical or sexual violence can create a significant barrier to women attempting negotiation and implementation of safe sexual practices (Farmer et al., 1996; Kalichman et al., 1998; Wingood & DiClemente, 1997) thereby potentially increasing their likelihood of future HIV infection. Recent research has shown that African-American women who report being in a physically abusive relationship are significantly less likely to attempt to negotiate condom use or use condoms with their partner, compared with women whose partners were not abusive (Wingood & DiClemente, 1997). Molina & Basinait-Smith (1998) conducted a study in which women who were temporarily residing in battered women's shelters were interviewed about their abusive partners and HIV risk. They found that 60% of the women reported that their abusive partner used illicit drugs, 63% reported their partner had other sex partners, 98% reported their partner either never or rarely used a condom, and 50% reported their partner had infected them with at least one STD. In another study in Kigali, Rwanda, researchers found that women who were infected with HIV-1 experienced significantly more sexual coercion by male sex partners than did women who were not infected (van der Straten et al., 1995).

DRUGS AND ALCOHOL

Intravenous Drug Use and Needle Sharing

The intravenous use of drugs in the United States is one of the most devastating behaviours to threaten women's health in the country's history (see Chapter 20). American women's deaths resulting, both directly and indirectly, from the use of intravenous drugs compare with those of much more prevalent health risk behaviours such as smoking and alcohol abuse. For example, it is estimated that approximately 100 000 women in the United States die each year from cancers, heart disease, and strokes caused by smoking (Centers for Disease Control and Prevention/Office of Women's Health, 1998). In 1996–97, there were 92 242 reported AIDS cases among women (Centers for Disease Control and Prevention, 1998a,b). Of these women, 41 029 were intravenous drug users, and of the 35 760 reported heterosexually acquired cases, most were infected by a male injection drug user (Centers for Disease Control and Prevention, 1998a,b). An additional 11 823 of the AIDS cases among women did not identify an HIV risk factor in that reporting year (Centers for Disease Control and Prevention, 1998a,b), however, one could reasonably assume that many of these cases were also directly linked to needle-sharing behaviours. Women who use intravenous drugs, such as heroin or cocaine, are also at risk for many other serious health problems, including tuberculosis and hepatitis.

Sexual Risk, Alcohol, and Drugs

Drug and alcohol use are also related to sexual HIV risk behaviour among women. Several years ago, Leigh & Stall (1993) conducted a review of the research literature on the relationship between substance-use and high-risk sexual behaviour. They found that the co-occurrence of substance use and sexual behaviour was particularly predictive of high-risk sexual behaviour. In a subsequent large survey of adults in the United States, researchers found that alcohol use was related to increased rates of sexual activity, which was, in turn, related to a greater likelihood of having more than one sex partner (Leigh et al., 1994). In this study however, alcohol use, in general, was not related to lower levels of condom use. More recently, Wingood & DiClemente (1997) found, in a sample of 180 African-American women at high risk for HIV, that women who used alcohol daily were significantly more likely to not use condoms. In addition to potentially increasing women's sexual risk for HIV infection, the abuse of alcohol has shown to increase the likelihood of needle-sharing behaviour among women who inject drugs (Stein et al., 1998).

As mentioned earlier in this chapter, the use of crack cocaine is also an important predictor of sexual risk behaviour among women. In a sample of 337 crack using female sex workers recruited from the streets of three cities in the United States, fewer than half reported consistent condom use with paying sex partners during vaginal sex, and only 23% reported using condoms consistently with non-paying sex part-ners (Jones et al., 1998). Of the women participating in this study, 25% tested positive for HIV, 40% tested positive for syphilis, and 73% tested positive for herpes (HSV-2) (Jones et al., 1998).

Interaction of STDs and HIV

Sexually transmitted diseases, other than HIV, represent a growing health concern for women. Those such as gonorrhoea, chlamydia, syphilis, and herpes can lead to a multitude of adverse health conse-quences for women, including cervical cancer, pelvic inflammatory disease, ectopic pregnancy, and infertility [Institute of Medicine (US), 1997]. Women with a history of STDs also are at greater risk of HIV infection (Wasserheit, 1992). Perhaps the most direct explanation of the STD/HIV relationship is that these infections share many of the same risk behaviours, such as unprotected vaginal sex. In addition, some STDs cause ulcerative lesions on the cervix and genital tract, both of which facilitate acquisition and transmission of HIV (Wasserheit, 1992). Furthermore, an HIV-positive person with an STD is more infectious and thus more easily transmits the virus to others (Wasserheit, 1992). In a study of patients who received two HIV tests at an urban STD clinic in the United States, researchers found that 10% acquired syphilis and 4% acquired HIV during the testing interval (Otten et al., 1994). In an international study that statistically modelled the spread of all HIV infections in rural Uganda between 1980 and 1990, researchers found that over 90% of all recorded HIV infections could be attributed to the enhancing effect that STD infection has on the transmission of HIV (Robinson et al., 1997).

INDIVIDUAL AND PSYCHOLOGICAL CORRELATES OF HIV RISK AND PROTECTIVE BEHAVIOURS

Although many social, economic, and biological factors are related to women's risk for HIV, there are also individual determinants of HIV risk and infection. Many women, after all, make an individual choice to engage in behaviours that put them at risk for becoming infected, such as using intravenous drugs, sharing needles, or engaging in unprotected sexual behaviour with a high-risk partner. The extent to which these choices are made by the individual, their environment, or a combination of the two, can and will be argued by many. However, the success of many preventive interventions, including those targeting HIV, implemented with women to date has largely depended on the attitudinal and behavioural changes of individual women. Through the provision of interventions including AIDS education and resource referral, motivational enhancement, skills training, and access to clean needles and condoms, many women have overturned previous personal decisions and have started to implement protective strategies. Because women have many different reasons for not engaging in protective sexual behaviour, effective HIV behavioural intervention requires both an accurate understanding of the processes by which a woman makes a decision to engage in risky sexual behaviour, as well as those which do lead to protective sexual behaviour. For example, if a woman does not perceive herself to be at any sexual risk with her partner or believes that only gay men get AIDS, she may choose not to initiate condom use in her relationship. On the other hand, a woman may believe or know that she is at risk for HIV with her sex partner, and understand that women just like herself have AIDS, but may not be practised in communication about sex and therefore feel unsure about talking to her partner.

Large national surveys of the sexual behaviour of adults in the United States indicate that the majority are sexually experienced, but that their number of lifetime sex partners is not exceedingly high, with a median of three partners since the age of 18 (Ku et al., 1997). Although condom use was fairly infrequent among this representative sample of North Americans, about 20% of women reporting the use of condoms, among those with more than one sex partner in the last 12-month period, condom use was lower. Eleven percent reported condom use all of the time and 38% never used them (Ku et al., 1997). In a study investigating the reasons that adults report not using condoms, the most commonly cited reason among a sample of 260 male and female patients attending urban STD clinics in the United States was having trust in their sex partner (Jadack et al., 1997). Other reasons given for not using condoms in this study included the committed nature of the sexual relationship (i.e. monogamous or regular partner) and availability of condoms (Ku et al., 1997). Few gender-related differences emerged in this study assessing reasons for condom non-use. However women were more likely to report that they did not know why they did not use a condom with their partner, while men were more likely to cite reasons related to sexual sensation (Ku et al., 1997). St. Lawrence et al. (1998) observed similar results, finding that women who were monogamous perceived themselves to be at lower risk, had fewer intentions to use condoms, and used condoms less than did women in non-monogamous relationships.

The Health Belief Model suggests that accurate information and perceived susceptibility to a health problem are predictive of a reduction of risk-taking behaviour (Becker, 1974). Similarly, Social Cognitive Theory proposes that social norms have a strong influence on one's health behaviour (Bandura, 1994). Social norms, such as a pervasive community perception that certain groups are not at risk for HIV infection, may be an important influence on an individual group member's decisions about sexual risk taking. However, studies that have investigated the relationship between women's risk perception and HIV risk behaviour have produced mixed findings (Eldridge et al., 1995; Hobfoll et al., 1993). Eldridge et al. (1995) assessed minority women's perceptions of risk and found that women demonstrated what Weinstein (1982) refers to as Optimistic Bias in their appraisal of their personal susceptibility to HIV infection. Specifically, women in this sample perceived themselves to be at less risk for HIV than others who are similar to them. In a discussion of the findings, Eldridge et al. (1995) suggested that these results may lead to inaccurate conclusions that women are underestimating their HIV risk, when an equally plausible explanation for the observed discrepancy is that they may reflect their exaggeration of others' risk. Kalichman et al. (1992) also found that when compared with the seriousness of other social problems affecting the lives of women, such as drug abuse, unemployment, and child care, AIDS was rated relatively low as a social problem.

PREVENTION OF AIDS: AN INTERNATIONAL MULTIDISCIPLINARY EFFORT

Extensive research conducted in the past decade on the sociocultural, behavioural, and psychological factors associated with HIV risk behaviour and infection has led to the development and implementation of many HIV prevention efforts designed to help individuals change behaviours that put them at risk. Beginning in the early 1980s, research findings on individuals' AIDS knowledge, attitudes, and behaviours have been combined with well-developed theories of health behaviour and behaviour change in order to construct the most sophisticated and appropriate interventions possible. In the absence of an AIDS vaccine, work on the development of behavioural interventions continues as the ever-changing AIDS epidemic moves into its third decade. Behavioural scientists and intervention specialists are faced with new challenges in the light of medical treatment breakthroughs that provide hope for those affected by HIV/AIDS and yet may reduce public concern about the seriousness of HIV infection. In addition, there are important issues such as treatment compliance, resistant viral strains, and post-exposure therapy that will serve as the backdrop for AIDS prevention efforts in the new millennium. These emerging issues emphasise the need for the refinement of our existing behavioural intervention arsenal and continued rigorous evaluation of intervention effectiveness.

Interventions for AIDS prevention have been implemented at the individual, small group, community, and policy levels with varying degrees of coverage and success. Behavioural strategies to control the transmission of HIV began with educational programmes intended to inform people about disease prevalence, routes of transmission, and prevention techniques. Although most would agree that knowledge is probably a necessary component in changing sexual risk behaviour, it has not proved to be, by itself, sufficient to change risk behaviour. Furthermore, reviews of the literature on behavioural effects of receiving routine HIV antibody testing and counselling have produced mixed evidence for risk reduction impact (Higgins et al., 1991; Lemp et al., 1990). As a result, researchers became more sophisticated in their intervention approaches to the prevention of HIV infection. Employing theoretical behavioural approaches from public health and psychology, such as Social Cognitive Theory (Bandura, 1994) and Theory of Reasoned Action (Fishbein & Middlestadt, 1989), interventions were designed to change sexual risk behaviour by focusing on individuals' skills, intentions, and motivations.

Individual Counselling Interventions with Women

Relatively few studies have evaluated the effectiveness of interventions delivered in an individualised risk reduction counselling session format.

In a recent large intervention study (Kamb et al., 1998), 5700 hetero-sexual patients from five inner-city STD clinics were randomly assigned to one of three face-to-face interventions coupled with HIV testing: (1) *standard practice*; (2) *HIV prevention counselling* with two 20-minute, client-centred sessions aimed at increasing risk perception and negoti-ating a behaviour change step; and (3) *enhanced counselling*, consisting of four theory-based interactive sessions. The first 20-minute session occurred during the initial clinic visit and was identical to the HIV prevention counselling. The next three were approximately 1 hour each and designed to change key theoretical variables such as skills, atti-tudes, self-efficacy, and norms for condom use. All interventions focused on consistent condom use with all sex partners. Participants were followed at 3-month intervals for a year by gathering behavioural data and conducting STD examinations. Eighty-two percent of partic-ipants completed all intervention sessions. After 3 months, self-reported frequencies of consistent condom use were significantly higher for the enhanced and HIV prevention counselling groups than those who received standard practice messages. After 6 months, more participants in the standard practice group developed new STDs (10.4%) than in the enhanced (7.2%) or HIV prevention counselling (7.4%) groups. This trend was similar for men and women, across all five sites.

In a much smaller but similar intervention study, Belcher et al. (1998) employed motivational enhancement interviewing techniques (Miller & Rollnick, 1991) and a skills training intervention strategy with high-risk women living in inner-city Atlanta, Georgia (n = 74). In this study, women were randomised to receive either a one-on-one single-session (2 hours) motivational enhancement and skills training intervention or a one-on-one single-session (2 hours) AIDS education-only control condition. Results from this study demonstrated the potential promise of brief individualised behavioural intervention, as women in the exper-imental condition increased their self-reported frequency of condom use by 44%, while women in the AIDS education-only condition increased condom use by 28%, a significant group effect at 3-month follow-up.

Small Group Interventions with Women at High Risk for STD and HIV

Small groups involving the participation of 8–12 people in an inter-active session have been the most common HIV intervention format evaluated in the United States. Several review articles documenting the women's HIV intervention literature have been published (Wingood & DiClemente, 1996; Exner et al., 1997; Ickovics & Yoshikawa, 1998), in addition to a meta-analysis comparing the relative effectiveness of inter-vention formats among several high-risk populations (Kalichman et al., 1996). The largest of these small-group intervention studies was the

National Multisite HIV Prevention Trial sponsored by the National Institute of Mental Health. In this randomised controlled HIV prevention intervention trial, 3706 high-risk adults from 37 clinics across the United States were randomly assigned to attend either a seven-session (14 hours), small-group HIV risk reduction intervention or a single session AIDS education intervention (NIMH Multisite Prevention Trial Group, 1998). The results of this intervention provide further evidence to support the effectiveness of behavioural intervention techniques in reducing high-risk sexual behaviour. Across the 12-month follow-up period, those participants who attended the more intensive skills training intervention reported fewer unprotected sexual acts and higher levels of condom use.

Several other small-group intervention studies have evaluated the effectiveness of programmes designed specifically for women, although several of these studies are limited by small sample sizes and, in some cases, excessive attrition. Kelly et al. (1994) conducted an intervention trial with women visiting public health clinics in Milwaukee ($n = 197$). Women were randomised to attend either a four-session (6 hours) skills-training intervention which also included components on AIDS education, personal risk sensitisation, and problem solving, or a three-session general health and nutrition control condition. Three months following the intervention, women assigned to the skills-training condition reported a higher percentage of condom-protected intercourse compared to the health education control condition.

Hobfoll et al. (1994) found similar effects in an intervention study conducted in Akron, Ohio, with pregnant women visiting a prenatal care facility ($n = 206$). Six months following a four-session (6–8 hours) intervention, women in the experimental condition reported more frequent acquisition and use of condoms than those randomly assigned to attend either a four-session health behaviour intervention or to a wait-list control condition.

DiClemente & Wingood (1995) also demonstrated the effectiveness of small-group behavioural interventions for women at risk for STD and HIV infection in a community-based study targeting African-American women ($n = 128$). Women in this study were randomised to either a five-session intervention that included components on gender and ethnic pride, HIV education, sexual assertiveness, condom use skills, coping, and sexual control, or to one of two control conditions (four-session health education or wait list). In this study, participants in the skills training condition reported increases in their consistent use of condoms (100% condom use) from 35 to 46%, in the health education control condition from 20 to 37%, and in the wait-list control condition from 21 to 29%.

Carey et al. (1997) employed a combination of behavioural skills and motivational enhancement interviewing techniques with a community-based sample of African-American women ($n = 102$) in Syracuse, New York. The results from this study indicated that the combination of these intervention techniques may provide a promising new behavioural strategy, as women attending the intervention significantly increased their frequency of self-reported condom use as compared with a wait-list control condition 2 months following the intervention.

In an effort to compare interventions that were based on the differing theoretical models in these earlier studies, St Lawrence et al. (1998) tested all three of the theoretical models against one another and a control condition with low-income minority women (n = 435). They found that each intervention model produced modest, but comparable changes in behaviour. Change was greater for women entering new relationships than for women who remained in ongoing relationships, suggesting existing interventions may not confer adequate protection for women whose primary risk results from a partner's behaviour.

In another recent intervention study, Eldridge et al. (1997) compared the effectiveness of an educational intervention against a behaviour skills training intervention in reducing sexual risk behaviour among 117 women who were court-ordered into an inpatient drug treatment programme. Two months following the intervention, participants in the behaviour skills training condition reported increases in condom use for vaginal intercourse, whereas participants in the educational intervention reported minor decreases in condom use.

Similar intervention studies to those already mentioned have also been conducted with IDUs (Gibson et al., 1998). These interventions have the same ultimate goal of using behavioural methods in reducing HIV risk behaviour; however instead of targeting sexual risk behaviour they are designed around the outcome cf a reduction in drug use and needle-sharing behaviour. Rather than focusing on women in particular, these intervention studies have most often recruited participants from drug treatment centres where the incidence of needle-sharing behaviour is high, and groups can be convened based on the shared risks that each IDU faces in negotiating his or her addiction in the era of HIV/AIDS. These studies have further demonstrated the effectiveness of behavioural methods in a very challenging context as many have reported significant reductions in injection behaviours as well as increases in health-protective behaviours such as needle cleaning (Baker et al., 1993; Gibson et al., 1989).

Cost Effectiveness of Behavioural HIV Intervention

The cost implications of preventive behavioural HIV intervention have been the subject of recent empirical investigation, as the enormous public and private costs of managing HIV and AIDS becomes more evident to policy-makers. To date, cost effectiveness analyses are available for very few behavioural intervention studies. However those that have been reported indicate that a preventive public health approach to the AIDS epidemic borrowed from the social and behavioural sciences would save several thousand dollars for each HIV infection averted. Specifically, in an analysis of the intervention study conducted by Kelly et al. (1994), Holtgrave & Kelly (1994) reported that under base case assumptions, the total societal cost of the intervention was $26 914, or $269 per client. Based on estimates of the cost of treating a case of HIV disease and AIDS as being $56 000, Holtgrave & Kelly (1997) conclude that the cost–utility ratio of this behavioural intervention is at a level that is generally considered to be very cost-effective.

Dissemination of Successful Behavioural HIV Interventions

Although many well-controlled HIV intervention studies over the past decade demonstrated the effectiveness of behavioural strategies in reducing high-risk sexual behaviour, surprisingly few of these programmes were subsequently transferred to community-based organisations and health agencies for implementation on a much larger scale (Kalichman et al., 1997).

WOMEN LIVING WITH HIV/AIDS: PRESENT LIFE CHALLENGES AND THE FUTURE

Women who are infected with HIV, or are living with AIDS, face a multitude of challenges in their daily lives that range from the basic physical manifestation of their illness to the psychological and social consequences of their HIV infection. In addition to these challenges, women infected with HIV are often faced with very difficult decisions to make about the future care of their children, many of whom are also infected. Family relationships are often strained by the social stigma surrounding HIV/AIDS, and as a result, these women are often abandoned by those whom they have relied on for support in the past.

The most common clinical manifestations of HIV and AIDS among women are gynaecological in nature; however, women living with AIDS also suffer from other health compromises such as lymphadenopathy, weight loss, diarrhoea, severe fatigue, and oral candidiasis (Carpenter et al., 1991). Although the time from HIV infection to AIDS diagnosis varies widely from person to person, almost half of HIV-infected people develop AIDS within 10 years of the initial infection (Brettle & Leon, 1991). However, with the development of advances in treatment and the wider availability of medications, these numbers are changing rapidly, increasing survival expectancies for people with HIV and AIDS (Enger et al., 1996). The variable rates of disease progression among HIV-infected individuals have been associated with socio-demographic factors, general health status, illness history, nutrition, genetic–immune factors, and variations in viral strain (Cohen & Williamson, 1991). It has also been suggested that men infected with HIV live longer after an AIDS diagnosis than do infected women (Friedman et al., 1991). However, subsequent research failed to show that non-gynaecological manifestations of HIV infection differ among men and women, and it has become more widely agreed upon that there are no known gender differences in the rate of disease progression or AIDS prognosis (Brettle & Leen, 1991; Melnick et al., 1994).

Medically tested treatments for HIV infection are becoming widely used in the United States and other developed countries. These medical therapies, antiretrovirals, act to suppress or inhibit the AIDS virus by disrupting the viral replication cycle by interfering with key enzymes in this process. Reverse transcriptase inhibitors, drugs such as zidovudine (AZT) and zalcitabine (ddC), are often used in combination with another class of antiretrovirals called protease inhibitors. These drug combinations, sometimes referred to as "cocktails" or "combination therapies", can provide a powerful and effective response to the debilitating effects that HIV can have on one's immune system. In clinical trials, highly active antiretroviral therapy (HAART), has demonstrated dramatic declines in the amount of HIV present in blood, even a short time after the initiation of treatment (Katzenstein et al., 1996). However, these treatments have not been effective among all of those treated, and it is as yet unclear if the AIDS virus will eventually evade or withstand the long-term use of HAART (Chun et al., 1997; Wong et al., 1997).

The medical management of HIV and AIDS has provided hope for many of those who have suffered from the physical and psychological trauma of this disease. However, the existing treatment regimens are both expensive and physically demanding and the future remains unclear. In light of these advances, people who have survived many years of illness are being faced with a life ahead of them for which they may have lost hope. It is without a welcome second chance for some, and for others an almost overwhelming twist of fate. Still others will not live to see the availability of these treatment advances reach their country, and for them the future remains more painfully clear.

CONCLUSION: FUTURE DIRECTIONS

Many things have changed since AIDS first became a global reality. When the AIDS epidemic first emerged in the United States in the 1980s, research on sexual behaviour was so sparse that the US Public Health Service was forced to rely on Kinsey's data from 40 years earlier to assist them in transmission estimate calculations for homosexual men (Bayer, 1997). Clearly, the powerful and far-reaching effect of this epidemic has forced us to reconsider many policies and procedures regarding medical and behavioural research and practice. Although there is perhaps nothing that could have prepared us for the public health dilemmas that HIV/AIDS presented, it is probably reasonable to assume that we have learned some painful and valuable lessons from these two decades of AIDS. The once tediously slow and unpopular arena of AIDS research has now become one of the most aggressively funded areas in all of health research in the United States. Our understanding of the AIDS virus, and our subsequent responses to it, are becoming exponentially more sophisticated, as they must if they are to match what is one of the most sophisticated viruses in modern medical history.

Even with the recent remarkable and noteworthy accomplishments in both the medical treatment and behavioural prevention of HIV, the challenges facing the world in the new millennium are no less significant. These challenges will prove to be particularly relevant to women's health researchers and practitioners, and will determine the fate of many individuals, and possibly some countries. Attention in the United States related to HIV/AIDS will probably be focused on the consistently controversial policy issues that have characterised much of America's AIDS experience, such as needle exchange programmes, sex education in public schools, and condom availability in prisons. Other countries, particularly in Sub-Saharan Africa, will be afforded less time for politics and national debate as the epidemic moves into a crisis stage.

Women's social and political place in history has often been associated with adverse health outcomes. Unfortunately, consideration of the AIDS epidemic in the final years of the twentieth century leads to a similar finding. It is because of their greater physiological, social, and political vulnerability that women are most often at risk for HIV infection. These are the issues that shaped the past and continue to shape the future of women's health in the era of AIDS.

REFERENCES

Abbott, J., Johnson, R., Koziol-McLain, J., & Lowenstein, S. (1995). Domestic violence against women. Incidence and prevalence in an emergency department population. *Journal of the American Medical Association, 273*, 1763–1767.

Adler, N., Boyce, T., Chesney, M., Folkman, S., & Syme, L. (1993). Socioeconomic inequalities in health: no easy solution. *Journal of the American Medical Association, 269*, 3140–3145.

AIDSCAP/Family Health International, Harvard School of Public Health, & UNAIDS (1996). The status and trends of the global HIV/AIDS pandemic. Final Report of a Satellite Symposium of the Eleventh International Conference on AIDS, July 7–12, Vancouver, B.C., Canada.

Amaro, H. (1995). Love, sex, and power: considering women's realities in HIV prevention. *American Psychologist, 50*, 437–447.

Baker, A., Heather, N., Wodak, A., & Dixon, J. (1993). Evaluation of a cognitive behavioral intervention for HIV prevention among injection drug users. *AIDS, 7,* 247–256.

Bandura, A. (1994). Social cognitive theory and exercise of control over HIV infection. In DiClemente, R. & Peterson, J. (Eds.), *Preventing AIDS. Theories and Methods of Behavioral Interventions.* New York: Plenum.

Bayer, R. (1997). Science, politics, and AIDS prevention. *Journal of Acquired Immune Deficiency Syndromes and Human Retrovirology, 14,* 22–29.

Becker, M. (1974). The health belief model and HIV risk behavior change. In DiClemente, R., & Peterson, J. (Eds.), *Preventing Aids. Theories and Methods of Behavioral Interventions.* New York: Plenum.

Belcher, L., Kalichman, S., Topping, M., Smith, S., Emshoff, J., Norris, F., & Nurss, J. (1998). A randomized trial of a brief HIV risk reduction counseling intervention for women. *Journal of Consulting and Clinical Psychology, 66,* 856–861.

Brettle, R., & Leon, L. (1991). The natural history of HIV and AIDS in women. *AIDS, 5,* 1283–1292.

Carey, M., Maisto, S., Kalichman, S., Forsyth, A., Wright, E., & Johnson, B. (1997). Enhancing motivation to reduce the risk of HIV infection for economically disadvantaged urban women. *Journal of Consulting and Clinical Psychology, 65,* 531–541.

Carpenter, C., Mayer, K., Stein, M., Leibman, B., Fisher, A., & Fiore, T. (1991). Human immunodeficiency virus infection in North American women: Experience with 200 cases and a review of the literature. *Medicine, 70,* 307–325.

Centers for Disease Control and Prevention (1997). *International Projections/Statistics.* Atlanta, GA: Centers for Disease Control and Prevention.

Centers for Disease Control and Prevention (1998a). *HIV/AIDS Surveillance Report: Mid-year Edition.* Atlanta, GA: Centers for Disease Control and Prevention.

Centers for Disease Control and Prevention (1998b). Diagnosis and reporting of HIV and AIDS in states with integrated HIV and AIDS surveillance – United States, January 1994 – June 1997. *Morbidity and Mortality Weekly, 47,* 309–314.

Centers for Disease Control and Prevention/Office of Women's Health (1998). *Women's Health: Tobacco Use.* Homepage, <http://www.cdc.gov/od/owh/whtob.html>

Chun, T., Carruth, L., Finzi, D., Shen, X., DiGiuseppe, J., Taylor, H., Hermankova, M., Chadwick, K., Margolick, J., Quinn, T., Kuo, Y., Brookmeyer, R., Zeiger, M., Barditch-Crovo, P., & Siliciano, R. (1997). Quantification of latent tissue reservoirs and total body viral load in HIV-1 infection. *Nature, 387,* 183–188.

Cohen, S., & Williamson, G. (1991). Stress and infectious disease in humans. *Psychological Bulletin, 109,* 5–24.

Diaz, T., Chu, J., Buehler, J., Boyd, D., Checko, P., Conti, L., Davidson, A., Hermann, P., Herr, M., & Levy, A. (1994). Socioeconomic differences among people with AIDS: results from a multi-state surveillance project. *American Journal of Preventive Medicine, 10,* 217–222.

DiClemente, R., & Wingood, G. (1995). A randomized controlled trial of a community-based HIV sexual risk reduction intervention for young adult African-American females. *Journal of the American Medical Association, 274,* 1271–1276.

Edlin, B., Irwin, K., Faraque, S., McCoy, C., Word, C., Serrano, Y., Inciardi, J., Bowser, B., Schilling, R., & Holmberg, S. (1994). Intersecting epidemic: crack cocaine use and HIV infection among inner-city young adults. *New England Journal of Medicine, 331,* 422–427.

Eldridge, G., St. Lawrence, J., Little, C., Shelby, M., & Brasfield, T. (1995). Barriers to condoms use and barrier method preferences among low-income African-American women. *Women and Health, 23,* 73–89.

Eldridge, G., St. Lawrence, J., Little, C., Shelby, M., Brasfield, T., Service, J., & Sly, K. (1997). Evaluation of an HIV risk reduction intervention for women entering inpatient substance abuse treatment. *AIDS Education and Prevention, 9(A),* 62–76.

Enger, C., Graham, N., Peng, Y., Chmiel, J., Kingsley, L., Detels, R., & Munoz, A. (1996). Survival from early, intermediate, and late stages of HIV infection. *Journal of the American Medical Association, 275,* 1329–1334.

Exner, T., Seal, D., & Ehrhardt, A. (1997). A review of HIV interventions for at-risk women. *AIDS and Behavior, 1,* 93–124.

Farmer, P., Connors, M., & Simmons, J. (Eds.) (1996). Women, poverty, and AIDS: sex, drugs, and structural violence. Monroe, ME: Common Courage Press.

Finelli, L., Budd, J., & Spitalny, K. (1993). Early syphilis relationship to sex, drugs, and high risk behavior from 1987–1990. *Sexually Transmitted Diseases, 20,* 89–95.

Fishbein, M., & Middlestadt, S. (1989). Using the theory of reasoned action as a framework for understanding and changing AIDS-related behaviors. In Mays, V., Albee, G., & Schneider, S. (Eds.), *Primary Prevention of AIDS: Psychological Approaches.* Newbury Park, CA: Sage.

Fournier, A., & Carmichael, C. (1998). Socioeconomic influences on the transmission of human immunodeficiency virus infection: the hidden risk. *Archives of Family Medicine, 7,* 214–217.

Friedman, Y., Franklin, C., Freels, S., & Weil, M. (1991). Long-term survival of patients with AIDS, *Pneumocystis carinii* pneumonia, and respiratory failure. *Journal of the American Medical Association, 28,* 65–68.

Gibson, D., Wermuth, L., Lovelle-Drache, J., Ham, J., & Sorenson, J. (1989). Brief counseling to reduce AIDS risk in intravenous drug users and their sexual partners: preliminary results. Special issue: AIDS

Counseling: Theory, Research, and Practice. *Counseling Psychology Quarterly, 2,* 15–19.

Gibson, D., McCusker, J., & Chesney, M. (1998). Effectiveness of psychosocial interventions in preventing HIV risk behavior in injecting drug users. *AIDS, 12,* 919–929.

Higgins, D., Galavotti, C., O'Reilly, K., Schnell, D., Moore, M., Rugg, D., & Johnson, R. (1991). Evidence for the effects of HIV antibody counseling and testing on HIV risk behavior. *Journal of the American Medical Association, 266,* 2419–2429.

Hobfoll, S., Jackson, A., Lavin, J., Britton, P., & Shepard, J. (1993). Safer sex knowledge, behavior, and attitudes of inner-city women. *Health Psychology, 12,* 481–488.

Hobfoll, S., Jackson, A., Lavin, J., Britton, J., & Shepard, J. (1994). Reducing inner-city women's AIDS risk activities: a study of single pregnant women. *Health Psychology, 13,* 3979–4403.

Holtgrave, D. & Kelly, J. (1996). Preventing HIV/AIDS among high risk urban women: the cost-effectiveness of a behavioral group intervention. *American Journal of Public Health, 86,* 1442–1445.

Holtgrave, D.R., & Kelly, J.A. (1997). Preventing HIV/AIDS among high risk urban women: the cost-effectiveness of a behavioral intervention group intervention. *American Journal of Public Health, 86,* 1442–1445.

Ickovics, J., & Yoshikawa, H. (1998). Preventive interventions to reduce heterosexual HIV risk for women: current perspectives, future directions. *AIDS, 12(Suppl A),* 197–208.

Institute of Medicine (US) (1997). In Eng, T., & Butler, W. (Eds.), *The Hidden Epidemic: Confronting Sexually Transmitted Diseases.* Washington DC: National Academy Press.

Jadack, R., Fresia, A., Rompalo, A., & Zenilman, J. (1997). Reasons for not using condoms of clients at urban sexually transmitted disease clinics. *Sexually Transmitted Diseases, 24,* 402–408.

Jones, D., Irwin, K., Inciardi, J., Bowser, B., Schilling, R., Word, C., Evans, P., Faruque, S., McCoy, V., Edlin, B., & The Multicenter Crack Cocaine and HIV Infection Study Team (1998). The high risk sexual practices of crack-smoking sex workers recruited from the streets of three American cities. *Sexually Transmitted Diseases, 25,* 187–193.

Kalichman, S., Hunter, T., & Kelly, J. (1992). Perceptions of AIDS susceptibility among minority and non-minority women at risk for HIV infection. *Journal of Consulting and Clinical Psychology, 60,* 725.

Kalichman, S., Carey, M., & Johnson, B. (1996). Prevention of sexually transmitted HIV infection: meta-analytic review and critique of the theory-based intervention outcome literature. *Annals of Behavioral Medicine, 18,* 6–15.

Kalichman, S., Belcher, L., Cherry, C., & Williams, E. (1997). Primary prevention of sexually transmitted HIV infections: transferring behavioral research technology to community programs. *The Journal of Primary Prevention, 18,* 149–172.

Kalichman, S., Williams, E., Cherry, C., Belcher, L., & Nachimson, D. (1998). Sexual coercion, domestic violence, and negotiating condom use among low-income African-American women. *Journal of Women's Health, 7,* 371–378.

Kamb, M., Fishbein, M., Douglas, J., Rhodes, F., Rogers, J., Bolan, G., Zenilman, J., Hoxworth, T., Malotte, D., Iatesta, M., Kent, C., Lentz, A., Graziano, S., Byers, R., Peterman, T., & the Project Respect Study Group (1998). HIV/STD prevention counseling reduces high risk behaviors and sexually transmitted diseases: results from a multi-center, randomized controlled trial (Project RESPECT). *Journal of the American Medical Association, 280,* 1161.

Kelly, J., Murphy, D., Washington, C., Wilson, T., Koob, J., Davis, D., Ledezma, G., & Davantes, B. (1994). The effects of HIV/AIDS intervention groups for high-risk women in urban clinics. *American Journal of Public Health, 84,* 1918–1922.

Ku, L., Sonenstein, F., Turner, C., Aral, S., & Black, C. (1997). The promise of integrated representative surveys about sexually transmitted diseases and behavior. *Sexually Transmitted Diseases, 24,* 299–309.

Leigh, B., & Stall, R. (1993). Substance use and risky sexual behavior for exposure to HIV: issues in methodology, interpretation, and prevention. *American Psychologist, 48,* 1035–1045.

Leigh, B., Temple, M., & Trocki, K. (1994). The relationship of alcohol use to sexual activity in a U.S. national sample. *Social Science and Medicine, 39,* 1527–1535.

Lemp, G., Payne, S., Neal, D., Temelso, T., & Rutherford, G. (1990). Survival trends for patients with AIDS. *Journal of the American Medical Association, 263,* 402–406.

Lurie, P., Fernandes, M., Hughes, V., Arevalo, E., Hudes, E., Reingold, A., Hearst, N., & the Instituto Adolfo Lutz Study Group (1995). Socioeconomic status and risk of HIV-1, syphilis, and hepatitis B infection among sex workers in Sao Paulo State, Brazil. *AIDS, 9(Suppl 1),* 31–37.

Mann, J. (1992). AIDS – the second decade: a global perspective. *Journal of Infectious Diseases, 165,* 245–250.

Marx, R., Aral, S., Rolfs, R., Sterk, C., & Kahn, J. (1991). Crack, sex, and STD. *Sexually Transmitted Diseases, 18,* 92–101.

Melnick, S., Sherer, R., Louis, T., Hillman, D., Rodriguez, E., Lackman, C., Capps, L., Brown, L., Carlyn, M., Korvick, J., & Deyton, L. (1994). Survival and disease progression according to gender of patients with HIV infection. *Journal of the American Medical Association, 272,* 1915–1921.

Miller, W., & Rollnick, S. (1991). *Motivational Interviewing: Preparing People to Change Addictive Behavior.* New York: Guilford.

Molina, L., & Basinait-Smith, C. (1998). Revisiting the intersection between domestic abuse and HIV risk. *American Journal of Public Health, 88,* 1267–1268.

NIMH Multisite HIV Prevention Trial (1998). The NIMH Multisite HIV Prevention Trial: Reducing sexual HIV risk behavior. *Science, 280,* 1889–1894.

Otten, M., Zaidi, A., Peterman, T., Rolfs, R., & Witte, J. (1994). High rate of HIV seroconversion among patients attending urban sexually transmitted disease clinics. *AIDS, 8,* 549–553.

Padian, N., Shiboski, S., Glass, S., & Vittinghoff, E. (1997). Heterosexual transmission of human immunodeficiency virus in Northern California: results from a ten year study. *American Journal of Epidemiology, 146,* 350–357.

Pappas, G., Queen, S., Hadden, W., & Fisher, G. (1993). The increasing disparity in mortality rates between socioeconomic groups in the United States, 1960–1986. *New England Journal of Medicine, 329,* 103–109.

Robinson, N., Mulder, D., Auvert, B., & Hayes, R. (1997). Proportion of HIV infections attributable to other sexually transmitted diseases in a rural Ugandan population: simulation model estimates. *International Journal of Epidemiology, 26,* 180–189.

Shilts, R. (1987). *And the Band Played On.* New York: Penguin Books.

Sobo, E. (1993). Inner-city women and AIDS: the psycho-social benefits of unsafe sex. *Culture, Medicine & Psychiatry, 17,* 455–485.

Stein, M., Hanna, L., Natarajan, R., Clarke, J., Marisi, M., Sobota, M., Rich, J., & The ProMethIUs Study (1998). Alcohol use patterns predict high risk HIV behaviors among active injection drug users. *Journal of General Internal Medicine, 13,* 102.

St Lawrence, J., Eldridge, G., Reitman, D., Little, C., Shelby, M., & Brasfield, T. (1998). Factors influencing condom use among African-American women: implications for risk reduction interventions. *American Journal of Community Psychology, 26,* 7–28.

St Lawrence, J., Wilson, T., Eldridge, G., Brasfield, T., & O'Bannon, R. (1998). Evaluation of community-based interventions to reduce low income African-American women's risk of sexually transmitted diseases: a randomized controlled trial of three theoretical models. *American Journal of Community Psychology, 26,* 7–28.

UNAIDS (1997). *The Impact of HIV and Sexual Health Education on the Sexual Health of Young People: A Review (Updated).* Geneva: Joint United Nations Program on AIDS.

US Census Bureau (December 1998). *Resident Population Estimates of the United States: Estimates by Sex, Race, and Hispanic Origin, with Median Age.* Published 28 December, 1998, <http://www.census.gov/population/estimates/nation/intfile3–1.txt>

van der Straten, A., King, R., Grinstead, O., Serufilira, A., & Allen, S. (1995). Couple communication, sexual coercion, and HIV risk reduction in Kigali, Rwanda. *AIDS, 9,* 935.

Wasserheit, J. (1992). Epidemiologic synergy. Interrelationships between human immunodeficiency virus infection and other sexually transmitted diseases. *Sexually Transmitted Diseases, 9,* 61–77.

Weiner, A., Wallace, J., Steinberg, A., Hoffmann, B., & Fielding, C. (July, 1992). Intravenous drug use, inconsistent condom use, and fellatio in relationship to crack smoking are risky behaviors for acquiring AIDS in streetwalkers. International Conference on AIDS, Berlin.

Weinstein, N. (1982). Unrealistic optimism about susceptibility to health problems. *Journal of Behavioral Medicine*, *5*, 441–460.

Wingood, G., & DiClemente, R. (1996). HIV sexual risk reduction interventions for women: a review. *American Journal of Preventive Medicine*, *12*, 209–217.

Wingood, G., & DiClemente, R. (1997). The effects of an abusive primary partner on the condom use and sexual negotiation practices of African-American women. *American Journal of Public Health*, *87*, 1016.

Wingood, G., & DiClemente, R. (1998). Gender-related correlates and predictors of consistent condom use among young adult African-American women. *Health Psychology*, *12*, 481–488.

Wong, J., Hezareh, M., Gunthard, H., Havlir, D., Ignacio, C., Spina, C., & Richman, D. (1997). Recovery of replication-competent HIV despite prolonged suppression of plasma viremia. *Science*, *278*, 1291–1293.

World Bank (1997a). *Confronting AIDS: A World Bank Policy Research Report*. New York: Oxford University Press.

World Bank (1997b). *World Development Indicators 1997*. Washington DC: World Bank.

Chapter 18

Women, Cognition and the Menstrual Cycle

Louise Dye

Leeds University, UK

and

John T.E. Richardson

Brunel University, UK

In his *Dictionary of Psychology*, Drever (1964) explained that "cognition" was "a general term covering all the various modes of knowing–perceiving, imagining, conceiving, judging, reasoning" (p.42). Cognition is situated at the interface between biology and culture. On the one hand, the normal functioning of these intellectual capabilities depends upon the biological integrity of the brain and, ultimately, upon that of the entire organism. On the other hand, the contents of cognition (that is, our knowledge and beliefs) are acquired through experience of the social and physical world, and they are organised through complex social institutions and practices.

   The topic of cognition is important in understanding women and their health in two different ways. First, one can study the beliefs that people (including, obviously, women themselves) hold about women and their health and especially about the role (or roles) of women in contemporary society. Second, one can study differences between

Women, Health and the Mind
Edited by L. Sherr and J.S. St Lawrence. © 2000 John Wiley & Sons, Ltd

women and men in terms of their intellectual functioning. This has traditionally been interpreted in terms of differences with regard to their intellectual abilities and, especially, their performance on psychological tests. The evidence suggests that any such differences are relatively small and result from the different social experiences of men and women and not from biological differences (Caplan et al., 1997).

Each of these in itself represents a major field of inquiry, and it would be impossible to do justice to either in this fairly short chapter. Instead, we shall focus our discussion of these issues on the involvement of the menstrual cycle. In the first part of the chapter, we shall examine women's attitudes towards menstruation and how they are influenced by both cultural factors and women's menstrual experience. In the second part, we shall look at the influence of the menstrual cycle upon women's cognitive performance. In the final part, we shall consider attitudes to menopause and the influence of the menopause upon cognitive performance.

COGNITION AND MENSTRUATION

The menstrual cycle is a phenomenon that is patently biological in nature. Indeed, it is one of the very few biological processes that serve as a sexual marker by differentiating between male and female members of the human species. Moreover, the experience of the onset of menstruation (or menarche) has a major impact on the development of a woman's personal identity (Koff et al., 1978). The precise impact of menarche depends upon attitudes towards menstruation that girls acquire from their close relatives as well as from their friends, the media and society in general (see Fradkin & Firestone, 1986; Ruble & Brooks-Gunn, 1979), and these attitudes appear to be well established even in pre-menarcheal girls and young boys (Clarke & Ruble, 1978). In fact, culturally shared beliefs about the menstrual cycle influence the expectations of both men and women with regard to the role(s) of women in society (Brooks-Gunn & Ruble, 1986; Strauss et al., 1987).

Although some men and women hold positive views of menstruation, many regard it as having debilitating effects on women's performance, sexuality and psychological well-being, or else tend to deny that it has any effects whatsoever (Brooks-Gunn & Ruble, 1980). Negative attitudes to menstruation seem to be acquired by women mainly from their mothers, although there are also generational differences such that mothers are more likely than their daughters to see menstruation as constraining or disrupting their everyday activities in general and their sexual behaviour in particular (see Golub, 1992, p.20). Strauss et al. (1990) noted that, whilst daughters reported having had a more positive experience of menarche and greater preparation for menstruation, the differences in menstrual attitudes between mothers and daughters were relatively slight, and this confirms the importance of mothers in passing both information and cultural norms across successive generations. However, the meanings of reproductive phenomena vary between different societies (Frayser, 1985). Women will call on whatever cultural frameworks are available to make sense of their experience of menstruation (Furth & Ch'en, 1992), and consequently attitudes to menstruation tend to differ from one culture to another (Chandra & Chaturvedi, 1992). The menstrual cycle is essentially a continuous biological process, but people in most cultures characterise it as consisting of a sequence of discrete phases (see Foster, 1996). Apart from the menstrual phase itself, most women report a variety of symptoms in the week or so before the onset of bleeding, though the incidence, severity and meaning of these symptoms varies widely across different cultures (Dan & Monagle, 1994). Indeed, in industrialised countries both medical and lay people recognise a condition of "premenstrual tension" or "premenstrual syndrome", which has emotional, somatic and behavioural components (see Richardson, 1995). Nevertheless, this seems to be very much a twentieth-century phenomenon and one that is not regarded as a clinical condition by women in nonindustrialised countries.

MENSTRUATION AND COGNITIVE PERFORMANCE

A major theme in the menstrual attitudes held by women and men and by girls and boys across most cultures is that the premenstrual and menstrual phases of the menstrual cycle (that is, the few days both before and after the onset of bleeding) are associated with intellectual debilitation. This stereotype is apparently confirmed by women's own accounts of the symptoms that they experience during the premenstrual and menstrual phases, both in general daily life and in formal academic studying (see Richardson, 1992). However, research has shown that people are really very poor at estimating their own cognitive performance, and that subjective accounts of cognitive impairment may have very little objective validity (Herrmann, 1984; Martin & Jones, 1984). Consequently, personal reports and cultural stereotypes do not constitute adequate evidence of poor objective performance.

What does the research literature on women's intellectual performance across the menstrual cycle tell us? Sommer (1992) provided a very thorough examination of this literature and concluded that, in a wide range of cognitive tasks, there was quite simply no good evidence for the notion of premenstrual or menstrual debilitation. This survey even included research on the academic performance of female students as measured by examinations or class tests (see also Richardson, 1991). Contrary, then, to the reports of women and the expectations of both women and men, menstruation does not appear to impair women's intellectual capabilities at all. Indeed, using a detection task known to be a sensitive indicator of the brain's processing efficiency, Dye (1992) found that women's objective performance was better in the premenstrual phase than at any other time in the menstrual cycle. Reviews of changes in sensory function (for example, vision, smell, touch, taste and pain sensitivity) have indicated that there may be fluctuations across the normal menstrual cycle. However, the pattern of fluctuation is by no means consistent, even amongst studies examining the same sensory modality (Doty et al., 1981; Parlee, 1983).

More recent research has failed to demonstrate differences in cognitive performance during the menstrual cycle (e.g. Girdler & Light, 1994; Gordon & Lee, 1993). Some research studies have based hypotheses of menstrual-cycle variation on a theory put forward by Broverman et al., (1968) and developed by Kimura & Hampson (1994). This attempted to relate hormone levels to particular types of cognitive performance and, in particular, implied that raised oestrogen would lead to increased brain activation. Following this theory, some researchers have documented changes in functional cerebral asymmetry, but taken together their results are inconsistent. Sanders & Wenmoth (1998) argued that the inconsistency in results disappeared if the nature of the tasks was taken into account: they found a greater asymmetry on a verbal (left-hemisphere) task during the mid-luteal phase (characterised by high levels of oestrogen) but greater asymmetry on a musical (right-hemisphere) task during menstruation (characterised by low levels of oestrogen).

Why should cultural stereotypes regarding the supposed impact of the menstrual cycle on human cognition be maintained despite the lack of any supportive evidence? In fact, we know that people have very sophisticated strategies for maintaining their beliefs and for avoiding or discrediting evidence that conflicts with those beliefs (Evans, 1987; Hewstone, 1988). As a result, assumptions both about oneself and about general categories of people gain considerable inertia (Snyder, 1984). Several studies have shown in particular that both men and women tend to ascribe negative moods experienced by women during the premenstrual or menstrual phases to the process of menstruation, but that they tend to ascribe precisely the same negative moods experienced by women at other times in the menstrual cycle to external situational factors (e.g. Koeske & Koeske, 1975). Although there seems to be no direct evidence on the matter, it is likely that the same tendencies operate in the case of attributions of cognitive failure.

MENOPAUSE AND COGNITIVE PERFORMANCE

Strictly speaking, "menopause" refers to the point of total cessation of the menstrual cycle, usually defined in terms of an absence of periods for 1 year. The more general term, climacteric, refers to the gradual changes associated with the end of reproductive capability that occur over a period of several years. Menopause is often discussed solely with regard to physical and emotional symptoms (Golub, 1992, Chapter 9), and the serious debate has been concerned with whether such symptoms define a recognisable menopausal "syndrome" (see Studd et al., 1977). Surveys of menopausal symptoms may either omit cognitive symptoms altogether or view them simply as a consequence of physical or emotional symptoms. In fact, the latter appear to have no effect on cognitive performance in menopausal women (Polo-Kantola et al., 1997).

One survey of 135 menopausal and postmenopausal women from an urban population in the United States found that 25% reported "forgetfulness" as a symptom that they either were experiencing or had experienced because of the menopause (Polit & LaRocco, 1980). However, a recent survey involving more than 900 women in the United Kingdom found that the chance of their reporting an "inability to concentrate" as a symptom experienced over the previous 6 months was roughly 25% throughout the age range of 37 to 58 years (Quine & Rubin, 1997; Rubin & Quine, 1995). The only exception arose in a small number of respondents aged between 55 and 58 who were not receiving hormone replacement therapy (HRT), of whom only 9% reported an inability to concentrate. Another study in Hong Kong found that memory disturbance was actually reported less often in women who had experienced a surgical menopause that resulted from hysterectomy (Haines et al., 1994).

The British survey found that more than a third of the 900 women felt that HRT was likely to relieve an inability to concentrate, once again regardless of whether they were receiving or had received HRT themselves. The evidence from clinical trials confirms that HRT tends to enhance both moods and cognition, but in both cases its effects are relatively modest (Halbreich, 1997; Sherwin, 1997). Some researchers have claimed that the menopause accelerates the intellectual decline associated with ageing and that HRT protects women against this process (Halbreich et al., 1995; Kimura, 1995; Resnick et al., 1997). However, such claims are based on studies that were correlational in nature and failed to include any comparison group of male participants.

In principle, it should be possible to address the issue of whether the menopause affects intellectual performance by administering a battery of tests to representative samples of men and women across the full adult age range. The evidence confirms that cognitive performance declines with age and that on many tasks the magnitude of this deficit accelerates with advancing age (Verhaeghen & Salthouse, 1997). However, the overall rate of intellectual decline is very similar in men and women (Herlitz et al., 1997; Meinz & Salthouse, 1998). Women appear to show a marginally faster decline on tests of perceptual speed or reasoning, but such effects depend on both the material and test procedure (Meinz & Salthouse, 1998). Herlitz et al. (1997) used a battery of tests with a sample of 1000 participants from the general population of a Swedish city. The latter had been chosen entirely at random, with the constraint that they defined 10 cohorts aged in multiples of 5 years between 35 and 80 years. Mean scores were presented by age and gender on three cognitive tests: the Mini-Mental State Examination (Folstein et al., 1975), verbal fluency and the Block Design sub-test of the Wechsler Adult Intelligence Scale – Revised (Wechsler, 1981). In none of the results of these tests was there any suggestion that the performance of women around the age of 50 years showed a specific reduction of the sort that would be associated with debilitation at the menopause.

CONCLUSIONS

On the one hand, the phenomenon of menstruation plays a major role in the establishment of women's identity. Both women and men acquire a set of attitudes and expectations about the role(s) of women in society, although the exact form taken by these stereotypes varies from culture to culture. These stereotypes appear to be successfully maintained despite the lack of any evidence that they are reflected in women's behaviour and performance. Indeed, on the other hand, the menstrual cycle is not associated with any reliable variations in women's intellectual capabilities, either in daily life or in the more cognitively demanding situations encountered in higher education. Moreover, there is no evidence for any intellectual impairment associated with the menopause. In short, the menstrual cycle plays a major role in the content of women's cognitions, yet at the same time it seems to have little or no impact upon the efficiency of cognitive processing.

REFERENCES

Brooks-Gunn, J., & Ruble, D.N. (1980). The Menstrual Attitude Questionnaire. *Psychosomatic Medicine, 42,* 503–512.

Brooks-Gunn, J., & Ruble, D.N. (1986). Men's and women's attitudes and beliefs about the menstrual cycle. *Sex Roles, 14,* 287–299.

Broverman, D.M., Klaiber, E.L., Kobayashi, Y., & Vowel, W. (1968). Roles of activation and inhibition in sex differences in cognitive abilities. *Psychological Review, 75,* 23–50.

Caplan, P.J., Crawford, M., Hyde, J.S., & Richardson, J.T.E. (1997). *Gender Differences in Human Cognition.* New York: Oxford University Press.

Chandra, P.S., & Chaturvedi, S.K. (1992). Cultural variations in attitudes toward menstruation. *Canadian Journal of Psychiatry, 37,* 196–198.

Clarke, A.E., & Ruble, D.N. (1978). Young adolescents' beliefs concerning menstruation. *Child Development, 49,* 231–234.

Dan, A.J., & Monagle, L. (1994). Sociocultural influences on women's experiences of perimenstrual symptoms. In Gold, J.H., & Severino, S.K. (Eds.), *Premenstrual Dysphoria: Myths and Realities* (pp.201–211). Washington DC: American Psychiatric Press.

Doty, R.L., Snyder, P.J., Huggins, G.R., & Lowry, D.D. (1981). Endocrine, cardiovascular, and psychological correlates of olfactory sensitivity changes during the human menstrual cycle. *Journal of Comparative and Physiological Psychology*, 95, 45–60.

Drever, J. (1964). *A Dictionary of Psychology* (revised by H. Wallerstein). Harmondsworth: Penguin Books.

Dye, L. (1992). Visual information processing and the menstrual cycle. In Richardson, J.T.E. (Ed.), *Cognition and the Menstrual Cycle* (pp.67–97). New York: Springer.

Evans, J. St. B.T. (1987). Beliefs and expectations as causes of judgemental bias. In Wright, G., & Ayton, P. (Eds.), *Judgemental Forecasting* (pp.120–137). Chichester: John Wiley & Sons Ltd.

Folstein, M.F., Folstein, S.E., & McHugh, P.R. (1975). Mini-Mental State: A practical method for grading the cognitive state of patients for the clinician. *Journal of Psychiatric Research*, 12, 189–198.

Foster, J. (1996). Menstrual time: the sociocognitive mapping of "the menstrual cycle". *Sociological Forum*, 11, 523–547.

Fradkin, B., & Firestone, P. (1986). Premenstrual tension, expectancy, and mother-child relations. *Journal of Behavioral Medicine*, 9, 245–249.

Frayser, S.G. (1985). *Varieties of Sexual Experience: An Anthropological Perspective on Human Sexuality*. New Haven, CT: Human Relations Area Files Press.

Furth, C., & Ch'en, S. (1992). Chinese medicine and the anthropology of menstruation in contemporary Taiwan. *Medical Anthropology Quarterly*, 6, 27–48.

Girdler, S.S., & Light, K.C. (1994). Hemodynamic stress responses in men and women examined as a function of female menstrual cycle phase. *International Journal of Psychophysiology*, 17, 233–248.

Golub, S. (1992). *Periods: From Menarche to Menopause*. Newbury Park, CA: Sage.

Gordon, H.W., & Lee, P.A. (1993). No difference in cognitive performance between phases of the menstrual cycle. *Psychoneuroendocrinology*, 18, 521–531.

Haines, C.J., Cung, T.K.H., & Leung, D.H.Y. (1994). A prospective study of the frequency of acute menopausal symptoms in Hong Kong. *Maturitas*, 18, 175–181.

Halbreich, U. (1997). Role of estrogen in postmenopausal depression. *Neurology*, 48(5, Suppl. 7), 16–20.

Halbreich, U., Lumley, L.A., Palter, S., Manning, C., Gengo, F., & Joe, S.H. (1995). Possible acceleration of age effects on cognition. *Journal of Psychiatric Research*, 29, 153–163.

Herlitz, A., Nilsson, L.-G., & Backman, L. (1997). Gender differences in episodic memory. *Memory and Cognition*, 25, 801–811.

Herrmann, D.J. (1984). Questionnaires about memory. In Harris, J.E., & Morris, P.E., (Eds.), *Everyday Memory, Actions and Absent-Mindedness* (pp.133–151). London: Academic Press.

Hewstone, M. (1988). Attributional bases of intergroup conflict. In Stroebe, W., Kruglanski, A.W., Bar-Tel, D., & Hewstone, M. (Eds.), *The Social Psychology of Intergroup Conflict: Theory, Research, and Applications* (pp.47–71). Berlin: Springer.

Kimura, D. (1995). Estrogen replacement therapy may protect against intellectual decline in postmenopausal women. *Hormones and Behavior, 29*, 312–321.

Kimura, D., & Hampson, E. (1994). Cognitive pattern in men and women is influenced by fluctuations in sex hormones. *Current Directions in Psychological Science, 3*, 57–61.

Koeske, R.K., & Koeske, G.F. (1975). An attributional approach to moods and the menstrual cycle. *Journal of Personality and Social Psychology, 31*, 473–478.

Koff, E., Rierdan, J., & Silverstone, E. (1978). Changes in representation of body image as a function of menarcheal status. *Developmental Psychology, 14*, 635–642.

Martin, M., & Jones, G.V. (1984). Cognitive failures in everyday life. In Harris, J.E., & Morris, P.E. (Eds.), *Everyday Memory, Actions and Absent-Mindedness* (pp.173–190). London: Academic Press.

Meinz, E.J., & Salthouse, T.A. (1998). Is age kinder to females than to males? *Psychonomic Bulletin and Review, 5*, 56–70.

Parlee, M.B. (1983). Menstrual rhythms in sensory processes: a review of fluctuations in vision, olfaction, audition, taste, and touch. *Psychological Bulletin, 93*, 539–548.

Polit, D.F., & LaRocco, S.A. (1980). Social and psychological correlates of menopausal symptoms. *Psychosomatic Medicine, 42*, 335–345.

Polo-Kantola, P., Portin, R., Koskinen, T., Polo, O., Irjala, K., & Erkkola, R. (1997). Climacteric symptoms do not impair cognitive performances in postmenopause. *Maturitas, 27*, 13–12.

Quine, L., & Rubin, R. (1997). Attitude, subjective norm and perceived behavioural control as predictors of women's intentions to take hormone replacement therapy. *British Journal of Health Psychology, 2*, 199–216.

Resnick, S.M., Metter, E.J., & Zonderman, A.B. (1997). Estrogen replacement therapy and longitudinal decline in visual memory: a possible protective effect? *Neurology, 49*, 1491–1497.

Richardson, J.T.E. (1991). The menstrual cycle and student learning. *Journal of Higher Education, 62*, 317–340.

Richardson, J.T.E. (1992). The menstrual cycle, cognition, and para-menstrual symptomatology. In Richardson, J.T.E. (Ed.), *Cognition and the Menstrual Cycle* (pp.1–38). New York: Springer.

Richardson, J.T.E. (1995). The premenstrual syndrome: a brief history. *Social Science and Medicine, 41*, 761–767.

Rubin, R., & Quine, L. (1995, December). Women's attitudes to the menopause and the use of Hormone Replacement Therapy. Paper presented at the conference of the British Psychological Society, London.

Ruble, D.N., & Brooks-Gunn, J. (1979). Menstrual symptoms: a social cognition analysis. *Journal of Behavioral Medicine, 2*, 171–194.

Sanders, G., & Wenmoth, D. (1998). Cerebral asymmetry and cognitive performance show complementary fluctuation across the menstrual cycle. In Ellis, L., & Ebertz, L. (Eds.), *Males, Females, and Behavior: Toward Biological Understanding* (pp.165–175). Westport, CT: Praeger.

Sherwin, B.B. (1997). Estrogen effects on cognition in menopausal women. *Neurology, 48(5, Suppl 7)*, 21–26.

Snyder, M. (1984). When belief creates reality. In Berkowitz, L. (Ed.), *Advances in Experimental Social Psychology*, Volume 18 (pp.247–305). Orlando, FL: Academic Press.

Sommer, B. (1992). Cognitive performance and the menstrual cycle. In Richardson, J.T.E. (Ed.), *Cognition and the Menstrual Cycle* (pp.39–66). New York: Springer.

Strauss, B., Appelt, H., Daub, U., & De Vries, I. (1990). Generationsunterschied im Menstruationserleben und in der Einstellung zur Menstruation. *Psychotherapie und Medizinische Psychologie, 40*, 48–56.

Strauss, B., Appelt, H., & Lange, C. (1987). Deutsche Neukonstruktion und Validierung des "Menstrual Attitude Questionnaire". *Psychotherapie und Medizinische Psychologie, 37*, 175–182.

Studd, J., Chakravarti, S., & Oram, D. (1977). The climacteric. In Greenblatt, R.B., & Studd, J. (Eds.), *Clinics in Obstetrics and Gynaecology*, Volume 4, No. 1, *The Menopause* (pp.3–29). London: W.B. Saunders.

Verhaeghen, P., & Salthouse, T.A. (1997). Meta-analyses of age–cognition relations in adulthood: estimates of linear and nonlinear age effects and structural models. *Psychological Bulletin, 122*, 231–249.

Wechsler, D. (1981). *Wechsler Adult Intelligence Scale – Revised*. New York: Psychological Corporation.

Section 5

WOMEN, HEALTH PROMOTION AND HEALTH LIFE-STYLES

Chapter 19

Physical Activity, Leisure, and Women's Health

Susan M. Shaw

University of Waterloo, Ontario, Canada

and

Karla A. Henderson

University of North Carolina, Chapel Hill, USA

In recent years many health professionals, as well as sports and recreation professionals, have directed their attention towards the health benefits of exercise and physical activity. In the United States, the 1996 report of the Surgeon General [United States Department of Health and Human Services (USDHHS), 1996] suggested that people who are usually inactive can improve their health and well-being by becoming even moderately active on a regular basis, and that greater health benefits can be achieved by increasing the amount or intensity of physical activity. In Canada, also, the Canadian Fitness and Lifestyle Research Institute (1998) has promoted the idea of "active living", and has funded research into the beneficial effects of physical activity. These reports and promotional programmes are based on the assumption that exercise not only reduces certain illnesses and diseases, but also that it is important in terms of gaining and maintaining health and well-being in general.

Women, Health and the Mind
Edited by L. Sherr and J.S. St Lawrence. © 2000 John Wiley & Sons, Ltd

The assumption that physical activity and exercise has beneficial outcomes for health is rarely disputed. Indeed, an increasing body of research points to particular health related benefits (Bouchard et al., 1990, 1994; USDHHS, 1996). However, explaining the reasons why such benefits accrue is a more difficult task. For example, although some of the biochemical mechanisms that lead to health-related change are known, other types of mechanisms are less well understood, and determining exactly what it is about physical activity that causes the change is difficult to determine. In other words, it is not always clear what types, frequencies, levels, or intensities of physical activities are the most advantageous and why. Clearly further theoretical, as well as empirical, research is needed.

One of the reasons why some aspects of the theoretical understanding of the health outcomes of physical activity remain incomplete may be related to the fact that such outcomes are not simply a result of the physiological changes brought about by exercise. Rather, exercise may lead to a complex mix of physiological, social, psychological, and attitudinal outcomes. For example, social interaction during physical activities, enjoyment of the activity itself, or the decision to take time out for oneself, may all have positive outcomes independent of the nature, intensity, or duration of the actual activity participation. Thus these kinds of impacts need to be taken into consideration and included in explanatory systems of health benefits, along with physiological impacts.

Furthermore, thinking about the social and psychological outcomes that are associated with the experience of participation in physical activity leads, logically, to consideration of other leisure activities as well. Positive health outcomes may arise out of a range of different leisure involvements, including both active and passive activities, if the experiences and social contexts of such activities are beneficial. Accordingly, a more complete understanding of the health benefits of activity may need to take into account the relationship between leisure and health, and the outcomes of leisure participation in general, as well as those of specific physical activities.

The focus of this chapter is on leisure, as well as on physical activity and exercise. This broader perspective suggests an emphasis on lifestyle, everyday activities, and factors affecting life-style decisions. We believe that this approach is particularly relevant to understanding women's health. Women's lives are affected by societal gender relations that influence their everyday leisure decisions and opportunities. Because of gender structures in society, women participate less than men in sports and physical activities (Bonen & Shaw, 1995; Robinson & Godbey, 1993; USDHHS, 1996) and have less time for and greater constraints regarding leisure in general (Deem, 1986; Green et al., 1990; Henderson, 1991; Henderson et al., 1996). Thus, to understand the importance of activity and leisure for women's health implies understanding women's gendered lives as well.

The chapter begins by examining the research on physical activity and health, with particular reference to women's health. We then broaden the discussion to an examination of the relationship between health and leisure in general, with particular attention focused on women. This focus leads to the issue of life-style and women's lives, with an examination of the factors that constrain women's participation in physical activities and leisure. At the end of the chapter suggestions are made about strategies for changing women's life-styles, increasing opportunities for their participation, and enhancing women's health.

PHYSICAL ACTIVITY AND HEALTH

Researchers have shown that physical activity has a direct and positive effect on health. It reduces the risk of disease, offsets the impact and severity of various diseases and health problems, and seems to increase perceptions of health and well-being in general (Bouchard et al., 1990, 1994; USDHHS, 1996).

Some specific diseases in which there is a strong and consistent benefit as a result of exercise include cardiovascular disease and diabetes (Froelicher, 1990; Vranic & Wasserman, 1990). Exercise is recommended by health professionals both as a preventive strategy for cardiovascular disease and as part of the recovery process following a heart attack or heart surgery (Blair, 1994; Quaglietti & Froelicher, 1994). Similarly, exercise is believed to reduce the risk of diabetes, and to reduce the severity of symptoms for people who have already been diagnosed with this disease (Gudat et al., 1994).

High blood pressure and obesity can also be controlled, at least to some extent, through an active life-style that includes regular physical activity and exercise (Bouchard et al., 1994). These underlying health problems are associated with higher risk for heart disease and diabetes, as well as a range of other health problems such as stroke and cancer (Colditz et al., 1990). In addition, exercise seems to relieve psychological stress and to alleviate some sleeping disorders (Sime, 1990). Stress, anxiety, and insomnia are also disorders that are known to be risk factors for or precursors of various illnesses.

Some of the health-related problems thought to benefit from physical exercise are problems specific to or particularly prevalent among women. These include premenstrual syndrome, osteoporosis, and difficulties associated with menopause. Exercise as a remedy or a preventive measure for these problems has been promoted by advocates of women's health because it is a natural solution and avoids the potential side-effects of long-term drug use (The Boston Women's Health Book Collective, 1998). For example, for those women who experience health difficulties associated with menopausal changes, exercise as a solution is much less controversial than the long-term use of hormone replacement therapy.

Despite evidence of the health benefits of exercise, we suggest that more attention still needs to be directed towards the theoretical explanations for these outcomes. Some of the research studies that show a causal relationship between exercise and disease reduction do not explicitly address the issue of theory. Other researchers have examined the underlying mechanisms thought to be involved in the exercise and health relationship. For some disease processes, the molecular or biochemical reactions that result from exercise have been well established. For example, researchers have shown how exercise influences fat metabolism, produces molecular changes in the heart muscle, causes biochemical reactions that affect plasma and cholesterol levels, and increases insulin sensitivity and glucose tolerance (Bouchard et al., 1990). These changes explain why exercise is associated with reduced risk for cardiovascular disease, diabetes, and other illnesses. Similarly, exercise is associated with mechanisms that increase bone mass, showing the link between activity and reduced risk for osteoporosis (Drinkwater, 1994).

It is less clear why exercise might be beneficial in reducing stress and stress-related diseases. More information is needed about the mechanisms that underlie this relationship, as well as the relationship between depression and activity (Brown, 1990; Mazzeo et al., 1997). The reasons why exercise might alleviate symptoms associated with premenstrual syndrome or menopausal complications are also not well understood.

Another weakness of the research done to date is the relative lack of attention that has been directed towards understanding the type and quantity (for example, the intensity and duration) of physical activity that is optimal for health. As a result, it is difficult for health or exercise professionals to provide exercise "prescriptions" or to advise about the kind or level of activity participation that is needed (Bouchard et al., 1994). Another issue relates to why individuals have difficulty in adhering to exercise programmes. Despite the gains made in recognizing the value of leisure and physical activity, little progress has been made in understanding and modifying physical activity and exercise behaviour (Dubbert, 1992).

One of the reasons why explanations for the relationship between exercise and health are incomplete may be the emphasis placed on physiological or biochemical theories. While these have proven to be useful in understanding the impact of exercise on particular disease processes, social and psychological mechanisms may also play a role in explaining the impact of activity on health. Researchers have known for a long time that there is a mind–body connection that needs to be taken into account in understanding health and illness, and this connection may be particularly relevant in understanding the health benefits of active life-styles.

Physical activity may have a direct and positive impact on psychological well-being, and thus on physical well-being as well. Another possibility is that exercise may indirectly influence health through the alleviation of psychological stress or distress. Yet another line of inquiry that needs further attention relates to the experience of participation in physical activity. That is, it may not be the activity *per se* that influences health, or that is the sole factor that influences health. Rather, the total experience associated with participation, including the quality of that experience and the social context of the activity, may also have health-related implications. This line of thinking has implications for understanding the type of activity that is likely to result in positive health outcomes. That is, the quality of experience may be one factor, along with other factors such as intensity and duration. Further, consideration of experiential aspects of participation suggests the potential significance of leisure, in that leisure experiences may have impacts on health above and beyond the physiological impact of exercise. In other words, because of the role of experiential factors, health benefits may accrue from physically passive as well as active forms of participation. The next section of this chapter looks at the research that has been carried out in the leisure studies field on the leisure and health relationship.

LEISURE AND HEALTH

A number of leisure researchers have suggested that there is a causal relationship between leisure and health. To understand this claim, though, it is important to know what researchers mean by the term "leisure".

Leisure can include all types of free-time activities, or activities that individuals participate in that are not part of employment, household, or other obligatory aspects of their lives. Leisure, therefore, potentially includes a range of social activities, such as visiting friends or being with family, media activities, such as television watching, and cultural and artistic activities, as well as sports and physical activities. However, most researchers do not define leisure according to activity type. Rather, they focus on the experiential aspects of participation. That is, the defining characteristics of leisure are that such activities are freely chosen, self-determined, intrinsically motivated, and done for their own sake, or for the intrinsic purposes of relaxation, enjoyment, and fun (Henderson et al., 1996; Mannell & Kleiber, 1997). In addition, leisure is often, though not always, interactional in nature, and the social context – whether it is with family members, with a romantic partner, with friends, or even with work colleagues – is an important component of the total leisure experience (Kelly, 1983). Even choosing to be alone or take time for self is a significant context that influences the quality of the leisure experience (Henderson et al., 1996).

Leisure is thought to benefit health in a number of ways. These include improving physical health, improving mental or psychological health, and reducing stress. These benefits are similar to some of the outcomes that medical researchers have suggested result from participation in physical activity and exercise. Leisure research, however, is different from physiological research on this topic in two fundamental ways. First, leisure researchers typically include in their analyses the benefits of physically inactive as well as active participation. In other words, they are more inclusive or broader in their definition of activity. Second, and perhaps more importantly, their explanations for the leisure and health relationship focus on the experiential or social–psychological aspects of activity rather than on the physical aspects. While not denying the clear physiological benefits that result from participation in exercise, leisure researchers argue that there may be additional psychological benefits from the leisure experience itself.

Various explanations have been proposed to explain the leisure and health relationship. One explanation is that participation in leisure acts as a form of stress reduction that reduces susceptibility to disease and increases psychological well-being (Iso-Ahola, 1980; Iwasaki & Mannell, 1998). Such stress reduction may come about from the enjoyment, pleasure, and relaxation components of leisure. Wankel (1993), for example, asserted that enjoyment is a crucial factor in realizing the psychological benefits of exercise. Further, it is thought that these experiential aspects of leisure, such as enjoyment, not only improve the quality of the moment, but may have a cumulative effect as well, and that the promotion of positive moods may influence general health and well-being (Hull, 1991). Stress reduction may also be related to the "escape" or diversionary possibilities of leisure (sometimes called the palliative leisure coping hypothesis), in that participation in leisure may allow people to temporarily forget about or put aside the problems they face in their everyday lives (Sharp & Mannell, 1996).

Another explanation for the health benefits of leisure focuses on the social interactional aspects of these experiences. The social component of leisure not only has the potential to provide pleasure but it is also thought to promote and facilitate social support for individuals, and the perception of social support is also an important component of psychological well-being. Coleman & Iso-Ahola (1993) suggest that the social support outcomes of leisure act as a buffer for individuals facing increased levels of life stress, and that this buffer serves to prevent the onset of physical and mental health problems that might otherwise result from these high stress levels. Thus their theory of "leisure coping" links the stress reduction and social support mechanisms of leisure.

Another component of leisure, also thought to buffer stress and to enhance health and well-being, is that of self-determination. Because leisure includes individual decision-making and active free choice to a greater extent than many obligatory or work-like activities, it may enhance feelings of control, autonomy and self-determination in life in general. Again, a sense of personal control, or self-efficacy, is associated with both physical and mental health (Brown, 1990; Wankel, 1993), and one empirical study has shown a link between perceived control in leisure and reduced ill health, especially for individuals who are highly stressed (Coleman, 1993). Self-determination and control are also associated with increased empowerment and with a developed sense of entitlement (Henderson & Bialeschki, 1991). These changes are thought to enable people to challenge, and perhaps overcome, the restrictions and constraints in their everyday lives (Freysinger & Flannery, 1992).

Although most of the research on health, as with the research on exercise and health, has not been focused specifically on women's health, some components of leisure are particularly relevant to women. Many women, and especially employed mothers, have high stress levels because of their double (or triple) work day, that includes their paid job, their household labour, and their responsibilities for the care of children (Hochschild, 1989; Shank, 1986). Women caring for elderly parents, sometimes at the same time as caring for young children, also experience high levels of stress. In addition, single parents and low-income women suffer considerable financial as well as workload and other stresses (Streather, 1979). Thus, if leisure has stress reduction functions, it may play a particularly salient role in health maintenance and health enhancement for women.

Social support is also important for women as well as for men. While the research indicates that women tend to find it easier to make and maintain friendships (Bate, 1988), there is also evidence that women have a particular need for friendships with other women in order to affirm themselves and one another (Green, 1998). Indeed, social inter-action appears to be one of the most important motivations underlying women's involvement in physical recreation as well as other leisure practices (Henderson & Bialeschki, 1994). Some women, though, may have difficulty finding female friends. For example, women whose paid work places them in a male-dominated environment may feel isolated and devalued (Caplan, 1993), and women who are full-time home-makers in communities where most women are employed may find that they have few options for social contact during the day.

Of all the health benefits of leisure, the potential for enhancing self-determination and empowerment is probably the most important for women. Numerous researchers have examined the low level of personal power that some women feel in their daily lives, their higher levels of dependency compared with men, and their adherence to an ethic of care that can lead to them caring for others' needs while neglecting their own (Henderson & Allen, 1991; Henderson & Bialeschki, 1991). Increases in self-determination can help to overcome these feelings of dependency and lead to a healthier perspective on life.

The particular needs of women, including the need for leisure, indi-cate the importance of taking women's total lives into account when considering their health and well-being. Thus, while the benefits of exercise and leisure may be recognized and supported by research, the reasons why women do not participate more in such activities need to be understood in terms of the material and social contexts of their lives.

CONSTRAINTS ON WOMEN'S PARTICIPATION

Societal gender relations and continued inequities between women and men mean that women face particular constraints in terms of their participation in physical activities and other forms of leisure. Some of the constraints they face are "structural" (sometimes referred to as "intervening", see Crawford et al., 1991), in that women would like to increase their leisure participation but are prevented by lack of resources, lack of opportunities, or other factors. Other constraints are more "subtle", and may relate to a lack of expressed desire for certain forms of leisure, arising for example out of social disapproval or perceived inappropriateness for a specific activity (often referred to as types of interpersonal or intrapersonal constraints; Crawford et al., 1991).

Despite progress in recent years, gender roles continue to be narrowly defined, with particular activities deemed by many to be "masculine" or inappropriate for women (Shaw, 1994). The impact of these gender-based beliefs and ideologies are particularly evident in the area of sports, which in many ways continues to be a male preserve (Messner & Sabo, 1990). Many high profile sports, for example American football in the United States, ice hockey in Canada, and soccer in the United Kingdom, continue to be primarily male activities. Other sports have opened their doors to women to a somewhat greater extent, but participation rates generally remain far from equal (Hall et al., 1991).

The relatively low level of women's participation in sports and physical activities is clearly related to societal beliefs about the gendered nature of these activities (Koivula, 1995), and the constraining nature of these beliefs on women's behaviours. Structural constraints reduce women's participation through the lack of facilities, opportunities, teams or leagues, and through the lack of financial support for women's sports. The disapproval of women's family members, friends, or partners for extensive sports participation may also constrain these behaviours. At the same time, expectations about women's family responsibilities and household duties mean that sports activities generally do not fit easily into the home-based leisure styles of the majority of women (Deem, 1987). Thus a range of intrapersonal constraints are evident as well. For example, social expectations and social disapproval of some activities may mean that women are less likely than men to learn to enjoy sports and physical activities: they may also fail to learn the skills required for enjoyment.

Other constraints that particularly affect participation in sports and physical activities include social embarrassment, low body image, and fear of violence. Research studies have consistently found that women, and especially young women, tend to have negative images of their own bodies (Jackson et al., 1986), and this can make them reluctant to participate in activities in which their bodies are "on display", such as dance, gymnastics, or swimming (Frederick & Shaw, 1995). Women also experience higher levels of fear of violence compared to men (Statistics Canada, 1993). Although this fear can constrain participation in a range of activities that take them out of the comfort of their home environment, it may be particularly damaging to participation rates in outdoors physical activities, such as jogging, walking, or hiking (Whyte & Shaw, 1994).

Apart from constraint in sports and physical activities, participation in general is constrained by lack of financial resources and lack of time. Clearly not all women lack the economic means to participate in leisure, but their lower levels of personal income compared to men, and their higher risk of poverty (Statistics Canada, 1995) make them more susceptible to financial constraints. In addition, not all women lack time for leisure, but research has shown that, on average, women have less leisure than men, and higher levels of obligatory activity (Shaw, 1985). This is due, in large part to the "double day" (Hochschild, 1989), as women have increased their participation in the labour market without reducing, to any great degree, their primary responsibility for the household and the care of children and other family members. The ethic of care also plays a constraining role here (Harrington et al., 1992) in that women care for the leisure needs of their children and other family members, rather than looking after their own needs. Moreover, they may lack a sense of entitlement and feel guilty if they take time out for themselves (Henderson & Bialeschki, 1991).

The constraints on women's leisure vary across their life span. For example, concerns about fitting in, and about body image and appearance, appear to be particularly prevalent among adolescents and young women. At this age, women are less likely to go against social conventions (Shaw et al., 1996). These constraints, though, may have long-term implications for participation, because women may not learn the skills, especially sports and physical activity skills, that are required for later participation.

Lack of time, lack of entitlement and the ethic of care particularly constrain women in their early to mid adulthood (Harrington et al., 1992). This stage of life is when women are most likely to have young children to care for, and when they may also be trying to develop a career path at the same time (Freysinger, 1995).

Older women may face fewer of these constraints, and may experience a re-emergence of leisure as their children grow older and become independent (Bialeschki & Michener, 1994). However, older women often lack the skills and confidence to take up new activities. They may also lack the economic resources to do so, and health problems can also emerge as leisure constraints at this stage of life.

Overall, it can be seen that women face numerous constraints in accessing leisure, and perhaps especially in accessing opportunities to participate in physically active leisure. Many of these constraints are considered to be gendered in that they apply primarily or uniquely to women as a result of their gender. Finding solutions to these constraints, and finding ways to enhance women's participation require an understanding of, and attention to, the impact of gender relations on women's lives.

CHANGING LIFE-STYLES AND ENHANCING HEALTH

Given the constraints that women face, it is not surprising that studies show that physical inactivity is more prevalent among women than men. Nor is it surprising that disadvantaged women, including women of colour, older women, and poorer women continue to have particularly high rates of inactivity (USDHHS, 1996; Wells, 1996). Thus, despite the gains made in recognizing the value of leisure and physical activity, there has been relatively little progress in changing patterns of participation (Dubbert, 1992).

A number of models have been proposed for predicting changes in activity level, such as social cognitive theory and stages of change models (Marcus, 1995; Marcus et al., 1994), but more research is needed. The most promising approaches are those that focus on women's relationship to family and community, as well as those which recognize the inter-relatedness of work, family, and leisure in women's lives. These approaches suggest that increasing participation in leisure and/or physical activities requires a fundamental change in life-style. Any change in leisure behaviour will affect, and be affected by, patterns of behaviour in other life spheres. Thus it does not appear to be useful to provide information about the benefits of increased participation without also understanding, and seeking to overcome, the constraints that women face in their daily lives in general. Moreover, changing lifestyles and patterns of participation also implies challenging gender beliefs and ideologies that underlie many of the leisure constraints that they encounter.

Overcoming leisure constraints and traditional ideologies about gender can take different forms. Women and girls could be encouraged into activities that challenge dominant gender role prescriptions. This encouragement could be part of the educational and policy development of schools as well as recreation and sports organizations. Encouraging non-traditional activities could lead to greater participation of girls and women in sports and physical activities. Moreover, such participation would constitute a form or "resistance" (Shaw, 1994; Wearing, 1990) to dominant gender relations, and, as such, would also tend to enhance feelings of self-determination, control, and entitlement (Freysinger & Flannery, 1992).

Although health, sports, and recreation professionals could do more to promote women's participation in leisure, most of the pathways to change involve women taking actions and making decisions over their own lives. One potential avenue for change is for women to take time for themselves. Many women would benefit, and their health and well-being would also be enhanced if they were able to take at least some time away from their household and family responsibilities. Mothers of young children, or women caring for dependent parents or other family members, may particularly benefit from some self-focused leisure (Wimbush, 1988). Some writers have suggested that one way to concep-tualize this change would be for women to think about caring for self rather than thinking only about caring for others (Bialeschki & Michener, 1994). Such self care could include women looking after their own health needs as well as their leisure and recreational needs. It could also involve seeking to overcome the feelings of guilt that some women experience when they attend to their own needs and desires, and seeking to replace such guilt with feeling of entitlement to sports, physical activities, and other forms of leisure.

In attempting to change life-styles and to enhance women's activity and leisure participation, attention also needs to be paid to the possi-bility that not all leisure is beneficial. Some activities, such as drug taking or gambling, are generally recognized as harmful rather than beneficial to the individual. However, other leisure activities can also have negative as well as positive outcomes. For example, television programmes, movies, women's and teen's magazines, as well as fashion shows, beauty pageants, and pornographic representations have all been widely criticized by feminist researchers for reproducing tradi-tional ideologies of femininity, and for reinforcing gender based inequities (Shaw, 1996). Some physically active leisure pursuits, too, can reinforce harmful aspects of these traditional ideologies. For example, activities that focus on appearance and weight loss, and espe-cially activities that are promoted as a means of obtaining the "ideal body" for women, can have negative rather than positive health outcomes.

In some sports, such as ballet and figure skating, coaches often encourage or require female participants to obtain an "ideal" body weight (Brooks-Gunn et al., 1988). Aerobics, too, has been criticized for encouraging women and girls to focus on their appearance and body shape rather than on their health and fitness (Frederick & Shaw, 1995; Shaw & Kemeny, 1989). While obesity is a health problem for many people, obsession with weight loss is not healthy either and can lead to various eating disorders, such as anorexia nervosa or bulimia, as well as to body image distortions – health problems that are wide-spread among young women (Garfinkel et al., 1987). Indeed, exercise obsession of any kind can have negative health outcomes (Polivy, 1994), including physical and psychological "disbenefits".

The possibility of negative health outcomes of some activities means that efforts to change life-styles and to enhance health through physical activity and leisure need to take both negative as well as positive outcomes into account. Exercise and leisure cannot be seen as a panacea for good health, and specific activities and activity contexts need to be critically evaluated by health promoters and by individual participants.

SUMMARY

This chapter has explored the many health benefits, both physical and mental, that can result from participation in physical activity and leisure. The physiological benefits to women from participation in physical exercise are numerous and have been extensively documented by researchers. In addition, though, researchers have also suggested that participation in leisure, whether physically active or not, can lead to stress reduction and other benefits that also enhance women's health.

Despite knowledge of the benefits of exercise and leisure, participation rates for women remain low, especially their participation in sports and physical activities. This lack of participation is the result of the multiple constraints that women face, including constraints related to traditional gender ideologies. The promotion of active life-styles, therefore, should include not only the provision of more opportunities and resources, but also finding ways to encourage women and girls to challenge narrow gender role prescriptions. Such promotion should also take into consideration the possibility of negative health outcomes of some activities, thus emphasizing the need for a critical approach to the question of exercise, leisure and health.

Given the constraints in women's lives, enhancing women's health through physical activity and leisure implies the need for a life-style change based on new and emerging ideologies and images of femininity. Life-style change is easier to promote during childhood and adolescence when opinions, attitudes, and behavioural patterns start to become established. Accordingly, particular attention needs to be directed towards this age group. Nevertheless, life-style change can be accomplished at other stages of life as well. Awareness of the various benefits and constraints, as well as critical assessments of leisure, exercise and life-style, can facilitate such change.

REFERENCES

Bate, B. (1988). *Communication and the Sexes*. New York: Harper & Row.

Bialeschki, M.D., & Michener, S. (1994). Re-entering leisure: transition within the role of motherhood. *Journal of Leisure Research, 26,* 57–74.

Blair, S.N. (1994). In Bouchard, C., Shephard, R.J., & Stephens, T. (Eds.), *Physical Activity, Fitness, and Health: International Proceedings and International Consensus Statement* (pp. 579–590). Champaign, IL: Human Kinetics.

Bonen, A., & Shaw, S.M. (1995). Recreation exercise participation and aerobic fitness in men and women: analysis of data from a national survey. *Journal of Sports Sciences*, 13, 297–303.

Boston Women's Health Book Collective (1998). *Our Bodies, Ourselves: For the Next Century*. New York: Simon & Schuster.

Bouchard, C., Shephard, R.J., Stephens, T., Sutton, J.R., & McPherson, B.D. (Eds.) (1990). *Exercise, Fitness, and Health: A Consensus of Current Knowledge*. Champaign, IL: Human Kinetics.

Bouchard, C., Shephard, R.J., & Stephens, T. (Eds.) (1994). *Physical Activity, Fitness, and Health: International Proceedings and International Consensus Statement*. Champaign, IL: Human Kinetics.

Brooks-Gunn, J., Burrow, C., & Warren, M.P. (1988). Attitudes towards eating and body weight in different groups of female adolescent athletes. *International Journal of Eating Disorders*, 7, 749–757.

Brown, D.R. (1990). Exercise, fitness, and mental health. In Bouchard, C., Shephard, R.J., Stephens, T., Sutton, J.R., & McPherson, B.D. (Eds.), *Exercise, Fitness, and Health: A Consensus of Current Knowledge* (pp. 607–626). Champaign, IL: Human Kinetics.

Canadian Fitness and Lifestyle Research Institute (1998). *The 1997 Physical Activity Benchmarks Report*. Ottawa, ON: Canadian Fitness and Lifestyle Research Unit.

Caplan, P.J. (1993). *Lifting a Ton of Feathers: A Woman's Guide to Surviving in the Academic World*. Toronto: University of Toronto Press.

Colditz, G.A., Willett, W.C., Stampfer, M.J., Manson, J.E., Hennekens, C.H., Arky, R.A., & Speizer, F.E. (1990). Weight as a risk factor for clinical diabetes in women. *American Journal of Epidemiology*, 132, 501–512.

Coleman, D. (1993). Leisure based social support, leisure dispositions and health. *Journal of Leisure Research*, 25, 350–361.

Coleman, D., & Iso-Ahola, S.E. (1993). Leisure and health: the role of social support and self-determination. *Journal of Leisure Research*, 25, 111–128.

Crawford, D., Jackson, E., & Godbey, G. (1991). A hierarchical model of leisure constraints. *Leisure Sciences*, 9, 119–127.

Deem, R. (1986). *All Work and No Play? The Sociology of Women and Leisure*. Milton Keynes: Open University Press.

Deem, R. (1987). Unleisured lives: sport in the context of women's leisure. *Women's Studies International Forum*, 10, 423–432.

Drinkwater, B.L. (1994). In Bouchard, C., Shephard, R.J., & Stephens, T. (Eds.), *Physical Activity, Fitness, and Health: International Proceedings and International Consensus Statement* (pp.724–736). Champaign, IL: Human Kinetics.

Dubbert, P.M. (1992). Exercise in behavioural medicine. *Journal of Consulting and Clinical Psychology*, 60, 613–618.

Frederick, C.J., & Shaw, S.M. (1995). Body image as a leisure constraint: examining the experience of aerobic exercise classes for young women. *Leisure Sciences*, 17, 57–73.

Freysinger, V.J. (1995). The dialectics of leisure and development for women and men in mid-life: an interpretive study. *Journal of Leisure Research, 27,* 61–84.

Freysinger, V.J., & Flannery, D. (1992). Women's leisure: affiliation, self-determination, empowerment and resistance? *Loisir et Société, 15,* 303–322.

Froelicher, V.F. (1990). In Bouchard, C., Shephard, R.J., Stephens, J.R., Sutton, J.R., & McPherson, B.D. (Eds.), *Exercise, Fitness, and Health: A Consensus of Current Knowledge* (pp.429–450). Champaign, IL: Human Kinetics.

Garfinkel, P., Garner, D., & Goldbloom, D. (1987). Eating disorders: implications for the 1990s. *Canadian Journal of Psychiatry, 32,* 624–630.

Green, D., Hebron, S., & Woodward, E. (1990). *Women's Leisure: What Leisure?* Basingstoke: Macmillan.

Green, E. (1998). 'Women doing friendship': an analysis of women's leisure as a site of identity construction, empowerment, and resistance. *Leisure Studies, 17,* 171–185.

Gudat, U., Berger, M., & Lefebvre, P.J. (1994). In Bouchard, C., Shephard, R.J., & Stephens, T. (Eds.), *Physical Activity, Fitness, and Health: International Proceedings and International Consensus Statement* (pp.669–683). Champaign, IL: Human Kinetics.

Hall, A., Slack, T., Smith, G., & Whitson, D. (1991). *Sport in Canadian Society.* Toronto: McClelland & Stewart.

Harrington, M., Dawson, D., & Bolla, P. (1992). Objective and subjective constraints on women's enjoyment of leisure. *Loisir et Société, 15,* 203–222.

Henderson, K.A. (1991). The contributions of feminism to an understanding of leisure constraints. *Journal of Leisure Research, 23,* 363–377.

Henderson, K.A., & Allen, K.R. (1991). *Loisir et Société, 14,* 97–113.

Henderson, K.A., & Bialeschki, M.D. (1991). A sense of entitlement to leisure as constraint and empowerment for women. *Leisure Sciences, 12,* 51–65.

Henderson, K.A., & Bialeschki, M.D. (1994). The meaning of physical recreation for women. *Women in Sport and Physical Activity Journal, 3,* 22–38.

Henderson, K.A., Bialeschki, M.D., Shaw, S.M., & Freysinger, V.J. (1996). *Both Gains and Gaps: Feminist Perspectives on Women's Leisure.* University Park, PA: Venture.

Hochschild, A. (1989). *The Second Shift.* New York: Viking.

Hull, R.B. (1991). Mood as a product of leisure: causes and consequences. In Driver, B.L., Brown, P.J., & Peterson, G.L. (Eds.), *Benefits of Leisure* (pp.249–262). State College, PA: Venture.

Iso-Ahola, S.E. (1980). *The Social Psychology of Leisure and Recreation.* Dubuque: William C. Brown.

Iwasaki, Y., & Mannell, R.C. (1998). In Bialeschki, M.D., & Stewart, W.P. (Eds.), *Symposium on Leisure Research.* Miami: National Recreation and Park Association.

Jackson, L.A., Sullivan, L.A., & Rostker, R. (1986). Gender, gender role, and body image. *Sex Roles, 19*, 429–443.

Kelly, J.R. (1983). *Leisure Identities and Interactions*. London: Allen & Unwin.

Koivula, N. (1995). Ratings of gender appropriateness of sports participation: effects of gender-based schematic processing. *Sex Roles, 33*, 543–557.

Mannell, R.C., & Kleiber, D.A. (1997). *A Social Psychology of Leisure*. Venture, State College, PA.

Marcus, B.H. (1995). Exercise behavior and strategies for intervention. *Research Quarterly for Exercise and Sport, 66*, 319–323.

Marcus, B.H., Pinto, B.M., Simkin, L.R., Audrain, J.E., & Taylor, E.R. (1994). Application of theoretical models to exercise behavior among employed women. *Journal of Health Promotion, 9*, 49–55.

Mazzeo, R.S., Cavanagh, P., Evans, W.J., Fiatarone, M., Hagberg, J., McAuley, E., & Startzelli, J. (1997). *Medicine and Science in Sports and Exercise, 29*, 992–1008.

Messner, M.A., & Sabo, D.F. (Eds.) (1990). *Sport, Men and the Gendered Order: Critical Feminist Perspectives*. Champaign, IL: Human Kinetics.

Polivy, J. (1994). In Bouchard, C., Shephard, R.J., & Stephens, T. (Eds.), *Physical Activity, Fitness, and Health: International Proceedings and International Consensus Statement* (pp.883–898). Champaign, IL: Human Kinetics.

Quaglietti, S., & Froelicher, V.F. (1994). In Bouchard, C., Shephard, R.J., & Stephens, T. (Eds.), *Physical Activity, Fitness, and Health: International Proceedings and International Consensus Statement* (pp.591–608). Champaign, IL: Human Kinetics.

Robinson, J.P., & Godbey, G. (1993). Sport, fitness, and the gender gap. *Leisure Sciences, 15*, 291–307.

Shank, J. (1986). An exploration of leisure in the lives of dual career women. *Journal of Leisure Research, 18*, 300–319.

Sharp, A., & Mannell, R.C. (1996). Participation in leisure as a coping strategy among bereaved women. In *Eighth Canadian Congress on Leisure Research* (pp.241–244). Ottawa: University of Ottawa.

Shaw, S.M. (1985). Gender and leisure: inequality in the distribution of leisure time. *Journal of Leisure Research, 17*, 266–282.

Shaw, S.M. (1994). Gender, leisure and constraint: towards a framework for the analysis of women's leisure. *Journal of Leisure Research, 26*, 8–22.

Shaw, S.M. (1996). The gendered nature of leisure: individual and societal outcomes of leisure practice. *World Leisure and Recreation Association Journal, 28*, 4–6.

Shaw, S.M., & Kemeny, L. (1989). Fitness promotion for adolescent girls: the impact and effectiveness of promotional material which emphasizes the slim ideal. *Adolescence, 24*, 677–687.

Shaw, S.M., Caldwell, L.L., & Kleiber, D.A. (1996). Stress and social control in the daily lives of adolescents. *Journal of Leisure Research, 28*, 274–292.

Sime, W.E. (1990). In Bouchard, C., Shephard, R.J., Stephens, T., Sutton, J.R., & McPherson, B.D. (Eds.), *Exercise, Fitness, and Health: A Consensus of Current Knowledge* (pp.627–633). Champaign, IL: Human Kinetics.

Statistics Canada (1993). *Changing the Landscape: Ending Violence – Achieving Equality*. Ottawa: Ministry of Supply and Services.

Statistics Canada (1995). *Women in Canada: A Statistical Report*. Ottawa: Statistics Canada.

Streather, J. (1979). In Coalter, F. (Ed.), *Freedom and Constraint: The Paradoxes of Leisure* (pp.175–186). New York: Routledge.

United States Department of Health and Human Services (USDHHS) (1996). *Physical Activity and Health: A Report of the Surgeon General*. Atlanta: US Department of Health and Human Services, Center for Disease Control and Prevention, and National Center for Chronic Disease Prevention and Health Promotion.

Vranic, M., & Wasserman, D. (1990). In Bouchard, C., Shephard, R.J., Stephens, J.R., Sutton, J.R., & McPherson, B.D. (Eds.), *Exercise, Fitness, and Health: A Consensus of Current Knowledge* (pp.467–490). Champaign, IL: Human Kinetics.

Wankel, L.M. (1993). The importance of enjoyment to adherence and psychological benefits from physical activity. *International Journal of Sport Psychology, 24*, 151–169.

Wearing, B. (1990). Beyond the ideology of motherhood: leisure as resistance. *Australian and New Zealand Journal of Sociology, 26*, 36–58.

Wells, C.L. (1996). Physical activity and women's health. *Physical Activity and Fitness Research Digest*, 1–8.

Whyte, L., & Shaw, S.M. (1994). Women's leisure: an exploratory study of fear of violence as a leisure constraint. *Journal of Applied Recreation Research, 19*, 5–21.

Wimbush, E. (1988). Mothers meeting. In Wimbush, E., & Talbot, M. (Eds.), *Relative Freedoms: Women and Leisure* (pp.60–74). Milton Keynes: Open University Press.

Chapter 20

Substance Abuse in Women: Biological, Psychological and Social Issues Related to Treatment

Gloria D. Eldridge

Jackson State University, USA

and

James M. Fitterling

G.V. (Sonny) Montgomery VA Medical Center, USA

Substance abuse has profound biological, psychological, and social consequences in the lives of women and in the lives of those close to them. Substance abuse includes illicit substances (e.g. heroin, inhalants, hallucinogens, cocaine, marijuana), and licit substances (e.g. alcohol, tobacco, prescription and over-the-counter medications). While tobacco use among women is a growing problem in many countries, this chapter will not address the problems of nicotine dependence. The chapter will first focus on key gender-specific aspects of substance abuse in women:

Women, Health and the Mind
Edited by L. Sherr and J.S. St Lawrence. © 2000 John Wiley & Sons, Ltd

prevalence, health and social consequences, treatment, and special issues such as stigma, pregnancy and parenting, relationships with men, childhood sexual abuse, violence, and co-morbid psychiatric disorders. The chapter will then describe several model programs for treatment of substance abuse in women. The chapter will conclude with a brief summary and analysis of substance abuse as a health concern for women. This chapter is based largely on research from the United States, but includes research from other countries to provide cross-cultural comparisons on key issues.

PREVALENCE OF SUBSTANCE USE, ABUSE, AND DEPENDENCE IN WOMEN

While cocaine abuse is the primary problem identified by most women in substance abuse treatment (Nardi, 1997; Wickizer et al., 1994), the most widely used and abused substance is alcohol (Substance Abuse and Mental Health Services Administration, 1993; 1995). In the United States, 79% of women report at least one-time use of alcohol (Substance Abuse and Mental Health Services Administration, 1993) and lifetime prevalence for alcohol dependence is 9.2% (Kandel et al., 1998). Lifetime use rates are markedly lower for other substances: 28% for marijuana, 10% for cocaine, and 15% for all other substances (Substance Abuse and Mental Health Services Administration, 1993). For women, substance use peaks between 18 and 25 years of age and then declines. Past year use of illicit substances is reported by 12% of females aged 12–17, 25% aged 18–25, 14% aged 26–34, and 4% over 34 years of age. At some point in their lives, one-fifth of females meet criteria for a diagnosis of substance abuse or dependence (Kandel et al., 1998). Once a woman has used any illicit drug, her risk of developing dependence is estimated at 1 in 7.5 (Anthony et al., 1994).

For all substances except legal psychoactive medications (e.g. tranquilizers, sedatives, and analgesics), men are more likely to be users and heavy users. For example, 39 longitudinal studies from 15 countries have shown that men are more likely to use alcohol, more likely to drink heavily, and more likely to have alcohol-related problems than women (Wilsnack et al., 1994). However, among women, lifetime use and abuse of legal psychoactive medications is twice that of men (Riska et al., 1993) and women are more likely to acquire these pharmaceuticals illegally if available. In Europe, compared with the United States, epidemiological studies of substance use seldom include legal psychotropic medications, resulting in an apparent disparity between female:male ratios of substance abuse in Europe and the United States. In Europe, the ratio of female:male substance abuse is estimated at 1:2, whereas female:male rates are estimated at 1:1.5 in the United States (Vogt, 1998).

HEALTH AND SOCIAL CONSEQUENCES OF SUBSTANCE USE

Health and social consequences of substance abuse are substantial for males and females; however, there are unique manifestations for females. For example, women are more vulnerable physiologically (Frezza et al., 1990) and cognitively (Acker, 1986) to the effects of alcohol. The negative physiological consequences of alcohol abuse, including hepatic disease, hypertension, obesity, anemia, malnutrition, reproductive dysfunction, gastrointestinal hemorrhage, and ulcers, appear earlier and are more severe in women (Lex, 1994; Schliebner, 1994; Schmidt et al., 1990). Alcohol interferes with the endocrine system and affects reproductive hormones such as progesterone and estrogens (Gavaler, 1991). Excessive alcohol consumption can reduce fertility, although the impact is less pronounced in women classified as "social drinkers" (Possati, 1992).

Substance use is linked to increased risk for sexually transmitted infections (STIs) and HIV infection in women. Women who abuse substances are more likely to have regular partners who also abuse substances, conferring added risk for STIs, HIV, and drug relapse (Lex, 1994). Among women in the United States, 44% of AIDS cases are attributed to injecting drug use and needle sharing; sex with an injecting drug user accounts for most of the 39% of cases attributed to heterosexual transmission (Centers for Disease Control and Prevention, 1997). Use of crack cocaine also increases risk for HIV and STIs among women, due to the frequent sex-for-drug transactions, with multiple, unknown, and high-risk partners, that are a staple of women's efforts to procure crack cocaine (Hser et al., 1999). In the United States, 91% of cases of pediatric AIDS are attributed to "mother with/at risk for HIV" (Centers for Disease Control and Prevention, 1997).

In the United States, a major consequence of the "war on drugs" is the increasing number of women in the criminal justice system (US Department of Justice, 1995). The proportion of women incarcerated for drug offenses is rising dramatically (Karan, 1989; Lex, 1994). Women who abuse crack cocaine are likely to have repeat criminal histories and to have committed their offenses, including prostitution and soliciting, to get money for drugs (El-Bassel et al., 1996). In contrast, in some European countries, prostitution is legal. Women who use substances in those countries can employ prostitution legally to procure money for drugs, and consequently, spend less time incarcerated and compelled to attend substance abuse treatment programs in the criminal justice system (Vogt, 1998).

Some European countries (e.g. The Netherlands, the United Kingdom, Switzerland) and Canada have begun to transform their public health and criminal justice policies and systems to approximate a harm-reduction model for addressing substance abuse. Although definitions and applications vary, harm reduction is a public health approach to

substance abuse intervention that places priority on reducing the negative effects of substance abuse rather than on eliminating substance use
entirely or enforcing abstinence (Marlatt, 1998). Examples of applications emanating from a harm reduction perspective include needle
exchange, drug decriminalization, prescription of abusable substances
for hard-core addicts, and moderation (as opposed to abstinence) treatment goals. Harm reduction goals and strategies are not inherently
gender-focused; however, they have the potential to ameliorate many
of the negative consequences associated with substance abuse in
women. For example, rates of AIDS and HIV-infection among injecting
drug users and their sex partners have been reduced dramatically by
needle-exchange programs (e.g. Buning et al., 1992) and maintenance
prescriptions of abusable drugs for hard-core addicts (e.g. Riley, 1994).

Relative to male substance abusers, women have more family problems associated with substance use, including distressed marriages and
relationships and problems with children (Schmidt et al., 1990).
Children of parents who abuse substances are at high risk for a variety
of medical and social problems, including vulnerability to substance
abuse, abuse and neglect, sexual abuse, hyperactivity, and conduct
disorder and delinquency (Deren, 1986; Kumpfer, 1987, 1998; Schuckit,
1992; Tarter & Mezzich, 1992).

In community samples, maternal substance abuse is common,
affecting over 10% of many obstetric populations (Glantz & Woods,
1993). Between 11 and 24% of pregnant women in the United States
use one or more illicit substances during pregnancy (Jansson et al.,
1996). Most drugs cross the placenta, leading to concerns about fetal
damage (Nardi, 1997). Despite an array of neurological and physiological deficits observed in infants born to women who used drugs
during pregnancy, it is difficult to attribute those deficits to prenatal
exposure to specific substances because of the confounding effects of
other substances, maternal malnutrition, stress, poverty, and poor
prenatal care (Day & Richardson, 1994; Jansson et al., 1996; van Baar
& de Graaff, 1994).

Contrary to popular wisdom, women who abuse substances come
from all races and socio-economic classes and, despite differences in
patterns of use, substance abuse occurs at similar rates among women
whether they are white or of color, well-resourced or impoverished
(Goldberg, 1995). However, substance abuse exerts a more negative
effect on the health and social functioning of low-income women and
women of color because they already have more health problems
and fewer resources.

SUBSTANCE ABUSE TREATMENT FOR WOMEN

Despite high lifetime prevalence and problems associated with substance abuse, women are under-represented in treatment (Schliebner,

1994). One reason for this may be that women are more likely to "self-change" and the majority of women who recover from substance abuse do so without treatment (Copeland, 1997). Yet, for women in traditional substance abuse treatment programs, retention rates are low and failure rates are high (Nelson-Zupko et al., 1995). Although one might conclude that women who abuse substances are unmotivated and resistant to treatment, another explanation is that traditional substance abuse treatment programs do not address the unique circumstances and needs of women (Hagan et al., 1994; Mondanaro, 1989). Of the more than 80 000 women in substance abuse treatment in the United States in 1990, only one-third were in treatment programs that offered special services for women (Wallen, 1998). Women typically receive substance abuse treatment – if at all – as a single component of a fragmented "system" of health and social services (Finkelstein, 1993). Wide gaps remain between services that are available and services that are needed by women who abuse substances.

Prior to the 1970s, the prevailing view among substance abuse researchers and treatment providers was that few females abused substances and those who did had no special needs or distinguishing features – aside from gender – from males who abused substances (Rosenbaum & Murphy, 1990). Virtually all substance abuse research and treatment was directed toward males. For example, early work by Jellinek (1946, 1952) was based on questionnaires from male members of Alcoholics Anonymous (AA). Questionnaires from female members of AA were not included because their responses differed markedly from the males (Fingarette, 1988; Jellinek, 1946, 1952, 1960).

In the 1970s, the "War on Drugs", the women's movement, and recognition of the health impact of prenatal drug exposure focused research, treatment, and funding on the problem of substance abuse in women (Finkelstein, 1993; Rosenbaum & Murphy, 1990). However, despite considerable strides in research and program development, most treatment programs in the United States are still based on methods and content developed for males (Duckert, 1987; Woodhouse, 1992) and many treatment providers still maintain that women who abuse substances do not differ from their male counterparts (Pursley-Crotteau & Stern, 1996). Male-oriented treatment models tend to be individualist medical or disease models that focus solely on addiction and exclude family and other system factors (Finkelstein, 1993, 1994). Often, other problems such as sexual abuse and ongoing family violence are considered distractions from the goal of recovery (Goldberg, 1995; Wallen, 1998; Zweben, 1996). Methods tend to be aggressive and confrontational, devoted to breaking down denial so the client can assume individual responsibility for her problem (Grella, 1996). However, aggressive confrontational models mimic patterns of dominance and victimization to which many women have been subjected (Kauffman et al., 1995). Consequently, many women are reluctant to enter confrontational treatment programs (Copeland, 1997), and many drop out (Zweben, 1996).

SPECIAL ISSUES FOR WOMEN IN SUBSTANCE ABUSE TREATMENT

Although special needs for women in substance abuse treatment are myriad, we will focus on several that have powerful effects on recruitment, retention, process, and outcome of treatment for women.

Stigmatization and Marginalization

Substance abuse is more stigmatizing for women than for men. Most societies disapprove more of alcohol consumption by females than by males (Gomberg, 1993) and women who use drugs are considered more deviant then men who use drugs (Sutker, 1987). For women, the social stigma surrounding substance abuse is associated with moral laxity, sexual promiscuity, and failure in prescribed feminine roles (Gomberg, 1993; Pursley-Crotteau & Stern, 1996). Intoxication in women runs counter to acceptable female roles and is perceived to be more disruptive of family life than intoxication in men (Schmidt et al., 1990). Women who drink too much are viewed as "tramps" who deserve to be used sexually (Goldberg, 1995). Even after treatment, female addicts are stigmatized more than their male counterparts (Rosenbaum & Murphy, 1990).

Friends and family members often support and help men who are seeking treatment for substance abuse (Robles et al., 1998). In contrast, friends and family members are more likely to fear reflected shame and social rejection and oppose women who are seeking treatment (Beckman & Amaro, 1986; Schliebner, 1994). In addition, health care and substance abuse treatment providers hold more negative perceptions of women who abuse substances, particularly those who are poor or homeless (Finkelstein, 1993). Women who abuse substances are viewed as dangerous, manipulative, and criminal. Their lack of education and resources is more likely to be seen as a consequence of addiction rather than as a contributing factor to addiction (Mason, 1996). When providers believe that substance abuse is "a hopeless condition of helpless people", "more a crime than a disease", and "a problem of the poor", they are less motivated to provide treatment to poor women who abuse substances (Woods, 1995, p.41). Even women who abuse substances share negative views of female intoxication (Gomberg, 1993) and view female addicts as more disgusting than male addicts (Goldberg, 1995). Many women avoid seeking treatment because of fear of stigmatization and feelings of guilt and shame (Copeland & Hall, 1992; O'Conner et al., 1994).

Stigmatization is more dramatic for pregnant women and women with children (Finkelstein, 1993). Women who use substances during pregnancy are viewed with repugnance. Treatment providers and society in general are powerfully "affected by the concept of an 'innocent baby' being 'abused' in utero by an 'unfeeling' or 'monstrous' mother" (Mason, 1996, p.29). This powerful distaste may result in legal sanctions (e.g. child custody loss, incarceration, or civil commitment) rather than treatment and assistance (Garcia, 1993, 1997; Paltrow, 1998; Robertson, 1991).

The extent to which female substance abusers are stigmatized and marginalized varies across cultures and may be related to prevalence rates of substance abuse among women in different countries (Vogt, 1998). European countries that have higher prevalence rates of substance abuse among women (e.g. Germany, Switzerland, The Netherlands) attend more to gender-specific issues than countries with lower prevalence rates (e.g. Spain). In different societies, views of women in general influence the stigmatization and marginalization of women who abuse substances. The extent of stigmatization is most dramatic in societies where women already have low status. For example, in Nigeria, traditional and contemporary views of women are characterized by rigid, narrow role expectations focused on fulfilling domestic responsibilities. Women are expected to "keep a humble and modest social outlook, and be more dedicated to making the home than anything else" (Ikuesan, 1994, p.941). While problem drinking among men may be condoned, drinking among women is viewed with opprobrium. Similarly, in Lesotho, women are responsible for managing households while men travel to neighboring South Africa for work. However, women are hostage to marriage laws that regard them as "children of their husbands" (Mphi, 1994). Married women who become problem drinkers can be discarded by their husbands and left without resources for economic survival. In these and other developing countries, women who abuse substances suffer more dramatically because of greater stigmatization and the corresponding dearth of treatment and social resources provided for them.

Pregnancy and Parenting

The peak years of substance use by women coincide with the peak years of child bearing (Kandel et al., 1998). Thirty-five percent of women in alcohol treatment programs are between 25 and 34 years of age, with 25% between 35 and 44 (Gomberg, 1994). Most women who seek treatment have children, many are pregnant, and many are single heads of household (Hagan et al., 1994; Schmidt et al., 1990). Most active female street addicts are mothers or are of child bearing age (Anglin et al., 1987).

Despite the prevailing view that women who abuse substances are uncaring mothers, many female substance abusers view their relationships with their children as their closest, most supportive, and most caring (Robles et al., 1998). Substance abuse may cause some women to neglect their children or divert resources from them (Woodhouse,

1992); however, most women who abuse substances are concerned for the welfare of their children (Nyamathi & Flaskerud, 1992) and want to create a better life for them. They fear their children may emulate their behavior (Woodhouse, 1992) and they feel guilty, ashamed, and inadequate as mothers (Nyamathi & Flaskerud, 1992; Wallen, 1998).

Children can be powerful motivators to seek and to remain in treatment (Wallen, 1998), and pregnancy is an especially powerful motivator (Baldwin et al., 1995). Many women want to "clean up" their addictions during pregnancy to avoid harm to their babies (Rosenbaum & Murphy, 1990). Pregnancy – a time when motivation is high and women may feel that a "new life" is possible for themselves and their children – can be an excellent time to recruit women into treatment (Pursley-Crotteau & Stern, 1996). However, it is unfortunate and ironic that most substance abuse treatment programs actually discourage pregnant women from entering treatment. For example, Chavkin (1990) reported that 54% of drug treatment programs in New York City did not accept pregnant women, 67% refused to treat pregnant women on Medicaid, and 87% refused to treat pregnant women on Medicaid who were addicted to cocaine. Pregnancy and responsibility for children, which otherwise could motivate treatment seeking, actually deter many women from seeking treatment for fear of precipitating child protection or custody actions (Copeland, 1997). In addition, many do not seek treatment because they cannot find safe child care while they are in treatment (Metsch et al., 1995; Nyamathi & Flaskerud, 1992). Few treatment centers accept pregnant women or accommodate needs for child care (Beckman & Kocel, 1982; Copeland et al., 1993; Goldberg, 1995). All of these barriers reduce treatment access for pregnant women and women with children (Klee et al., 1991).

Concern for the welfare of their children is strongly associated with positive treatment outcomes for women. Making provision for the children of women in substance abuse treatment has profound advantages. Services for children reduce stress and depression for women, facilitate recovery, and reduce relapse (Kumpfer et al., 1996). Treatment retention is enhanced by admitting children into residential treatment with their mothers (Wobie et al., 1997) and by providing free babysitting and transportation to the treatment program (Szuster et al., 1996). For many mothers, having their children with them decreases substance abuse and criminal behavior, increases employment, and improves parenting and parent–child relationships (Kumpfer, 1998). Conversely, after losing custody of their children, many women lose hope and drop out of treatment.

Pregnant women who abuse substances have less access to pharmacological treatment for substance abuse and other psychiatric disorders. Until 1993, pregnant women and women of child bearing age were excluded as subjects in medication research, in part because of fears of liability. Consequently, little information exists about bioavailability, metabolism, and clearance of medications and their relationship to pregnancy, menstruation, menopause, and hormone use. Yet, medications that have not been tested with pregnant women and women of child bearing potential are prescribed routinely (Zweben, 1996). Access to detoxification is also limited for pregnant women because of fears about the negative effects of detoxification and detoxification medications on the fetus. Since detoxification is a major point of entry into the substance abuse treatment system, limiting access to detoxification keeps many pregnant women out of treatment (Finkelstein, 1993).

There is great concern for the potential negative effects of intrauterine drug exposure, especially with respect to crack cocaine. However, other than Fetal Alcohol Syndrome (FAS), there is no clear relationship between drug use in pregnancy and poor outcomes for drug-exposed children (Day & Richardson, 1994). Many early deficits improve with time and adequate parenting (Black et al., 1993). Quality of the community and home environment, postnatal support of the mother, role of the father, maternal responsiveness to the child's needs, and personality and health characteristics of the mother may be more powerful in shaping child development than prenatal exposure to drugs (Wetherington et al., 1996). Indeed, there is growing evidence that a supportive and challenging environment may have a measurable positive effect on the development of drug-exposed infants (Wobie et al., 1997).

Nevertheless, women who use substances during pregnancy are assumed to be guilty of child neglect or abuse (Goldberg, 1995), and pregnant women and their fetuses have been forced to become legal adversaries. Although apparently well-intentioned, there is some question whether charging women with child abuse or neglect serves more to punish the woman for substance abuse than to protect her fetus (Garcia, 1993, 1997; Paltrow, 1998; Robertson, 1991). In the United States, more than 200 women in 30 states have been prosecuted for "fetal abuse", delivery of drugs through the umbilical cord, assault with a deadly weapon (cocaine), and contributing to the delinquency of a minor. Pregnant women face the threat of civil commitment and incarceration for minor offenses for the sole purpose of protecting their fetuses from potential harm. Ironically, the health of a woman and her child may be jeopardized more by putting her in jail where drugs are more available than treatment and prenatal care. In most cases, these judgments have been deemed to violate the woman's right to privacy and due process and appeal judges have ruled that states can protect fetal health through less restrictive means, including education, medical care, and drug treatment for pregnant women. However, the unintended effect of using legal sanctions to prevent drug use in pregnancy has been to make pregnant women avoid prenatal or medical care and drug treatment for fear of being detected and prosecuted (Paltrow, 1998; Robertson, 1991; Robles et al., 1998).

Urine toxicology at delivery shows little variation in rates of substance use by white women, women of color, or women in public and private health facilities (Goldberg, 1995). Indeed, most women who use illicit drugs while pregnant are white (Paltrow, 1998). However, women of color and women delivering in public hospitals serving poor and minority women are more likely to be tested for drugs (Robertson, 1991) and more likely to be subject to criminal charges and child protection interventions (Goldberg, 1995). In one Florida county, Black women were 10 times more likely than White women to be reported to authorities following a positive urine toxicology (Chasnoff et al., 1990). In many areas of the United States, newborns have been apprehended after a single positive drug test, without evaluation of the mother's ability to care for the child (Garcia, 1993, 1997; Paltrow, 1998).

Relationships with Men

Women have less access to social and economic resources and often depend on other individuals (e.g. husband, boyfriend) or institutions (e.g. welfare) for economic survival. Dependency gives rise to a lack of empowerment, problem-solving and decision-making skills, and self-confidence. Substance abuse exacerbates the dependency-related problems that many women face. Women who abuse substances are more impoverished personally and economically than men who abuse substances (Hagan et al., 1994).

Most drug-abusing women are introduced to drugs by men and get their drugs from men (Amaro & Hardy-Fanta, 1995; Woodhouse, 1992). Most are introduced to hard drugs by male partners in the context of new relationships, dating, and parties. Many women seek male partners who can supply them with drugs, and drug-related activities are a major source of connection with their partners (Amaro & Hardy-Fanta, 1995). Having a partner who abuses substances is more likely to lead to substance abuse in women than it is in men (Wilsnack & Wilsnack, 1991). Women are more tolerant of the behavior of men who use substances and less likely to divorce alcoholic husbands than husbands are to divorce alcoholic wives (Lex, 1994). Partner support is important in recovery (Anglin et al., 1987), yet few women get support from partners, and many get strong and persistent opposition. Male partners are more likely than female partners to oppose treatment (Beckman & Amaro, 1986), and relapse is more likely if women return to non-supportive partners (Amaro & Hardy-Fanta, 1995).

Drug abuse often takes place in relationships where needs for love, caring, and intimacy conflict with desires to stop substance use. Women who abuse substances often come from families filled with "conflict, chaos, inconsistency, unpredictability, anger, violence, and incest". Consequently, "many women feel powerlessness, depression, anxiety, low self-esteem and isolation, and describe their lives ... filled with many losses or disconnections" (Finkelstein & Piedade, 1993, p.9). Women who abuse substances often view themselves as dependent on men, without an identity except in their relationships with men

(Woodhouse, 1992). Letting go of even non-supportive relationships is difficult, and even if women recognize the harm in those relationships, they feel connected to partners who fathered their children and with whom they shared hard times (Amaro & Hardy-Fanta, 1995).

For many women, access to drugs is through men who have access to money, power, and drugs. Women attempt to manipulate this uneven relationship to their best advantage (Murphy & Rosenbaum, 1992), often by using sex in exchange for drugs and money. The toll in humiliation, abuse, and rape which they suffer from partners, customers, and men on the streets is a central theme in substance abuse treatment for women and a challenge to recovery (Amaro & Hardy-Fanta, 1995).

Childhood Sexual Abuse

Childhood sexual abuse (CSA) is an important risk factor for substance abuse in women (Miller & Downs, 1993; Miller et al., 1993). Women with a history of CSA are more likely to report substance abuse (Wilsnack et al., 1997). Women in substance abuse treatment have higher rates of CSA than women in the general population (Miller et al., 1987). Compared with women who were not sexually abused, women who have been sexually abused start using drugs at an earlier age (12.6 versus 17 years) and are more likely to have family members who were also addicted (Teets, 1995). Lifetime rates of substance abuse and dependence are higher for women who have experienced sexual assault (18.4 and 20.4%, respectively) than for women who have not experienced sexual assault (13.8 and 5.5%; Burnam et al., 1988).

If CSA is not addressed in substance abuse treatment, women experience more anxiety and depression early in recovery, have more problems maintaining early sobriety, and are more vulnerable to relapse (Kovach, 1986; Zweben, 1996). Yet, fewer than 20% of substance abuse treatment programs offer specialized services for CSA (Yandow, 1989). Women with histories of CSA may not be identified because their symptoms are not severe enough for a diagnosis of post-traumatic stress disorder (Pearce & Lovejoy, 1995), and many women do not disclose CSA unless queried directly (Bollerud, 1990). Often, treatment programs avoid mention of CSA because of concern that the client will be distracted from dealing with her addiction. However, deferring therapy for the consequences of CSA until abstinence is achieved actually increases the likelihood of treatment failure. Beginning early in treatment, women should be encouraged to address CSA with a goal of managing their feelings about CSA without reverting to drugs or alcohol (Zweben, 1996).

Violence

Higher lifetime rates of alcohol abuse and dependence are associated with severe traumatic events, including criminal victimization (Kilpatrick et al., 1998). Women in alcohol treatment experience higher levels of severe partner violence than women in the general population (Miller & Downs, 1993). A woman's risk of violent assault while pregnant doubles if her partner uses illicit drugs, and for women who exchange sex for money or drugs, the risk of violence is greater from partners than from "clients" (Amaro et al., 1990). Eighty percent of women in substance abuse treatment have experienced severe violence at the hands of their partners, with 26% of women experiencing severe partner violence in the preceding 6 months. For many women who abuse substances, severe partner violence occurs even while they are in treatment, affecting the course of treatment and increasing the probability of relapse (North et al., 1996).

The illicit drug culture is particularly dangerous for women (Kilpatrick et al., 1997). For example, procuring crack cocaine often involves sex-for-drugs exchanges where women experience rape, other physical and sexual abuse, and victimization (Fullilove et al., 1992). Women may use crack as their only available and effective means to relieve depression or trauma. Yet, in the course of their efforts to procure the drug, they become further victimized, leading to a vicious cycle of trauma, depression, substance use, and victimization (Nyamathi & Flaskerud, 1992).

Does substance abuse make women more vulnerable to victimization and violence, or do victimization and violence make women more vulnerable to substance abuse? In a prospective study, Kilpatrick et al. (1997) examined the temporal relationship between violent assault and substance use. Among women with no previous history of substance use or assault, being assaulted increased the probability of subsequent alcohol and drug abuse. Among women with a history of substance abuse, current drug use – but not current alcohol use – increased the probability of a subsequent assault. The risk of assault was greatest for women who used drugs and who had already been assaulted.

Screening and treating women for assault-related psychological problems might enhance the impact of substance abuse treatment (Kilpatrick et al., 1998) and reduce the likelihood of future victimization (Kilpatrick et al., 1997). Assault victims, especially those with a family history of substance abuse, are at high risk for substance abuse. Women who abuse substances are at high risk for assault, further increasing risk for alcohol and drug problems. Despite this relationship between substance abuse and violence, few substance abuse treatment facilities address the problem of violence and most shelters for abused women do not serve women with active alcohol or drug problems (Robertson, 1991).

Co-morbid Psychiatric Disorders

Co-morbid psychiatric disorders are common in males and females who abuse substances. However, women are more likely to present with affective disorders, and men are more likely to be diagnosed with anti-social personality disorder (Kessler et al., 1994). Low self-esteem, depression, suicide attempts, and hospitalization for other psychiatric problems are common in women with substance abuse disorders (Klee et al., 1991; Schmidt et al., 1990). Among women, depression precedes drinking problems in 66% of cases of co-morbid depression and alcoholism (Helzer et al., 1991). Depression is cited by 88% of women as a reason for entering substance abuse treatment (Gomberg, 1993), and untreated depression increases treatment attrition (Williams & Roberts, 1991). More than half the drug-related suicide attempts seen in Emergency Rooms are among women, and, in these circumstances, women are more likely than men to complete a suicide attempt (National Institute on Drug Abuse, 1992).

MODEL PROGRAMS FOR WOMEN WHO ABUSE SUBSTANCES

The previous sections of the chapter have illustrated the range of consequences – biological, social, and psychological – associated with substance abuse in women, as well as the special strengths, constraints, and needs that women bring to substance abuse treatment. Substance abuse has serious physical, emotional, and reproductive health consequences for women. Women who abuse substances are at greater risk for STIs and HIV infection. The social consequences of substance abuse – disrupted families, vulnerable children, and increased risk for incarceration – are enormous, as are the psychological consequences. Women who abuse substances are often survivors of CSA and are vulnerable to assault and violence, frequently from their partners.

Although the majority of women recover from substance abuse problems without treatment, many women require treatment. Unfortunately, most substance abuse treatment models are based on the experiences and needs of male substance abusers, and women face formidable barriers getting access to appropriate treatment. Barriers range from the stigma faced by women who abuse substances, to lack of support from friends and family members and partners, to a scarcity of resources for pregnant women and women with children. However, in response to a growing recognition of these special needs of women who abuse substances, efforts have begun to develop gender-specific programs for the treatment of substance abuse. One area of particular focus has been on an especially vulnerable subset of women who abuse substances – women who have children and/or are pregnant. As one example of the response to this need, the Center for Substance Abuse Treatment

(CSAT) and the National Institute on Drug Abuse (NIDA) in the United States co-sponsored a series of demonstration projects focusing on substance abuse treatment for pregnant and perinatal women and their drug-exposed children (Rahdert, 1996). These and other funding initiatives have led to a growing number of model programs for women who abuse substances. Table 20.1 summarizes the essential components of four model programs developed in the United States.

The most significant feature of these programs is the recognition that substance abuse, while a central focus of treatment, is only one aspect of a constellation of problems faced by women who abuse substances. Effective treatment for substance abuse requires a holistic approach with diverse services integrated into programs tailored for the needs of individual women. A second significant feature is the recognition that the majority of women who abuse substances are of child bearing age, have children, or are pregnant. For many women who abuse substances, responsibility for children is a central and vitally important feature of their lives. Consequently, these model programs make provision for care and services for children in addition to substance abuse treatment for the mother. Family-oriented programs must deal with additional – and often more complex – problems than those encountered with other substance abuse treatment populations. Problems included child custody, intensive child care in the event of the mother's hospitalization, child abuse reporting, and determining the range and degree of illnesses of the mother and child(ren) that the program can accommodate. These additional considerations serve as formidable barriers to making a family-oriented treatment program a realistic option for this needy population (Metsch et al., 1995).

A third significant feature of these model programs is the development of strong collaborative agreements and partnerships with a wide variety of public and private agencies. A single program would have difficulty in meeting the diverse needs of women who abuse substances; therefore, aggressive collaboration is necessary to provide the diversity and magnitude of resources to address their needs adequately. Thus, an important focus of intervention is coordinating an array of diverse and often disconnected agencies and other resources to address problems that comprise the social context in which women substance abusers and their families live.

CONCLUSIONS

Progress is being made in basic research and the development and evaluation of gender-specific treatment programs for women who abuse substances. In recent years, there has been a dramatic increase in research and community demonstration projects focusing on this important and historically overlooked population. Some studies have identified the specific and varied biopsychosocial needs of this special

Table 20.1   Model programs for women substance abusers

Program and reference	Description
Dena A Coy (Namyniuk et al., 1997)	Clients are pregnant and parenting Alaskan native women and their children Goals centered on family preservation: decrease substance abuse, improve physical and mental health of mothers and children, enhance socio-economic resources of the family, decrease criminal activity, improve mother–child relationship, prevent similar problems among children Women and children live on-site in a therapeutic community Culturally-sensitive treatment is ensured by recruiting and training staff for cultural sensitivity and diversity Program is family-oriented; parenting education and support are provided Physical and mental health needs of mother and child are addressed Childhood sexual abuse and violence are addressed in psychotherapy Special treatment, such as self-esteem groups to address women's dependency-related problems, is offered Service barriers reduced by aggressive outreach and collaboration with other community agencies
PROTOTYPES (Mosley, 1996)	Clients are dually diagnosed perinatal drug abusers in Los Angeles Urban model for reducing barriers to treatment: (a) diverse services are located in a central facility for "one-stop shopping", and (b) program is located in an urban area with convenient access by public transportation Ongoing cross-training of staff (e.g. HIV/AIDS, domestic violence) to integrate treatment for diverse problems in addition to substance abuse
Fresno County Mental Health Department (Ryland & Lucas, 1996)	Clients are pregnant and parenting dually diagnosed women and their children Rural model for reducing service access barriers due to poverty, minimal public transit, and geographical dispersion of services in a sparsely populated area Case managers co-ordinate a system of services from contracted agencies Program provides home visits and transportation of women and children to services Access barriers reduced by a major revision to the clinic-based model of health care reimbursement by the state; new policies allow payment for transportation and home visits
Options For Recovery (Brindis et al., 1997a,b)	Clients are pregnant and parenting women and their children Goals: decrease substance abuse, connect women with essential services, increase family reunification, enhance perinatal recovery and child health Used trained, culturally appropriate foster care parents for infants with special needs to reduce multiple foster care placements until family reunified Model designed through collaboration with service providers, experts and policy makers

population. Other studies have identified and described gender-based treatment barriers across individual, cultural, economic, and social domains. Still others have provided promising results attesting to the efficacy of model treatment programs for various subpopulations of women substance abusers.

These developments represent significant breakthroughs in understanding and addressing the problem of substance abuse among women. However, much remains to be accomplished. Despite their efficacy, model programs are resource intensive. The high cost of such care will be a significant impediment to these programs becoming realities for this population. The applications learned from these treatment efficacy studies must be implemented in ways that are available, accessible, and able to survive in the context of prevailing health care systems. Cost-effectiveness research is needed to assess and measure the cost of treatment relative to savings in costs for health-care, criminal justice, child welfare, and social assistance. Once cost-effectiveness is established, legislative action and agency policy formulation will be necessary to redefine "the system" and reallocate resources to support its operation. (Unfortunately, it is hard to place a monetary value on many of the more significant costs of substance abuse, such as family disruption and misery.)

Assuming that gender-specific programs will be funded and will survive in the real world, comprehensive, family-focused programs alone will still be insufficient for addressing the problem of substance abuse in women. Some visionary program developers and administrators have seen the value in providing cross-training to their clinical staff in domains outside their own area of training (e.g. substance abuse and mental health). Similar "cross-training" and education of policy makers and agency officials is needed to provide a better understanding of the complexity and breadth of the problems facing this population, of which substance abuse is only one aspect. Substance abuse treatment must be considered as only one part of a larger, comprehensive initiative that includes prevention at individual, familial, and social levels. Such an initiative must identify and address the social, economic, and legal factors that contribute to the development and persistence of this major public health problem. For this to occur, the problem of substance abuse among women must attain sufficient political, social, economic, and cultural importance to be accorded the level of attention and corresponding commitment of resources to make a real impact. Given the degree of stigma directed toward women who abuse substances, this will be a formidable task for the years ahead.

ACKNOWLEDGEMENTS

This work was supported by grant DA10418 from the National Institute on Drug Abuse at the National Institutes of Health to Gloria D. Eldridge, Ph.D., and in part, by a Veterans Integrated Service Network 16 Mental

Illness Research Education and Clinical Center Award for James M. Fitterling, Ph.D. Address correspondence to Gloria D. Eldridge, Ph.D., Community Health Program, Jackson State University, P.O. Box 17005, Jackson, MS USA 39217. E-mail: eldridge@netdoor.com.

REFERENCES

Acker, C. (1986). Neuropsychological deficits in alcoholics: the relative contributions of gender and drinking history. *British Journal of Addiction*, *81*, 395–403.

Amaro, H., Fried, L., Cabral, H., & Zuckerman, B. (1990). Violence during pregnancy: the relationship to drug use among women and their partners. *American Journal of Public Health*, *80*, 575–579.

Amaro, H., & Hardy-Fanta, C. (1995). Gender relations in addiction and recovery. *Journal of Psychoactive Drugs*, *27*, 325–337.

Anglin, M.D., Hser, Y., & Booth, M.W. (1987). Sex differences in addict careers. IV. Treatment. *American Journal of Drug and Alcohol Abuse*, *13*, 253–280.

Anthony, J., Warner, L., & Kessler, R. (1994). Comparative epidemiology of dependence on tobacco, alcohol, controlled substances, and inhalants: Basic findings from the National Comorbidity Survey. *Experimental and Clinical Psychopharmacology*, *2*, 244–268.

Baldwin, D.M., Brecht, M.L., Monahan, G., Annon, K., Wellisch, J., & Anglin, M.D. (1995). Perceived need for treatment among pregnant and nonpregnant women arrestees. *Journal of Psychoactive Drugs*, *27*, 389–399.

Beckman, L., & Amaro, H. (1986). Personal and social difficulties faced by women and men entering alcoholism treatment. *Journal of Studies on Alcohol*, *47*, 220–228.

Beckman, L., & Kocel, K. (1982). The treatment delivery system and alcohol abuse in women: social policy implications. *Journal of Social Issues*, *38*, 139–152.

Black, M., Schuler, M., & Nair, P. (1993). Prenatal drug exposure: neurodevelopmental outcome and parenting environment. *Journal of Pediatric Psychology*, *18*, 605–620.

Bollerud, K. (1990). A model for the treatment of trauma-related syndromes among chemically dependent inpatient women. *Journal of Substance Abuse Treatment*, *7*, 83–87.

Brindis, C.D., Berkowitz, G., Clayson, Z., & Lamb, B. (1997a). California's approach to perinatal substance abuse: toward a model of comprehensive care. *Journal of Psychoactive Drugs*, *29*, 113–122.

Brindis, C.D., Clayson, Z., & Berkowitz, G. (1997b). Options for recovery: California's perinatal projects. *Journal of Psychoactive Drugs*, *29*, 89–99.

Buning, E.C., Brussel, G.V., & Santen, G.B. (1992). The impact of harm reduction drug policy on AIDS prevention in Amsterdam. In O'Hare,

P., Newcomb, R., Matthews, A., Buning, E.C., & Drucker, E. (Eds.), *The Reduction of Drug Related Harm* (pp.30–38). London: Routledge.

Burnam, J.A., Stein, J.A., Golding, J.M., Siegel, J.M., Sorenson, S.B., Forsythe, A.B., & Telles, C.A. (1988). Sexual assault and mental health disorders in a community population. *Journal of Consulting and Clinical Psychology, 56*, 843–850.

Centers for Disease Control and Prevention (1997). *HIV/AIDS Surveillance Report, 9*, 12.

Chasnoff, I.J., Landress, H.J., & Barrett, M.E. (1990). The prevalence of illicit-drug or alcohol use during pregnancy and discrepancies in mandatory reporting in Pinellas County, Florida. *New England Journal of Medicine, 322*, 1202–1206.

Chavkin, W. (1990). Drug addiction and pregnancy: policy crossroads. *American Journal of Public Health, 80*, 483–487.

Copeland, J. (1997). A qualitative study of barriers to formal treatment among women who self-managed change in addictive behaviours. *Journal of Substance Abuse Treatment, 14*, 183–190.

Copeland, J., & Hall, W. (1992). A comparison of women seeking drug and alcohol treatment in a specialist women's and two traditional mixed-sex treatment services. *British Journal of Addiction, 87*, 1293–1302.

Copeland, J., Hall, W., & Didcott, P. (1993). Comparison of a specialist women's alcohol and other drug service with two traditional mixed-sex services: client characteristics and treatment outcome. *Drug and Alcohol Dependence, 32*, 81–92.

Day, N.L., & Richardson, G.A. (1994). Comparative teratogenicity of alcohol and other drugs. *Alcohol Health and Research World, 18*, 42–48.

Deren, S. (1986). Children of substance abusers: a review of the literature. *Journal of Substance Abuse and Treatment, 3*, 77–94.

Duckert, F. (1987). Recruitment into treatment and effects of treatment for female problem drinkers. *Addictive Behavior, 12*, 137–150.

El-Bassel, N., Gilbert, L., Schilling, R., Ivanoff, A., & Borne, D. (1996). Correlates of crack abuse among drug-using incarcerated women: Psychological trauma, social support, and coping behavior. *American Journal of Drug and Alcohol Abuse, 22*, 41–56.

Fingarette, H. (1988). *Heavy Drinking: The Myth of Alcoholism as a Disease.* Berkeley, CA: University of California Press.

Finkelstein, N. (1993). Treatment programming for alcohol and drug-dependent pregnant women. *The International Journal of the Addictions, 28*, 1275–1309.

Finkelstein, N. (1994). Treatment issues for alcohol- and drug-dependent pregnant and parenting women. *Health and Social Work, 19*, 7–15.

Finkelstein, N., & Piedade, E. (1993). The relational-model and the treatment of addicted females. *The Counselor Magazine*, May–June, 8–11.

Frezza, M., DiPadova, C., Pozzato, G., Terpin, M., Baraona, E., & Lieber, C. (1990). High blood alcohol levels in women: the role of decreased gastric alcohol dehydrogenase activity to first-pass metabolism. *New England Journal of Medicine*, 322, 95–99.

Fullilove, M.T., Lown, E.A., & Fullilove, R.E. (1992). Crack 'hos and skeezers: traumatic experiences of women crack users. *The Journal of Sex Research*, 29, 275–287.

Garcia, S.A. (1993). Maternal drug abuse: laws and ethics as agents of just balances and therapeutic interventions. *The International Journal of the Addictions*, 28, 1311–1339.

Garcia, S.A. (1997). Ethical and legal issues associated with substance abuse by pregnant and parenting women. *Journal of Psychoactive Drugs*, 29, 101–111.

Gavaler, J.S. (1991). Effects of alcohol on female endocrine function. *Alcohol Health & Research World*, 15, 104–108.

Glantz, J.C., & Woods, J.R. (1993). Cocaine, heroin, and phencyclidine: Obstetric perspectives. *Clinical Obstetrics and Gynecology*, 36, 279–301.

Goldberg, M. (1995). Substance-abusing women: false stereotypes and real needs. *Social Work*, 40, 789–798.

Gomberg, E. (1993). Women and alcohol: use and abuse. *The Journal of Nervous and Mental Disease*, 181, 211–219.

Gomberg, E. (1994). Risk factors for drinking over a woman's life span. *Alcohol Health and Research World*, 18, 220–227.

Grella, C. (1996). Background and overview of mental health and substance abuse treatment systems: meeting the needs of women who are pregnant or parenting. *Journal of Psychoactive Drugs*, 28, 319–343.

Hagan, T.A., Finnegan, L.P., & Nelson-Zlupko, L. (1994). Impediments to comprehensive treatment models for substance-dependent women: treatment and research questions. *Journal of Psychoactive Drugs*, 26, 163–171.

Helzer, J., Burnam, A., & McEvoy, L. (1991). Alcohol abuse and dependence. In Robins, L., and Regier, D. (Eds.), *Psychiatric Disorders in America: The Epidemiologic Catchment Area Study* (pp.81–115). New York: Free Press.

Hser, Y., Chou, C., Hoffman, V., & Anglin, M. (1999). Cocaine use and high-risk sexual behavior among STD clinic patients. *Sexually Transmitted Diseases*, 26, 82–86.

Ikuesan, B.A. (1994). Drinking problems and the position of women in Nigeria. *Addiction*, 89, 941–944.

Jansson, L.M., Svikis, D., Lee, J., Paluzzi, P., Rutigliano, P., & Hackerman, F. (1996). Pregnancy and addiction: a comprehensive care model. *Journal of Substance Abuse Treatment*, 13, 321–329.

Jellinek, E. (1946). Phases in the drinking history of alcoholics – analysis of a survey conducted by the official organ of Alcoholics Anonymous. *Quarterly Journal of Studies in Alcohol*, 7, 1–88.

Jellinek, E. (1952). The phases of alcohol addiction. *Quarterly Journal of Studies in Alcohol*, 13, 673–684.

Jellinek, E. (1960). *The Concept of Alcoholism*. New Haven: Hilhouse Press.

Kandel, D.B., Warner, L.A., & Kessler, R.C. (1998). The epidemiology of substance use and dependence among women. In Wetherington, C., & Roman, A. (Eds.), *Drug Addiction Research and the Health of Women* (pp.105–130). Rockville, MD: National Institute on Drug Abuse.

Karan, L.D. (1989). AIDS prevention and chemical dependence treatment needs of women and their children. *Journal of Psychoactive Drugs*, *21*, 395–399.

Kauffman, E., Dore, M.M., & Nelson-Zlupko, L. (1995). The role of women's therapy groups in the treatment of chemical dependence. *American Journal of Orthopsychiatry*, *65*, 355–363.

Kessler, R.C., McGonagle, K.A., Zhao, S., Nelson, C.B., Hughes, M., Eshleman, S., Wittchen, H.U., & Kandler, K.S. (1994). Lifetime and 12-month prevalence of DSM-III-R psychiatric disorders in the United States. *Archives of General Psychiatry*, *51*, 8–19.

Kilpatrick, D.G., Acierno, R., Resnick, H.S., Saunders, B.E., & Best, C.L. (1997). A 2-year longitudinal analysis of the relationships between violent assault and substance use in women. *Journal of Consulting and Clinical Psychology*, *65*, 834–847.

Kilpatrick, D., Resnick, H., Saunders, B., & Best, C. (1998). Victimization, post traumatic stress disorder, and substance use and abuse among women. In Wetherington, C., & Roman, A. (Eds.), *Drug Addiction Research and the Health of Women* (pp.285–307). Rockville, MD: National Institute on Drug Abuse.

Klee, L., Schmidt, C., & Ames, G. (1991). Indicators of women's alcohol problems: what women themselves report. *The International Journal of the Addictions*, *26*, 879–895.

Kovach, J. (1986). Incest as a treatment issue for alcoholic women. *Alcoholism Treatment Quarterly*, *3*, 1–15.

Kumpfer, K.L. (1987). Special populations: etiology and prevention of vulnerability to chemical dependency in children of substance abusers. In Brown, B., & Mills, A. (Eds.), *Youth at High Risk for Substance Abuse* (pp.1–71). Washington, DC: National Institute on Drug Abuse.

Kumpfer, K.L. (1998). Links between prevention and treatment for drug-abusing women and their children. In Wetherington, C., & Roman, A. (Eds.), *Drug Addiction Research and the Health of Women* (pp.417–437). Rockville, MD: National Institute on Drug Abuse.

Kumpfer, K.L., Molgaard, V., & Spoth, R. (1996). Family interventions for the prevention of delinquency and drug use in special populations. In de Peters, R.V., & McMahon, R. (Eds.), *Preventing Childhood Disorders, Substance Abuse, and Delinquency* (pp.241–267). Thousand Oaks, CA: Sage.

Lex, B.W. (1994). Alcohol and other drug abuse among women. *Alcohol Health and Research World*, *18*, 212–219.

Marlatt, G.A. (Ed.) (1998). *Harm Reduction: Pragmatic Strategies for Managing High-risk Behaviors*. New York: The Guilford Press.

Mason, E. (1996). Conducting a treatment research project in a medical center-based program for chemically dependent pregnant women. In Rahdert, E. (Ed.), *Treatment for Drug-Exposed Women and Their Children: Advances in Research Methodology (NIDA Research Monograph 166)*. Rockville, MD: US Department of Health and Human Services.

Metsch, L.R., Rivers, J.E., Miller, M., Bohs, R., McCoy, C.B., Morrow, C.J., Bandstra, E.S., Jackson, V., & Gissen, M. (1995). Implementation of a family-centered treatment program for substance-abusing women and their children: barriers and resolutions. *Journal of Psychoactive Drugs, 27*, 73–83.

Miller, J. (1986). *Toward a New Psychology of Women*, 2nd Edition. Boston, MA: Beacon Press.

Miller, B.A., & Downs, W.R. (1993). The impact of family violence on the use of alcohol by women. *Alcohol Health and Research World, 17*, 137–143.

Miller, B.A., Downs, W.R., Gondoli, D.M., & Keil, A. (1987). The role of childhood sexual abuse in the development of alcoholism in women. *Violence and Victims, 2*, 157–171.

Miller, B.A., Downs, W.R., & Testa, M. (1993). Interrelationships between victimization experiences and women's alcohol use. *Journal of Studies on Alcohol, (Suppl 11)*, 109–117.

Mondanaro, J. (1989). *Chemically Dependent Women*. Lexington, MA: Lexington Books.

Mosley, T.M. (1996). PROTOTYPES: an urban model program of treatment and recovery services for dually diagnosed perinatal program participants. *Journal of Psychoactive Drugs, 28*, 381–388.

Mphi, M. (1994). Female alcoholism problems in Lesotho. *Addiction, 89*, 945–949.

Murphy, S., & Rosenbaum, M. (1992). Women who use cocaine too much: smoking crack vs. snorting cocaine. *Journal of Psychoactive Drugs, 24*, 381–388.

Namyniuk, L., Brems, C., & Carson, S. (1997). Southcentral Foundation – Dena A Coy: a model program for the treatment of pregnant substance-abusing women. *Journal of Substance Abuse Treatment, 14*, 285–295.

Nardi, D.A. (1997). Risk factors, attendance, and abstinence patterns of low-income women in perinatal addiction treatment: lessons from a 5-year program. *Issues in Mental Health Nursing, 18*, 125–138.

National Institute on Drug Abuse (1992). Annual Emergency Room Data, 1991. Series 1, No. 11A. DHHS Pub. No.(ADM) 92–1955. Washington, DC: US Government Printing Office.

Nelson-Zlupko, L., Kauffman, E., & Dore, M.M. (1995). Gender differences in drug abuse and treatment: implications for social work intervention with substance abusing women. *Social Work, 40*, 45–54.

North, C., Thompson, S., Smith, E., & Kyburz, L. (1996). Violence in the lives of homeless mothers in a substance abuse treatment program: a descriptive study. *Journal of Interpersonal Violence, 11*, 234–249.

Nyamathi, A., & Flaskerud, J. (1992). A community-based inventory of current concerns of impoverished homeless and drug-addicted minority women. *Research in Nursing and Health, 15,* 121–129.

O'Conner, L., Berry, J., Inaba, D., Weiss, J., & Morrison, A. (1994). Shame, guilt, and depression in men and women in recovery from addiction. *Journal of Substance Abuse Treatment, 11,* 503–510.

Paltrow, L.M. (1998). Punishing women for their behavior during pregnancy: an approach that undermines the health of women and children. In Wetherington, C., & Roman, A. (Eds.), *Drug Addiction Research and the Health of Women* (pp.467–501). Rockville, MD: National Institute on Drug Abuse.

Pearce, E.J., & Lovejoy, F.H. (1995). Detecting a history of childhood sexual experiences among women substance abusers. *Journal of Substance Abuse Treatment, 12,* 283–287.

Possati, G. (1992). Chronic alcohol intake and infertility. *Alcologia, 4,* 11–12.

Pursley-Crotteau, S., & Stern, P. (1996). Creating a new life: dimensions of temperance in perinatal cocaine crack users. *Qualitative Health Research, 6,* 350–367.

Rahdert, E.R. (1996). Introduction to the Perinatal-20 Treatment Research Demonstration Program. In Rahdert, E.R. (Ed.), *Treatment for Drug-Exposed Women and Their Children: Advances in Research Methodology (NIDA Research Monograph 166)* (pp.1–4). Washington, DC: US Government Printing Office.

Riley, D. (1994). *The Harm Reduction Model: Pragmatic Approaches to Drug Use from the Area Between Intolerance and Neglect.* Ottawa: Canadian Centre on Substance Abuse.

Riska, E., Kühlhorn, E., Nordlund, S., & Skinhoj, K.T. (Eds.) (1993). *Minor Tranquilizers in the Nordic Countries.* Helsinki: Nordic Council for Alcohol and Drug Research.

Robertson, M. (1991). Homeless women with children: The role of alcohol and other drug abuse. *American Psychologist, 46,* 1198–1204.

Robles, R., Marrero, C., Matos, T., Colon, H., Cancel, L., & Reyes, J. (1998). Social and behavioral consequences of chemical dependence. In Wetherington, C., & Roman, A. (Eds.), *Drug Addiction Research and the Health of Women* (pp.355–364). Rockville, MD: National Institute on Drug Abuse.

Rosenbaum, M., & Murphy, S. (1990). Women and addiction: process, treatment, and outcome. In Lambert, E. (Ed.), *The Collection and Interpretation of Data from Hidden Populations (NIDA Research Monograph 98)* (pp.120–127). Rockville, MD: US Department of Health and Human Services.

Ryland, S.A., & Lucas, L. (1996). A rural collaborative model of treatment and recovery services for pregnant and parenting women with dual disorders. *Journal of Psychoactive Drugs, 28,* 389–395.

Schliebner, C.T. (1994). Gender-sensitive therapy: an alternative for women in substance abuse treatment. *Journal of Substance Abuse Treatment, 11,* 511–515.

Schmidt, C., Klee, L., & Ames, G. (1990). Review and analysis of literature on indicators of women's drinking problems. *British Journal of Addictions*, 85, 179–192.

Schuckit, M. (1992). Advances in understanding the vulnerability to alcoholism. In O'Brien, C., & Jaffe, J. (Eds.), *Advances in Understanding the Vulnerability to Alcoholism* (pp.93–108). New York: Raven Press.

Substance Abuse and Mental Health Services Administration (1993). *National Household Survey on Drug Abuse: Population Estimates*. Rockville, MD: Substance Abuse and Mental Health Services Administration.

Substance Abuse and Mental Health Services Administration (1995). *National Household Survey on Drug Abuse*. Rockville, MD: US Department of Health and Human Services.

Sutker, P. (1987). Drug dependent women. In Bescher, G., Reed, B., & Monderano, J. (Eds.), *Treatment Services for Drug Dependent Women*, Vol. 1 (pp.25–51). Washington, DC: US Government Printing Office.

Szuster, R., Rich, L., Chung, A., & Bisconer, S. (1996). Treatment retention in women's residential chemical dependency treatment: the effect of admission with children. *Substance Use and Misuse*, 31, 1001–1013.

Tarter, R., & Mezzich, A. (1992). Ontogeny of substance abuse: perspectives and findings. In Glantz, M., & Pickens, R. (Eds.), *Vulnerability to Drug Abuse* (pp.149–177). Washington, DC: American Psychological Association.

Teets, J.M. (1995). Childhood sexual trauma of chemically dependent women. *Journal of Psychoactive Drugs*, 27, 231–238.

US Department of Justice (1995). *Prisoners in 1994*. Washington, DC: Office of Justice Programs.

van Baar, A. & de Graaff, B.M.T. (1994). Cognitive development at preschool-age of infants of drug-dependent mothers. *Developmental Medicine and Child Neurology*, 36, 1063–1075.

Vogt, I. (1998). Gender and drug treatment systems. In Klingemann, H., & Hunt, G. (Eds.), *Drug Treatment Systems in an International Perspective: Drugs, Demons, and Delinquents* (pp.281–297). Thousand Oaks, CA: Sage.

Wallen, J. (1998). Need for services research on treatment for drug abuse in women. In Wetherington, C., & Roman, A. (Eds.), *Drug Addiction Research and the Health of Women* (pp.229–236). Rockville, MD National Institute on Drug Abuse.

Wetherington, C.L, Smeriglio, V.L., & Finnegan, L.P. (1996). *Behavioral Studies of Drug-exposed Offspring: Methodological Issues in Human and Animal Research (NIDA Research Monograph 164)*. Washington, DC: US Department of Health and Human Services.

Wickizer, T., Maynard, C., Atherly, A., Frederick, M., Koepsell, T., Krupski, A., & Stark, K. (1994). Completion rates of clients discharged from drug and alcohol treatment programs in Washington State. *American Journal of Public Health*, 84, 215–221.

Williams, M., & Roberts, C. (1991). Predicting length of stay in long-term treatment for chemically dependent females. *The International Journal of the Addictions*, 26, 605–613.

Wilsnack, S.C., & Wilsnack, R.W. (1991). Epidemiology of women's drinking. *Journal of Substance Abuse*, 3, 133–158.

Wilsnack, S.C., Wilsnack, R.W., & Hiller-Sturmhöfel, S. (1994). How women drink: epidemiology of women's drinking and problem drinking. *Alcohol Health and Research World*, 18, 173–181.

Wilsnack, S.C., Vogeltanz, N.D., Klassen, A.D., & Harris, T.R. (1997). Childhood sexual abuse and women's substance abuse: national survey findings. *Journal of Studies on Alcohol*, 58, 264–271.

Wobie, K., Eyler, F.D., Conlon, M., Clarke, L., & Behnke, M. (1997). Women and children in residential treatment: outcomes for mothers and their infants. *Journal of Drug Issues*, 27, 585–606.

Woodhouse, L. (1992). Women with jagged edges: voices from a culture of substance abuse. *Qualitative Health Research*, 2, 262–281.

Woods, J. (1995). Clinical management of drug dependency in pregnancy. In Chiang, C., & Finnegan, L. (Eds.), *Medications Development for the Treatment of Pregnant Addicts and Their Infants* (pp.39–57). Rockville, MD: US Department of Health and Human Services.

Yandow, V. (1989). Alcoholism in women. *Psychiatric Annals*, 19, 243–247.

Zweben, J.E. (1996). Psychiatric problems among alcohol and other drug dependent women. *Journal of Psychoactive Drugs*, 28, 345–366.

Index

Related titles of interest from Wiley. . .

Treating Postnatal Depression
A Psychological Approach for Health Care Practitioners
JEANNETTE MILGROM, PAUL R. MARTIN and LISA M. NEGRI

Outlines a 10-week treatment programme with clinical guidelines and detailed intervention procedures.

0–471–98645–3 292pp 1999 Paperback

The Healing Journey Through Menopause
Your Journal for Reflection and Renewal
PHIL RICH and FRAN MERVYN

An inspirational workbook which draws on the power of writing to help women work through the life change.

0–471–32691–7 282pp 1999 Paperback

Stress in Health Professionals
Psychological and Organisational Causes and Interventions
Edited by JENNY FIRTH-COZENS and ROY L. PAYNE

Takes approaches from organisational and clinical psychology to focus on key staff groups, considering wider issues such as team work, burn-out, training and counselling services, and investigating the effectiveness of both organisational and individual interventions.

0–471–99876–1 286pp 1999 Paperback

Clinical Handbook of Marriage and Couples Intervention
Edited by KIM HALFORD and HOWARD MARKMAN

Provides a comprehensive, analytic overview of research on marriage and marital interventions, with the unifying theme of the concept of a healthy marriage.

0–471–95519–1 748pp 1997 Hardback

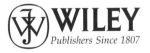

WILEY
Publishers Since 1807